CONSUMING PLEASURES

Australia and the
International Drug Business

J O H N   R A I N F O R D

FREMANTLE PRESS

First published 2009 by
FREMANTLE PRESS
25 Quarry Street, Fremantle
(PO Box 158, North Fremantle 6159)
Western Australia.
www.fremantlepress.com.au

Cover design: Tracey Gibbs
Cover photograph: Pidjoe/istockphoto.com

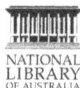

A catalogue record for this
book is available from the
National Library of Australia

NATIONAL
LIBRARY
OF AUSTRALIA

ISBN 9781921361432 (paperback)

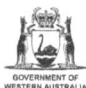

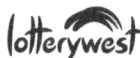

GOVERNMENT OF
WESTERN AUSTRALIA

lotterywest

Fremantle Press is supported by the Western Australian State Government through
the Department of Cultural Industries, Tourism and Sport.

Contents

Introduction: Sighs of the oppressed   5

1.   Doctors, quacks and self-healers:
     Drug use and the medical profession   12
2.   Pills, potions and pharmaceuticals   46
3.   The food drugs, tobacco and alcohol   78
4.   Stimulants for work and pleasure:
     Cocaine and amphetamines   107
5.   Hallucinogenic dreaming:
     Cannabis, LSD and ecstasy   143
6.   Opium and the masses   194
7.   Drug laws and changes in supply   215
8.   The Cold War and the CIA   227
9.   Australia's heroin market   254
10. The triumph of the market?   279

Epilogue: The defeat of communism and
          the revenge of religion   315
Endnotes   332
Bibliography   379
Acknowledgements   389
Index   391

For Stephen

Introduction
Sighs of the oppressed

Religion is the sigh of the oppressed creature, the heart of a heartless world and the soul of soulless conditions. It is the opium of the people.

These words were first published in Paris in 1844 in a journal as obscure as it was short-lived. They were part of a critique of the philosophy of Georg Hegel, and while writing this, the 25-year-old author continued his development of a theory called communism. This theory would shape the global political divide and profoundly affect world affairs for more than 100 years after his death in London in 1883. Yet for many, Dr Karl Marx is simply remembered for the epigram: 'Religion is the opium of the people.'[1] As a vituperative one-line appraisal of the befuddling nature of religion, its place in history seems guaranteed.

But what of the analogy with opium? If people — the 'masses' — were in need of religion to make life bearable, who was using the opium? How would Marx's contemporaries have understood the expression? Much better than most of us today, it turns out, as a great many citizens of the mid-19th century used opium on a fairly regular basis. Indeed its use then was so prevalent as to warrant the considered view of one of the more distinguished scholars of the period, Virginia Berridge, that 'opium itself was the opiate of the people'.[2]

In England in 1844 almost 15 tonnes of opium was consumed and, during the 19th century and beyond, yearly consumption reached far higher levels.[3] Given that a medical analgesic dose was 1–2 grains every six hours,[4] and each imported tonne contained 15,432,358 grains, opium use measured in tonnes represents consumption of considerable significance. By the first year of the 20th century the amount of opium legally imported into England, mainly from Turkey, had reached 378 tonnes.[5]

Opium was readily available and readily used throughout the 19th century, commonly in the form of laudanum, a preparation made by mixing opium with distilled water and alcohol. Its primary use among the working class was as self-medication. According to a contemporary observer, working people did not go to skilled physicians when they were ill because they were unable to pay the high fees the doctors charged. The result was high use of quack remedies and patent medicines prepared with opiates, such as Godfrey's Cordial.[6] The huge quantities consumed suggest that dependence and addiction were not uncommon,[7] although, with the exception of references to celebrities, evidence seems largely anecdotal.

Recreational use (known in the 19th century as 'luxurious' or 'stimulant' use)[8] wasn't unknown, but it appears to have been much more the preserve of the well-to-do than of the working class.

The distinction between self-medication, recreational use and dependence wasn't always clear cut. The opium use of Thomas De Quincey is a case in point. Born in 1785, the son of a Manchester merchant, De Quincey first used opium as a 19-year-old to alleviate a painful gastric condition and recurring anxiety states.[9] He went on to use it recreationally and became dependent on it. In 1821, an account of his early life and opium addiction was serialised in *The London Magazine*; it was published as a book, *Confessions of an English Opium-Eater*, the following year. The book aroused considerable interest and is credited with both popularising and demonising the recreational use of opium.

The 'luxurious' use of opium in the 19th century was particularly prevalent among writers and poets. Byron, Keats and Shelley were all recreational users. Samuel Taylor Coleridge was an opium addict in denial, and his famous poem 'Kubla Khan' is said to have been the creative product of his taking two grains of the drug.[10] The poet laureate, Robert Southey, took opium for sleeplessness, as did Elizabeth Barrett Browning.

Sir Walter Scott, author of the Waverley novels, partook of both laudanum and opium, initially prescribed for a stomach complaint. The novelist Wilkie Collins similarly began taking laudanum for a rheumatic condition and continued its use throughout his life. Opiate use was central to a number of his novels, including what is perhaps his best known, *The Moonstone*, said to be the first English detective novel.

Sir Edward Bulwer-Lytton, who famously gave us the line 'the pen is mightier than the sword', was, somewhat unusually for the time, an opium smoker. Both Charles Dickens and Oscar Wilde were users of opium who went on to write about the drug in a sensationalist way in, respectively, *The Mystery of Edwin Drood* and *The Picture of Dorian Gray*.

The English monarch George IV, who died in 1830, was a big consumer of opiates, as was the anti-slavery campaigner William Wilberforce. The famed nurse and hospital reformer Florence Nightingale was a more moderate consumer. Among politicians, the four-time British Prime Minister William Gladstone was a user of laudanum who thought that the drug assisted his public-speaking demeanour, while across the Channel the former French Prime Minister Louis Molé died of opiate addiction in 1855.

So there was certainly enough opium about when Marx first wrote of it, and it is not implausible that he was aware of the class dimensions of its use. For the proletariat it was a self-administered medicine; for the bourgeoisie, or some of them at least, it was also a recreational drug that, like religion, was capable of disguising the reality of the present.

Further reference points for Marx were the Opium Wars between Britain and China, the first of which was fought between 1839 and 1842. Marx wrote about the opium trade for the *New York Daily Tribune* during the second Opium War (1856–60). The wars were about the prohibition of the opium trade in China (see Chapter 6). The way in which the trade was carried on — monopoly production and restrictions on wholesale purchase and transportation — meant that it was dominated by a small number of large players. Had the trade been legalised at this point these interests could have been expected to dominate given their entrenched position, but others would have been able to enter the trade if they had enough capital and were prepared to risk it. A legal trade would have invited competition, which could have resulted in reduced prices. The larger companies would have resisted this, but it would certainly have been preferable for them not to trade at all.

These wars were among British imperialism's more shameful episodes, being fought in the name of 'free trade' at the urging of the first drug barons, William Jardine and James Matheson, so that Indian cultivators could be kept in penury and forced to grow opium for the Chinese, whose government had declared its importation illegal. Free trade in opium was about profit, pure and simple. There was more money to be made in the opium trade than in any other, particularly in China, because it was illegal.

Jardine and Matheson made their fortunes smuggling Indian

opium into China from early in the 19th century. By the 1830s their opium imports amounted to something like one-third of all China's foreign trade.[11] At the conclusion of the first Opium War, Jardine was well pleased that the Chinese authorities still refused to make the trade legal. This meant that 'men of small capital'[12] would continue to be excluded from 'the safest and most gentleman-like speculation that I am aware of', leaving the companies that dominated the trade, including his, safe from competition.[13] Both Jardine and Matheson eventually took themselves and a considerable amount of their accumulated capital back to Britain. Jardine became a landowner in Scotland and a member of parliament in London. Matheson also became a landowner in Scotland, spending over half a million pounds buying the island of Lewis in 1844. After Jardine's death, Matheson took over Jardine's parliamentary seat, sparing himself the inconvenience of having to find one of his own, and was made a baronet some years later.[14]

The political history of opium since Marx first wrote about it in 1844 is replete with irony. The British doctrine of free trade pressed opium on the Chinese and created an addict population of more than 13 million who were smoking their way through more than 39,000 tonnes of opium at the beginning of the 20th century. The political fragmentation of China, in which opium played an important part, spawned a nationalist movement, the Kuomintang, whose leader, Chiang Kai-shek, fought his communist allies to take control of Shanghai in 1927. The Kuomintang also took control of the opium industry. By this time opium had long met modernity and given us morphine and heroin, as well as the syringe with which to administer them more efficiently.

In the late 1930s, there were some 40 million opiate addicts in China. After the communist victory of Mao Tse-tung in 1949, Kuomintang insurgents who had fled to Burma captured the opium-producing industry in the region which has become known as the Golden Triangle. Chinese gangsters who had flourished in Shanghai before fleeing to Hong Kong turned that opium into high-grade heroin. From 1970, this was consumed in large quantities by US troops fighting in South Vietnam. They took the habit home with them, and heroin from the Golden Triangle supplanted that supplied to the United States by the 'French Connection' in Marseille. The Marseille trade itself had been made possible by the defeat of communists in that city from 1947 to 1950 in one of the earlier struggles of the Cold War.[15]

In the 1980s and 1990s, what began as a war against communism in Afghanistan fuelled the expansion of that country's opium and heroin industries and led to the rise of a terrorist organisation called al-Qaeda, whose opium is religion of a particularly virulent and fundamentalist sort. One of the most fascinating aspects of the drug trade from the second half of the 20th century on is the regularity with which wars fought against communism coincided with rising levels of heroin and cocaine use.

The most obvious difference between the use of opiates and other recreational drugs today and in 1844 is their legal status. With the noticeable early exception of China, opiates and other drugs that have come to be used recreationally, such as cannabis and cocaine, were legally available and widely advertised in most countries in the 19th century. Today these drugs are almost universally classed as illicit. But just as it did in China in the mid-19th century, the illicitness of drugs today increases their profitability. The international illicit drug trade has an annual turnover in excess of US$400 billion, which, at 8 per cent of world trade, is on a par with the tourist and oil industries and greater than the world's iron and steel or motor vehicle industries.[16]

Consuming Pleasures traces the history of licit and illicit drug use, examining why we consume and what we consume, as well as the way in which consumption is regulated in the era of global free trade. It also looks at drug use from an Australian perspective, going back to our own opium-growing industry and the racist origins of our drug laws. In doing so it considers the paradox of contemporary white Australian identity: on the one hand an image of fit, sun-bronzed athletic types at home in the surf; on the other a nation of people whose per capita drug consumption often equals and more often than not surpasses that of most other nations.

The first two chapters link the origins of global drug control to the early development of the medical profession and the pharmaceutical industry, and examine the influence of each on the Australian and international drug markets as a consequence of the legislative limits placed on self-medication. The next three chapters describe the history and present market conditions for the licit drugs alcohol, tobacco, caffeine and sugar, as well as some of the more popular, and illicit, hallucinogens and stimulants. Chapters 6 to 9 look at opium and its derivatives, morphine and heroin, from a similar perspective, and examine the role of the Cold War in assisting the expansion of the world opiate and cocaine markets and the development of Australia's heroin market. The final chapters explore the dynamics of the drug market and the rationale for state intervention and control before drawing some conclusions about the collapse of communism and the role of religion in the 21st century.

If Marx were around today he would no doubt be intrigued to see how the drug market has developed, and fascinated by the insights its history from the mid-19th century provides — as well as a little perplexed about how it illustrates the efficiency of the free-market economies that defeated the command economies established in his name.

1
Doctors, quacks and self-healers: Drug use and the medical profession

In 1925 the International Opium Conference convened in Geneva by the League of Nations introduced the first effective global controls on drugs. The controlled substances were opium, morphine, heroin, cocaine and cannabis (described at the time as Indian hemp).

When the League of Nations became the United Nations following World War II, it extended its reach beyond the 36 nations that had attended the Geneva conference — most notably, it now includes the United States.[1] In the second half of the 20th century controls became more stringent and the controlled drugs more numerous.

The most striking outcome of the prohibitionist policies adopted at Geneva was an environment that allowed the growth of an illicit industry that was to become one of the most profitable the world has ever known. Along the way, prohibition put hundreds of millions of consumers on the wrong side of the law, incarcerated millions of them, created a new class of 'narco-rich' and corrupted law enforcement agencies, judicial officers, banking institutions and politicians at all levels of government. What were the circumstances that compelled a policy approach that has had such disastrous, and surely unintended, consequences? What exactly was 'the drug problem' in 1925?

The Opium Conference

On an international level, the most pressing problem was addiction arising from opium smoking. This had been a concern in China for the better part of 200 years. Chinese emigrants had taken their opium habit with them, so that its use was now common not only in expatriate Chinese communities but also in the various communities where they had settled, most notably in Southeast Asia.

Among the more economically advanced Western economies, the widespread use, from the mid-19th century onwards, of what were commonly called patent medicines that contained preparations of opium, cannabis and cocaine, was seen by some of the delegates to be a problem. But as early as 1916, almost all of these proprietary medicines sold in the United States (the nation pressing most strongly for international controls) were already free of narcotics as a result of legislation. Similar initiatives in Australia meant that the worst excesses of the industry had been curbed even earlier (by 1910).[2] In Britain the removal of morphine and opium from proprietary medicines had been evident from 1903:[3] in the late 19th century there was a movement to restrict some of the more dangerous patent medicines, largely as a result of Chlorodyne poisoning cases. A Privy Council Committee investigated the composition of patent medicines in 1903 and reported that some, but not all, of the manufacturers had dropped morphine and opium from their preparations. The British Medical Association's investigations in 1909 and 1912 confirmed the trend.

To the extent that cocaine and heroin use was a large-scale problem anywhere, it was a problem in the United States, but by 1925 recreational use had already been prohibited for more than a decade. Gone were the days when you could readily avail yourself of the 15 different forms of cocaine (which came with a cocaine kit complete with hypodermic syringe) marketed by the Parke-Davis company.[4] Laudanum at 10 cents a bottle, coca wine at 95 cents and as much opium as you like could no longer be conveniently bought by mail order from Sears, Roebuck and Company in Chicago.[5] Even possession of their nickel-plated syringes 'in a neat morocco case' was prohibited in several American states by the early 1930s.[6]

And despite the availability of 'Cigares de Joy' (cannabis cigarettes), the bulk of cannabis consumption occurred in those parts of the globe, such as India, where its use had been common for thousands of years. It would be several decades after the controls established at Geneva before the drug came into widespread popular use in other countries.

* * * * *

Opium smoking in Far Eastern countries, the revenue from which sustained much state expenditure in those countries, had been dealt with during the first stage of the Opium Conference, which began in November 1924: the supply of opium by private contractors was to be replaced by government monopoly and consumption was to be regulated by the registration of licensed smokers.

The 1925 conference was the second stage, and covered manufactured drugs, primarily heroin and cocaine. After long and sometimes acrimonious debate, the conference determined that participating countries would control the manufacture, sale and transport of designated drugs so as to ensure their 'legitimate' use.

The United States, which had refused to join the League of Nations but had attended the conference and earlier advisory committee meetings in an observer capacity, walked out in early February after failing to get agreement on heroin prohibition, stricter controls on coca production and a phasing-out of opium use for non-medical purposes.[7]

US prohibition initiatives

The Geneva Conference followed the International Opium Commission (Shanghai, 1909) and the International Conference on Opium (The Hague, 1911–12). Both were convened at the instigation of the United States — the one country outside China that readily identified a 'drug problem'. (There was, however, a belief in the British Foreign Office that the US motives in convening the Shanghai commission owed something to gaining trade advantages with China.[8])

Fifty years before the Geneva Conference, in San Francisco in 1875, local authorities passed the first anti-drug laws in the United States. They were aimed at opium smokers, who were mainly, but not exclusively, Chinese. The federal *Smoking Opium Exclusion Act 1909*, which prohibited opium from being imported or used in the United States except for medical purposes, was preceded by drug prohibition laws — which criminalised opium use by imposing fines and prison sentences on individuals who operated or used opium shops — enacted in 11 state jurisdictions between 1877 and 1890.[9] Similarly, the *Harrison Narcotic Act 1914* prohibiting the recreational use of morphine, heroin and cocaine was preceded by laws passed in 46 states regulating cocaine use from as early as 1897.[10]

Cannabis in the United States was commonly called marijuana, reflecting its popularity among Mexicans who migrated there in the early decades of the 20th century. As their marijuana consumption became conspicuous and was taken up by non-Mexicans, individual states legislated against its use for non-medical purposes, beginning with California and Utah in

1915.[11] Federal regulation came somewhat later, in the form of the *Marijuana Tax Act 1937*.

So the United States, by the time of the Geneva Conference, had a comprehensive set of legislative controls prohibiting all of the drugs under consideration at the conference. As well as opiates, cocaine and cannabis, the United States also had a prohibition on alcohol, established via a constitutional amendment, that took effect from 1920.

Attempting to contain international drug supply in the face of a measurably rising domestic demand (most notably in the United States) seemed doomed to failure, and the truth of this was recognised in 1933 when the prohibition on alcohol was lifted. At the time of the Geneva Conference there were some 200,000 heroin addicts in the United States, whose supply, as with alcohol, came from an illicit market. But the lesson learned from prohibition was limited to alcohol; there was no attempt to understand the dynamics of demand for other drugs.

The controls implemented at Geneva in 1925 and at the subsequent 1931 Limitation Convention did limit the production of heroin and opium.[12] But the most significant interruption to production, supply and consumption was World War II. After the war, illicit drug consumption continued to rise, even as prohibitionist legislation increasingly dominated the statute books of nations around the world.

Doctors and drugs

The international controls reflected in national legislation didn't prohibit the nominated drugs per se; rather they provided that their use by individuals be mediated by doctors. Typically, specific drugs were banned except for 'medical or scientific purposes'. The medical gaze now had to be accompanied by a medical scribble. In the United States heroin was at first the only exception: it was prohibited even for medical purposes in

1924.[13]

When doctors in England began to restrict their prescription of opium they 'became the custodians of a problem which they had helped to define'.[14] With the restrictions on the use of opiates and cocaine that came from national and international controls in the 20th century, doctors became a part of the proposed solution to a problem that was largely of their making.

From the latter part of the 19th century and into the 20th century, there was a clear gender divide with opiate addiction. Although addiction in Australia and the United Kingdom was almost insignificant compared to that in the United States, the pattern was the same. Morphine was the main drug of addiction, doctors were often the suppliers, and women represented the vast majority of those addicted. The morphine addiction described by Eugene O'Neill in his play *Long Day's Journey into Night* was based on the experience of his own mother, and was the story of many American women. According to a number of surveys, women represented between two-thirds and three-quarters of the total number of those addicted to opiates.[15] Of the 250,000 opiate addicts that US public health officials estimated in 1900, the great majority were 'genteel, middle-class women'.[16] Between self-medication and doctors' prescriptions, opiates had become both a sign of women's oppression and their attempt to gain relief from it. At the same time, a majority of male addicts were doctors, with some estimates suggesting that as many as 20 per cent of the profession were 'opium inebriates'.[17]

Around the end of the first decade of the 20th century, the over-prescribing of morphine was widely recognised (including by doctors themselves) as the main cause of addiction,[18] and there was a corresponding fall in the rate of prescriptions.[19] But it wasn't just morphine that doctors too frequently prescribed. Cocaine use was similarly popularised,[20] and although the percentage of medically addicted heroin addicts wasn't large, its use too, and the problem of addiction, came, initially at least, by way of the medical profession.[21]

From around 1910 in the United States, heroin started to become more popular than morphine with recreational consumers. New York became the heroin capital, although morphine was still the mainstay of addicts elsewhere. Among the 10,000 addicts in the United States in various institutions such as hospitals and sanatoria in the 1916–18 period, the overall majority were still morphine addicts. However, in institutions such as reformatories and prisons, heroin addicts were more numerous. These addicts were increasingly young, male and 'deviant' (a deviant was merely a member of a disliked group which at the time included poor Catholic immigrants, Chinese labourers, big-city delinquents and African-American men).[22] The medical profession now classified the older, morphine-addicted women as 'accidental addicts' (able to be treated to the benefit of patient and doctor alike), and the young male deviants as 'vicious addicts' who were beyond help.[23]

Following the enactment of the *Harrison Narcotic Act 1914*, recreational opiate and cocaine users could either abstain or seek their drugs on the illicit market. Addicts, however, could expect from their doctors a maintenance regime accompanied, where appropriate, by a program designed to bring their dependence to an end. In some cities, public health clinics catered specifically for addicts. But in 1919 the US Supreme Court determined that the maintenance of addicts violated the *Harrison Act*. The public clinics were closed down and any doctor prescribing to addicts was liable to prosecution and a possible prison sentence. This attack by the Supreme Court might have been expected to provoke a response from the doctors' professional body, the American Medical Association, commensurate with the threat that it represented to independent judgement and practice. In fact, the opposite occurred. The American Medical Association supported the Supreme Court's decision by policy resolutions adopted in both 1919 and 1924.[24] Still, many doctors continued to prescribe to addicts: figures show that in the 16 years following the Supreme Court decision, more than 25,000 doctors were indicted under the *Harrison Act* and 2500 were sentenced to prison.[25]

* * * * *

In Australia the recreational use of opiates didn't surface as a problem until the 1960s. But in many other ways our experience was similar to that in the United States. From the early 20th century, the typical Australian drug addict was a middle-aged, middle-class woman initially prescribed morphine or heroin by her doctor for some painful or chronic condition. And as in the United States, more than one-third of known addicts were doctors, nurses or other health professionals.[26]

Australia had an 'unofficial' policy of maintaining addicts under medical supervision. Various state regulations prohibited the supply or prescription of opiates to addicts, but in practice, Australia followed the British system, based on the Rolleston Report of 1926, which established the principle that it was solely a matter for doctors to determine the appropriate treatment for their addict patients. Supplying them with heroin or morphine therefore reflected a considered and respected medical judgement.[27]

Britain's addict population was similar in profile to Australia's. The known number of addicts was comparatively low; they were more likely to be female than male; a considerable number had become therapeutically addicted; and a disproportionately large number were doctors themselves. In 1938 there were just over 500 addicts, the majority of them women. Of the 383 known addicts in 1947, 219 were female and 82 were doctors.[28]

The problem of patients becoming addicted to prescription drugs that was evident before the Geneva Conference didn't go away as a result of any of the deliberations of the conference. Nor, for that matter, did the self-administered heroin addiction that was equally apparent in the United States at the time — drug consumption continued to increase. While the interruption of war led to a decrease in the non-medical consumption of opiates, it also led to many combatants consuming large quantities of amphetamines, drugs that were judged by the medical profession to be well suited for military purposes.

To see why the state vested the medical profession with the authority to mediate drug consumption, we need to look at the history of healthcare, and in particular at the role that the profession came to play in it.

The rise of the medical profession

That any sane nation, having observed that you could provide for the supply of bread by giving bakers a pecuniary interest in baking for you, should go on to give a surgeon a pecuniary interest in cutting off your leg, is enough to make one despair of political humanity.

George Bernard Shaw

On French philosopher Michel Foucault's account, 'modern medicine has fixed its own date of birth as being in the last years of the 18th century'.[29] This view from the heights of postmodernism notwithstanding, it was still possible, in the early decades of the 19th century, to set up in practice as a doctor in Britain (and in colonies such as Australia) by the simple expedient of purchasing, at the cost of less than £2, a medical degree granting its recipient, according to one contemporary complainant, 'a patent to slay thousands according to the law'.[30]

The American Medical Association's Council on Pharmacy and Chemistry would report early in the 20th century that the conditions of medical practice at the time when the first controls on opium were introduced in San Francisco, in 1875, were essentially the same as when Thomas Sydenham developed laudanum in the 1660s.[31] Medical practice as we know it today is indeed of quite recent origin.

When human activity began to change from hunter-gathering to settled agriculture and animal husbandry some 10,000 years ago, it brought with it the capacity to end starvation. Surplus food production led to population growth, permanent dwellings and the development of social hierarchies.[32] It also brought disease, much of it a result of our close relationship with animals. The disease-producing bacteria of cattle gave us tuberculosis and smallpox; pigs and ducks gave us influenza; horses, the common cold; and measles came to us from either cattle or dogs. Drinking water contaminated by animal faeces spread polio, cholera, typhoid, whooping cough and diphtheria. The productive agricultural environment attracted parasites, disease-carrying rodents and insects, such as mosquitoes that brought malaria.[33] With varying degrees of success, we have battled with these, and other more recent diseases, ever since.

In contrast to hunter-gatherer groups, who were more likely to abandon the sick than care for them, the more settled agricultural communities began to treat the sick and attempt to nurse them back to health.[34] Illness was primarily treated within the family, and as a body of knowledge covering various illnesses gradually increased, a division of labour emerged that led to specific healers identified and trusted with specialist treatment. What were considered less serious health problems were dealt with by folk healers such as herbalists, bone-setters and tooth extractors. Women birth attendants assisted with childbirth.[35] The more serious cases of ill-health were thought to have supernatural causes which required the intervention of clairvoyants, shamans, diviners, charmers and healer-priests.[36] This secular/religious divide continued in the practice of medicine in ancient Greece and the Roman Empire. The cult of Asclepius, son of Apollo and Greek god of healing, reached its zenith in Imperial Rome.

The more secular approach of Hippocrates (c. 450–370 BCE), which was carried on by Galen (130–c. 200 AD), centred on the doctrine of humoralism. According to this doctrine, ill-health was a result of an imbalance in the four bodily humours: blood, phlegm, yellow bile and black bile. These bodily humours were held to be analogous with the four basic elements of existence: earth, air, fire and water.[37] Restoring good health relied on techniques to rebalance the humours.

In the history of western medicine at least, there was little advance in medical knowledge for more than 1000 years after Galen's death.[38] It is testimony to his great influence that the anatomical and physiological doctrines he pioneered were not subject to critical challenge until the 16th and 17th centuries. For an even longer period, complex drug mixtures were known as 'Galenics'.[39]

Although medical knowledge was being disseminated through Benedictine monasteries at the end of the 6th century, it was another 600 years before the teaching of medicine found a place alongside law and theology in the medieval universities of Europe. The small number of learned graduates, licensed to practice on the ultimate authority of the Pope, had an equally small number of patients wealthy enough to afford their fees. The poor continued to rely on themselves and their families for medical care, with occasional recourse to folk healers.[40]

The professional identity of university-trained medical men (in most places women were excluded) was based on their education and on a church ruling which prohibited them from participating in any form of medical practice that involved either bloodshed or potential fatality.[41]

In the prevailing humoral doctrine, which held that good health was a product of the body functioning as an 'efficient throughput system' fuelled by food and drink, blockages were thought to cause illness by preventing natural evacuation. The courses of treatment used thus included vomiting, purging, sweating and bloodletting.[42] Not only was bloodletting common practice; according to Galen, the more serious the illness, the more blood should be let.[43]

As they were prohibited from bloodletting, graduate physicians saw themselves as teachers, observers and consultants — at some distance from the hands-on healing.[44] Bloodletting became the province of tradesmen barbers who began to organise in craft guilds. The Guild of Barbers of London was chartered in 1462 and a charter for surgeons was established in 1475. The Guild of Surgeons joined with the Company of Barbers to form the United Barber-Surgeon Company in 1540,[45] and developed an apprenticeship system aimed at controlling entry into a defined labour market. In northern Europe, guild members practised major surgery such as amputations. Surgeons were associated with barbers until the formation of the Royal Company of Surgeons in 1745; this became the Royal College of Surgeons in 1800.[46]

Colleges of physicians also emerged in Europe from the late 14th century. They were separate from the medical faculties and the guilds, and gained jurisdiction over examining and licensing, acting as specialist advisors to governments on issues of public health.[47] The college of physicians established in Florence in 1560, for example, had only 12 physicians, who were appointed for life. Its jurisdiction over examining and licensing of practitioners for the entire region superseded the authority of the local healing guild.

Apothecaries, druggists and chemists came to play a more prominent role in medicine following the wider use of chemical remedies (such as mercury, for syphilis) pioneered by the German physician Paracelsus (1493–1541). The discovery of blood circulation by William Harvey (1578–1657) seemed to open up the possibility of a more scientifically based and professionally organised practice of medicine, and thus an elevated social standing for its practitioners. However, the preference of these increasing numbers of groups of practitioners for self-regulation and control of the whole healing field eventually collided with the laissez-faire principles of late Enlightenment France.[48]

Laissez-faire, laissez-aller — let do, let go — was the slogan of a group of 18th-century French economists called the physiocrats,[49] whose principle of non-interference in the marketplace was seen to apply equally to medical practice, particularly since the surgeon-physician and founder of physiocracy, Dr Francois Quesnay (1694–1774) was also first physician to the French King Louis XV. Simple market principles would determine the choice of individuals to practise as either physicians or surgeons in a marketplace governed by patient demand.

These principles, as championed also by Adam Smith (1723–90) in Britain, meant open competition among physicians, surgeons, apothecaries, chemists and folk healers in what had become a healthcare market.[50] In his immensely influential work, An *Inquiry into the Nature and Causes of the Wealth of Nations*, Smith set out his criticism of the guild system (which was that monopoly control artificially raised prices) and his support for apothecaries making a 1000 per cent profit on their sale of drugs.[51]

* * * * *

This then was the state of medical practice immediately prior to its modern birth in France. Indeed, the deregulatory environment in which medicine was practised in the first decade of the French Revolution remains unparalleled in the history of Western medicine.[52]

According to Foucault, the French Revolution gave birth to two great myths: the first, that a nationalised medical profession could replace the clergy; and the second, that disease would disappear in a society restored to its original state of health by radical political change, where citizens would be free from the ills of oppression. The defeat of disease would begin with the demise of bad government, of the tyranny of wealth over poverty; the path to good health would be trod only by the liberated.[53] Such is the recorded mythology. But the medical revolution that came with the death of the old regime was no myth.

Clinical medicine wasn't a product of the revolution. It already had some standing in 1714 thanks to Hermann Boerhaave (1668–1738), the 'illustrious successor' to Franciscus Sylvius (1614–72) who had first used hospital beds for teaching at Leyden in 1658. Boerhaave's pupils were instrumental in setting up teaching hospitals at Edinburgh and Vienna, and at other European centres, including Oxford, Cambridge and Dublin. But in terms of professional medical education, these teaching clinics were limited to a privileged few students.[54]

In France the revolution changed this by dismantling all the old institutions of learning and re-erecting them. Universities, scientific academics and the old hospital structures were abolished. A new medicine took their place. It was based on the clinic, where teaching was communicated 'within the concrete field of experience'.[55] Medicine and surgery were formally unified and 'schools of health' were established in Paris, Montpellier and Strasbourg, providing a broad theoretical teaching for a medicine to be practised in hospitals for the benefit of the poor.[56] (A healthy labour force had emerged as a principal objective of political power.[57]) Hospitals, previously regarded as 'temples of death', were reinvented as modern 'temples of Asclepius', whose gates were shut to those would-be priests who lacked the requisite entry requirements.[58] A second level of medical officers working in the countryside was established, and the shape of future monopoly practice became evident with the appointment of medical magistrates to prosecute charlatans.[59]

Clinical medicine in the teaching hospitals profoundly altered what became known as the doctor–patient relationship. It brought the all-knowing gaze of a doctor confident that his training (except in rare instances, women didn't practise modern medicine until well into the 20th century) could categorise your ailment once you told him 'where it hurt'.[60] He'd seen it all on his hospital perambulations, or at least had the benefit of some learned consultant explaining it to him, prodding and pointing at these educational objects known as patients.[61]

What came with this new medicine was a new status and authority for doctors. Clinical knowledge could only be acquired in a hospital, and hospitals were reserved for doctors and doctors-in-training; they were not open to lay people. The power that came with this knowledge would enable doctors to control the relationship they had with their patients.[62] They could now deny the description given to them by Voltaire (1694–1778) as 'men who prescribe medicine of which they know little to cure diseases of which they know less in human beings of which they know nothing'.[63]

The hospital too had begun its transformation from an institution whose rarely treated inmates were the poor, the homeless, the destitute, the sick, mad, crippled and incurable into a place at the centre of a very specialised medicine.[64] Still, midway through the 19th century doctors and hospitals played a role of no great significance in the lives of most people.[65] The rise to prominence of both coincided with two events: modern surgery and professional organisation.

Modern surgery

Until the mid-19th century, surgical practice was limited in range, excruciatingly painful and extremely risky. At hospitals in London and Paris in the early decades of that century it was also something of a spectator sport. Crowds in the public gallery overlooking the operating table would applaud the skills of the star surgeons of the day, adding a special dimension to the idea of 'theatre'. Speed was of the essence, and the fastest surgeons could amputate a leg through the hip joint in a mere 90 seconds.[66]

But speed notwithstanding, the pain associated with surgery was so severe that death was considered preferable by many patients. Opium, hemlock, mandrake and alcohol were just a few of the many drugs used through history in the attempt to alleviate pain, but their application to surgery was limited by their unreliability.[67] Too small a dose wouldn't entirely eliminate the pain too large a dose would eliminate both pain and patient.[68]

Dr Oliver Wendell Holmes (1809–94), professor of anatomy at Harvard University, first suggested the term 'anaesthesia' to describe the effects of ether following the first use of ether inhalation by a Boston surgeon in the United States in October 1846.[69] The pent-up demand for anaesthetics was demonstrated by the speed with which they were diffused. Within months, ether anaesthesia had been used in surgical operations in England, France, Switzerland and Germany. By early 1847 chloroform and nitrous oxide were also in use as anaesthetic agents,[70] and in June of that year ether was first used as an anaesthetic in Australia.[71]

The use of chloroform to alleviate the pain of women in labour was initially objected to, in accordance with the biblical injunction that 'In sorrow thou shalt bring forth children'[72] — presumably interpreted by male clergy to mean that God intended childbirth to be painful. These objections were overcome when Queen Victoria sensibly opted for chloroform during the birth of Prince Leopold in 1853.[73] Given that he was her eighth child, she was in a good position to judge the efficacy of the chloroform. She must have approved, because she elected to use it again during the birth of her next child, Princess Beatrice, in 1857.[74]

Nitrous oxide or 'laughing gas' was the most important

of the three general anaesthetics that came into use in the mid-19th century. First produced in 1772 by Joseph Priestley (1733–1804), its use was pioneered by Sir Humphry Davy (1778–1829), who heroically, and enjoyably, self-experimented with it and introduced it to both Robert Southey and Samuel Taylor Coleridge as well as to Peter Mark Roget, the physician who gave his name to the thesaurus.[75]

Professional organisation

Occupational organisation was a natural progression for a profession that had long been monopolistic in intent, keen to define who was 'in' and who was 'out'.[76] As the 19th century progressed, an expanding middle class with an increasing disposable income created the conditions for market growth in specialist services.[77] At the same time, in both Britain and Australia, medicine became an attractive career choice for the middle classes.[78] Towards the end of the century this led to claims of 'overcrowding'; these were addressed by restricting entry and controlling competition.[79] But the more pressing problem for doctors in the mid-19th century was external competition — from pharmacists, quacks, untrained chemists and druggists, and even from shopkeepers.[80]

Professional organisation was the key to sustaining pressure on the state to enact legislation that would confer monopoly status and allow self-regulation, and doctors began to organise themselves in a number of countries. The American Medical Association was formed in 1847, the British Medical Association (BMA) in 1855, a French equivalent three years later and the Canadian Medical Association (CMA) in 1867.[81] In Australia, local medical associations tended to be mostly short-lived, and in consequence, BMA branches were established in Sydney, Melbourne and Adelaide in 1880, Queensland in 1894 and Tasmania in 1889. Western Australia, insulated by its isolation, had its medical association incorporated as a BMA branch in 1899. Not until 1962 was this umbilical cord of association with the BMA severed when the Australian Medical Association (AMA) came into being.[82]

The professionalisation of medicine involved the essential elements of autonomy, authority and sovereignty. Autonomy would give doctors the right to determine who would practice and the right to self-regulate the conditions of practice; authority would place doctors at the top of the healthcare pyramid, with para-professionals and other professionals (such as nurses) in a subordinate position; and sovereignty would reserve for doctors alone the right to decide on diagnosis and treatment of patients, institutionalising their dominant position in the relationship between the healthcare sector and the rest of society.[83]

The major hurdle in achieving this desired status was the reluctance of the legislature to break with the established traditions of laissez-faire. However, doctors in the United Kingdom benefited from parliamentary interventions that were becoming necessary to regulate an increasingly complex society and to meet the demands of a vocal, yet disenfranchised working class. Voting rights, the right to an education and labour rights, limited though they might be, were all established in a broader scheme of state intervention during the 19th century. In this environment the *Medical Act 1858* was passed, providing for the registration of approved practitioners who would have a monopoly on public employment. It specified entry qualifications and established the process of self-regulation with the creation of the General Medical Council.[84]

The rise of the medical profession had begun. By virtue of the *Pharmacy Act 1868*, pharmacists too were granted a system of registration that rested on an educational monopoly held by their professional body, the Pharmaceutical Society. Although subordinate to doctors, the society had also begun a process that would eventually eliminate competition and reserve for its members a niche market as the sole dispensers of prescriptions for doctors and as the monopoly suppliers of designated drugs. Following the UK example, pharmacists in Australia were also able to control their own destiny, courtesy of a legislative regime that began in 1876 with the establishment of pharmacy boards in New South Wales and Victoria, whose composition was determined by pharmacists themselves.[85]

In the United Kingdom in 1836 and 1837, Medical Witnesses Acts established a fee structure for expert medical testimony at inquests and criminal trials.[86] Similar legislation concerning medical witnesses was enacted in the colonies of Van Diemen's Land and New South Wales in 1836 and 1838.[87] Because the Australian colonies lacked the tradition of medical men trained at universities such as Oxford and Cambridge, it became necessary to define the character of these medical witnesses. The two colonies were obliged to enact legislation providing for the registration of 'legally qualified medical practitioners'. Van Diemen's Land had legislation allowing for the regulation of medical practice in 1837; New South Wales had a Medical Act by 1842 and South Australia by 1844. Other colonies previously administered by New South Wales duly enacted medical legislation during the century.[88]

Medical education

For most of the 19th century most doctors in Australia came, not surprisingly, from the United Kingdom and Ireland. The 1863 medical register of Victoria shows that doctors from these two locations accounted for 94 per cent of those registered. Not until the second decade of the 20th century were the majority of doctors in Victoria products of the Melbourne Medical School.[89]

Established in 1862, the Melbourne Medical School predated the Sydney school by 21 years and the Adelaide school by 23 years.[90] Entry requirements were restrictive from the start, and included things other than simple academic achievement. For instance, while Victoria was the first colony to provide for compulsory education, it didn't ordinarily provide for learning in Latin and Greek; this was much more the preserve of private schools. These subjects were, however, prerequisites for entry into the medical school.[91] Moreover the course offered was of five years' duration, as opposed to the four-year course in England, and the fees were impossible for all except the wealthy. For those without parents or benefactors who could afford a private education, and the capacity to provide financial support for a five-year period, the study of medicine was thus unavailable. Even the conservative Medical Association of Victoria was moved to complain that these requirements represented 'a virtual monopoly to the wealthy'.[92] Medicine was to be a reserved occupation.

In the early years of the 20th century, fees at the medical school were double the average wage in the manufacturing industry, a wage that was supposed to keep a man, his wife and three children in frugal comfort.[93] When student enrolments increased sharply after the end of World War I, the medical schools of Melbourne, Sydney and Adelaide reduced numbers by agreeing in 1920 to increase the length of the course and raise fees by 20 per cent. These measures were introduced in 1923 — in the following year enrolments were 65, compared to 202 in 1920.[94]

While the process for selecting students for university courses, including medicine, was by open entry, in 1948 only 2 per cent of 17-year-olds entered university. The 429 medical graduates of that year represented 16 per cent of all bachelor graduates. As the overall number of university students began to increase from 1956, the University of Melbourne limited entry to its medical school by the imposition of quotas; it was soon followed by the University of Sydney. By 1963, almost

30 per cent of students who were qualified to (in the sense of having the requisite marks in the end of high school exams) and had applied to study medicine were prevented from doing so by the quotas set by the universities. The University of Queensland was the only university without a quota system for entry into medicine. As the higher education system expanded to include more working-class students, medicine continued to maintain its elite status by using these quotas. In 1979 the 2510 graduates from medical schools represented only 3.8 per cent of all graduates.[95] In 2002 the total number of Bachelor of Medicine and Bachelor of Surgery graduates was 1264, less than 1.3 per cent of all students graduating at the bachelor level. The Australian Competition and Consumer Commission (ACCC) has accused the Royal Australian College of Surgeons (RACS), who have a monopoly on training, of operating a closed shop and three state governments have threatened action against them. The ACCC conducted a review of the RACS and other colleges because of concerns over their use of market power to restrict access to the medical workforce; this resulted in 'rapid assessment units' being established in order to facilitate the recruitment of overseas doctors. At the GP level, surgeries are now 'bursting at the seams' because of a 'GP shortage around the country', according to Health Minister Nicola Roxon. The problem of doctor shortages is being addressed at a number of levels and new medical schools have been established, but if there were a true free market economy, there would be mechanisms to ensure that supply is capable of meeting demand.[96]

Scientific medicine

In 1900 the average life expectancy in Australia was 56.5 years. In 2000 it was 79.8 years (for non-Indigenous Australians). For most advanced economies, life expectancy increased over the century by more than half, from a little more than

50 years to just over 78 (in the United Kingdom, 50.5 years and 77.7 respectively; the United States, 49.3 years and 77.1; in France, 47 years and 78.8).[97] In 1750, at the high point of the Enlightenment, the average Englishman lived for around 36 years, the average Frenchman for no more than 27.[98] Perhaps the only advance comparable to that of longevity in the last 120 years is that of science. It is here that a modern myth arises, one that has proved to be enduring, unlike the two great myths of the French Revolution. It can be dated from two events: Louis Pasteur's exposition of the effectiveness of the rabies vaccine in 1885 and the first use of the diphtheria antitoxin that Emil von Behring had discovered in 1890.[99]

Rabies is transmitted in the saliva of biting animals, most often infected dogs. It was invariably fatal, and since antiquity was feared as the 'epitome of terror and mystery'.[100] Pasteur had developed a vaccine treatment which showed promise in experiments he conducted with dogs, but in July of 1885 he wasn't yet confident of its application to humans. When a young boy suffering from rabid dog bites was brought to him he had serious reservations about whether or not to apply the vaccine. He eventually overcame his caution and the young boy survived, going on to become the gatekeeper at the Pasteur Institute. Saved from certain death as a child, he committed suicide in 1940 rather than open Pasteur's burial crypt for the Germans who had invaded and occupied France.

Immunisation came of age in 1885 and in less than 18 months almost 2500 people had been vaccinated against rabies in France. Pasteur was depicted in the popular press, replete with halo, as the saviour of children threatened by mad dogs.[101]

The breakthrough with diphtheria was just as dramatic. Diphtheria is a highly infectious disease that in the 19th century was responsible for the deaths of thousands of children. During epidemics it had a case fatality rate of between 30 and 50 per cent, and parents everywhere prayed that their children didn't succumb to its deadly embrace. Diphtheria inflames the mucous membrane of the throat and causes a false membrane to form; this often results in suffocation as the area around the neck swells. The Spanish called the disease 'the strangler'.

On Christmas Day 1891 at the Bergman Clinic in Berlin, Behring's antitoxin rescued a diphtheritic child from the arms of death. Like Pasteur, Behring was hailed as a saviour of children and a grateful German government raised him to the nobility.[102] As well as saving the lives of countless children, the diphtheria vaccine also became the model for proving the 'germ theory' of Robert Koch (1843–1910), which finally buried the age-old idea that miasmas and evil winds were responsible for disease.[103] Behring became the first recipient of the Nobel Prize in 'physiology or medicine' in 1901 'for his work on serum therapy, especially its application against diphtheria, by which he has opened a new road in the domain of medical science and thereby placed in the hands of the physician a victorious weapon against illness and disease'.[104]

It was from this point that, in the public mind, medicine became married to science in a union that no authority could annul. Medical practitioners were now invested with a dual character: doctor and scientist. Faith in the miracle of science and evidence of the wonders of scientific discoveries as they unfolded in the 20th century established and maintained a myth that doctors could, in fact, cure disease.[105]

Plato, who lived almost 2500 years ago, described medicine not as a science but an art, and its history from that time largely confirms his diagnosis.[106] Improvements in health and longevity since the late 19th century have in fact had little to do with doctors. As the eminent medical historian Roy Porter observed:

> the retreat of the lethal diseases (diphtheria, typhoid, tuberculosis and so forth) was due, in the first instance, more to urban improvements, superior nutrition and public health than to curative

> *medicine. The one early striking instance of the conquest of disease, the introduction first of smallpox inoculation and then of vaccination, came not through 'science' but through embracing popular medical folklore.*[107]

Credit for the reduction in mortality from infectious diseases belongs primarily to those social reformers whose action at a political level led to the provision of cleaner water, more efficient sewage disposal and improved living standards.[108]

Social conditions in mid-19th century London demonstrate the point. Squalid, overcrowded living conditions coupled with inhumane working conditions and inadequate nutrition meant that in some poorer areas of the city the average age of death among labourers was just 16, compared with 45 among the better off.[109] Cholera alone claimed some 40,000 lives from 1831 before a new sewer system was constructed following the 'Great Stink' of 1858.[110] A study examining the decline in typhoid deaths in Melbourne between 1870 and 1914 concluded that improved water supplies, drainage and sanitation made the difference, not scientific medicine.[111] The Professor of Social Medicine at Birmingham University, Thomas McKeown, concluded at the latter end of the 20th century that on the historical evidence, 'medical intervention has made, and can be expected to make, a relatively small contribution to prevention of sickness and death'. He argued that life expectancy statistics were misleading given that the increase was in the main attributable to higher living standards that enabled more people to survive childbirth and infancy. For those who reached adulthood, life expectancy was not much higher at the end of the 20th century than it was at the beginning.[112]

The association of medicine with the prestige of science was clearly evident in the United States, assisted in no small part by the thousands of American doctors who undertook postgraduate studies at what were the leading centres of science and medicine in Germany and Austria from around 1870 until the start of World War I. As a result, the study and practice of medicine in the United States moved from the least regulated system in the Western world to a model of corporate monopoly.[113] Medicine was transformed into 'the most sought after career and respected profession in the United States'.[114]

After World War II, the centre of scientific learning shifted to the United States, where it is now firmly — and, it seems, permanently — located. Advances in science and technology, the benefits of which were first felt in the United States, shifted medical practice from the homes of patients to the surgeries and private clinics of doctors. This increased the number of patients that doctors could profitably see and further shifted the power in the doctor–patient relationship towards the doctor.[115]

The new road in medical science that the Nobel Prize committee credited von Behring with opening up became something of a therapeutic maze as science went on to place antibiotics, and large numbers of synthetic drugs that weren't always victorious weapons against illness, in the hands of doctors. The specialisation of practice accelerated. This too was first evident in the United States: even before World War II ended, a majority of practitioners were specialists.[116] Only a few decades earlier, in 1900, less than 10 per cent of practicing physicians were even graduates of genuine medical schools.[117]

Medicine and the mind

While stamping their authority on the body, doctors were also turning their attention to the troublesome area of the mind.

We owe the word 'psychiatry' (from the ancient Greek for 'medicine of the mind') to Johann Reil (1759–1813), a German physician who first used the term in 1808.[118] Psychiatry began to be practised as a specialised form of medicine under the influence of Philippe Pinel (1745–1826), a physician who was given responsibility for the insane at the Bicêtre institution in Paris in 1793, during the French Revolution.[119] At the time, treatment for those considered mad was incarceration, frequently including manacled restraint. In Pinel's view, if people thus restrained could stand accused of behaving like animals it was primarily because that was the way they were treated.[120] His solution was a 'moral treatment' which involved managing a patient's problems with gentle, humanitarian optimism; the idea was to gain their confidence and respect in order to correct their muddled thinking.[121]

Commendable though 'moral treatment' undoubtedly was, it was plainly a non-medical technique. This seemed an altogether too difficult obstacle to a medical claim for monopoly of treatment.[122] In Britain the medical profession solved the problem by insisting that the insane could best be treated by both medical means (the humoral techniques of blistering, bleeding and purging) and moral treatment which, with their special knack of dealing with patients, doctors could perform better than most. In France, a student of Pinel's, Jean Etienne Dominique Esquirol (1772–1840), persuaded the state to construct new institutions for the insane, called asylums — places of refuge — staffed by doctors with a 'special expertise'. This regime commenced in France with a law passed in 1838, and with the passage in Britain of the *Lunatics Act 1845*, a similar process of specialist medical supervision was set in train.[123]

In the first half of the 19th century, asylum psychiatry worked on a simple view of insanity: either you were mad or you weren't. Asylum specialists were employed by the state and the confinement of their patients precluded the establishment of a more profitable private practice. This impediment receded when, from mid-century, the idea of being half-mad came into being. If you were psychotic you were so detached from reality that you had to be removed from society.[124] If, however, you were merely neurotic, you could still function in society provided that you received psychiatric treatment at a public outpatient clinic or as a paying customer at a private practice.[125] Jean-Martin Charcot (1825–93) established the first outpatient clinic at the women's asylum in Paris in 1879, 14 years after psychiatry had first linked itself to science — the Chair of Psychiatry and Neurology was established at the University of Berlin in 1865.[126]

But it was in the United States that the private practice of psychiatry was really pioneered. The Association of Medical Superintendents had first emerged in 1844, but membership was limited to those in charge of asylums. The American Neurological Association, founded in 1875, was, by contrast, an association with a membership in private practice that proclaimed allegiance to scientific medicine and challenged the expert status of the superintendents.[127] Private practice had received a considerable boost six years earlier when a New York electrotherapist, George Beard (1839–83), announced that he'd discovered a new disease called neurasthenia, physical exhaustion of the nerves.[128] Sometimes known as Beard's disease or 'American nervousness' after the title of one of his books, it was an odd disease. It was said to be organic yet it couldn't be detected by microscope; its existence was confirmed by the patient's symptoms, which in turn proved that it was real.[129] The profession had thus 'reduced the mind to the body' … and completed its reach of authority.[130] 'Nerves' was to be the future of the profession, not 'disorders of the brain', which remained relegated to asylums, which in turn degenerated into grossly overcrowded warehouses of the mad in the Age of Confinement.[131]

The 'nervous condition' was, like postmodernism, more defined by what it was not than what it might actually be. It was not insanity; it was not hereditary; it was not incurable. More importantly, it did not involve a custodial sentence at the feared asylum. As to what it might be, well — perhaps a reaction to overwork and overexertion, and, initially at least, held to be confined to some of the 'brain workers' of the middle class.

Fortunately for sufferers of neurasthenia, a cure was at hand courtesy of another American nerve doctor, Silas Weir Mitchell (1829–1914). By 1875 his rest cure had arrived, its therapeutic value derived from isolated bed rest, massage and electrical treatment supplemented by a milk diet. This rest cure usually took place (at considerable expense) in a private clinic for 6–12 weeks.[132]

It was 'nerves' that allowed psychiatrists in the United States to begin their move from the asylum to the consulting rooms in the city, alongside their medical peers. With psychoanalysis, even more doctors were able to leave the asylum.[133] The number of psychiatrists in private practice in the United States almost reached 10 per cent of the profession in the World War I period, and was closer to 40 per cent in the next great conflict; in Britain, as in Australia, psychiatrists were still firmly anchored in the asylums at the end of World War II. By 1970, private practitioner psychiatrists in the United States represented more than two-thirds of the total.[134]

The Freudian technique of psychoanalysis had crossed the Atlantic with US students returning from Germany and Austria, and later with psychoanalysts fleeing persecution in Europe. It rested on the premise that analysis resolved the 'unconscious conflicts over long-past events, especially those of a sexual nature'.[135] Like Pinel's moral therapy, it was a non-medical technique, yet the profession, protected by the American Psychoanalytic Association's monopoly on credentialing,[136] was successful in excluding others with counselling skills until the 1970s, by which time psychoanalysis was starting to go out of fashion.[137]

The therapeutic benefits of psychoanalysis, such as they were, were largely restricted to the well off. Those deemed mentally ill among the poor were more likely to be confined within the austere walls of the overburdened asylums, while the more seriously ill among the middle classes found themselves in the much more comfortable surrounds of private 'rest homes' and 'nerve clinics'.[138] Treatment in the asylums meant drugs such as morphine, chloral, bromides and barbiturates, whose primary purpose was to calm and subdue patients. Such 'cures' as were attempted ranged from sleep comas and convulsive therapies to frontal lobotomies. This last was an invasive procedure, first performed in Portugal in 1935, that involved the destruction of the nerve fibres of the brain's frontal lobes by inserting an instrument resembling an icepick above the patient's eye socket.[139] Said to be painless, it was certainly irreversible and, as a cure, probably far worse than the disease, reducing its recipients to 'unrecognisable automatons'.[140]

In the Medical Journal of Australia in September of 1949, John Cade (1912–80), superintendent at the Bundoora Repatriation Mental Hospital, published an article entitled 'Lithium Salts in the Treatment of Psychotic Excitement', in which he described the first psychotropic drug successful in managing what was then known as manic-depression.[141] From this beginning, pharmaceutical companies in the early 1950s started producing a variety of antipsychotic and antidepressant drugs, some of whose therapeutic effects were likened to a chemical lobotomy or the application of a 'liquid cosh'.[142] This form of drug treatment contributed to the rise of the antipsychiatry movement, whose leading lights included R D Laing, Thomas Szasz and Michel Foucault. These critics pointed out that the incarceration and treatment of the 'abnormal' was based on them being posited as the opposite of 'normal', without 'normal' ever being defined. And they had a point, as an experiment carried out by the psychologist David Rosenhan in the early 1970s demonstrated. Rosenhan had eight sane people fake admission to mental institutions by saying that they heard voices. Once they were admitted, the pseudo-patients, who were diagnosed as schizophrenic, behaved normally, yet this normal behaviour was deemed abnormal, and not one of the eight was identified by hospital staff as being sane. The only people who entertained the suspicion that the eight might be normal were other inmates at the institution.[143]

Psychopharmacology and the antipsychiatry movement played a large part in the deinstitutionalisation of the mentally ill, with the course of events in Australia being typical. A cycle of asylum-building, overcrowding, scandals and inquiries had been repeating itself ever since the first asylum opened in 1811, following the first 'lunatic' being officially declared in 1808. This cycle was interrupted when patients began to be discharged into the community from the late 1960s through the 1970s and into the 1980s.[144]

Deinstitutionalisation was attractive to governments, patients and reform activists alike, but the criticism that followed was an inevitable consequence of the lack of resources allocated to community care and the failure to recognise both the effects and the side effects of the powerful drugs now being prescribed. If, in an unsupervised environment, patients thought that the drugs were doing them some good, they might feel inclined to take more of them to make them feel even better. Or they might stop taking them altogether because they thought they had got things under control, or because they had gained a significant amount of weight or developed diabetes, two typical side effects of some antipsychotic drugs.[145] These were reason enough for some to stop taking the drugs, and why some simply swapped one institution, an asylum, for another, a prison. Ironically, there are now groups calling for a return to some form of institutional care.

Medicine and the state

From slow beginnings in the 19th century, the medical profession became an authoritative part of the bureaucratic mechanism of state governance. With scientific medicine came the promise of a disease-free, healthy population, and the prospect that discoveries in the laboratory, combined with the medicine practised in hospitals, would at least ameliorate, if not completely cure, the worst cases of ill-health among the populace. The claims of scientific medicine led to demand for its services, the supply of which the state was obliged to underwrite in one form or another. The state now had to provide for the health of its citizens, an obligation that was first established as a human right in France by the Committee on Salubrity in 1793, the same year Pinel was introducing his moral therapy at Bicêtre.[146]

Healthcare, like the supply of electricity and water, had become an essential service. The state now needed the medical profession to provide this essential service, just as the profession needed the state to guarantee its position as monopoly supplier. The profession's authority was extended as the state spent an increasing share of national income on health, and, in turn, doctors' authority extended further into society — in time, to access to hospitals, to certain drugs, to life insurance, to employment, to a driver's licence, to compensation arising from injury, to expert witness evidence in civil and criminal proceedings, though such evidence has often proved so contradictory as to make a mockery of scientific objectivity.[147]

Preventive medicine and self-care

By the 1920s it was already evident that more people were suffering and dying from chronic degenerative diseases than from infection and injury. As longevity increased in the next half-century, it became more expensive for the state to provide for the healthcare needs of an ageing population that was outside of the labour force and unable to contribute to overall productivity.[148] The state needed to shift resources from clinical medicine to preventive medicine, but this could only be achieved with the cooperation of doctors. It was impossible for the state to regulate the day-to-day relationship that doctors had with their patients, and by the 1970s some of the critics of medical practice were claiming that doctors had a vested interest in what was now the business of the profession — ill-health.[149] It also became clear that medicine's claim that it was improving the overall health of the community was, at the very least, problematic. By the mid-1970s, the Director General of the World Health Organization (WHO) was asserting that the medical profession had exploited its monopoly by mystifying medical practice and distancing healthcare from medical care.[150]

At the same time, Ivan Illich, one of the most trenchant of medicine's critics, was writing that the threat to health that came from the medical establishment itself had reached epidemic proportions.[151] The name for this new physician-induced epidemic was iatrogenesis. Examining the evolution of disease patterns over the preceding century, Illich concluded that doctors had no more affected epidemics than priests had done in earlier centuries. While not denying the usefulness of specific medical techniques, he pointed out that technical medical intervention was of itself responsible for high levels of morbidity. Like many others, he concluded that nutritious food, clean water, unpolluted air, stable populations and socio-political equality were 'decisive' in determining health patterns. The dramatic increase in life expectancy in advanced economies came from the reduction of infant mortality, which owed more to food, antisepsis, civil engineering and the changing attitude on child death than to medical intervention.

Illich argued that the autonomy of the medical profession had degenerated into a 'radical monopoly' exercising exclusive control and able to both create and shape the level of demand for the services which it alone could supply. Effective preventive measures, which would reduce the incidence of ill-health in the community, would, he said, also reduce the income of doctors.[152]

Illich's thesis is borne out by subsequent studies. In 1974 the US Senate reported that there were 2.4 million unnecessary operations performed in that country each year, costing US$3.9 billion and causing 11,900 deaths.[153] In Australia, a 1995 study found that 16.6 per cent of hospital admissions, involving 470,000 patients a year, resulted in an 'adverse event'. These caused 18,000 deaths and 50,000 cases of permanent disability.[154]

By the last quarter of the 20th century, medicine, although dependent on science, had become disconnected from its direct development. New surgical and diagnostic techniques owed much to a sophisticated engineering science that by 1969 had already landed men on the moon and was beginning to run communications from satellites located in space. In general practice, doctors were dependent for their knowledge of the therapeutic effects of new drugs not on the direct science of the academy but on the scientists and salespeople in the employ of the pharmaceutical companies. Just as these doctors mediated their patients' use of drugs, so was their own knowledge of these drugs mediated.

Criticism of monopoly medicine hasn't been confined to commentators such as Illich. It has found some resonance in the profession itself as doctors have withdrawn from their existing professional bodies and joined reform organisations. More importantly, significant numbers of people have turned away from contemporary medical practice and sought alternatives. Seventy-four per cent of Australians now take complementary or herbal medicines. It is an industry worth some $9 billion a year.[155] The same trend has been evident in the United Kingdom, where, by the early 1980s, the number of complementary practitioners was already greater than the number of GPs. In the following decade, Americans were making almost 50 million more visits a year to unconventional healers than to primary care physicians.[156]

Despite what the doctor might order, it is common for those who are prescribed drugs to determine the dosage themselves, and so to take more, less or none at all, of what is prescribed. The compliance rates for taking prescribed medicine range from 0 per cent to 100 per cent, with an average of 50 per cent.[157] The state and the spread of medicine may have turned 'mutual care' — illness being treated within the family — and self-medication into misdemeanours or felonies,[158] but they are both nevertheless commonplace, even among the medical profession. A US study published in 2002, for example, showed that 40 per cent of pharmacists self-reported illegally using some form of potentially addictive, mind-altering prescription drug. The study referred to other studies, going back to 1960, that also demonstrated drug use and abuse in the healthcare profession.[159] Habits stretching back many years are apparently hard to break.

2
Pills, potions and pharmaceuticals

Despite the international controls that emerged from Geneva in 1925, the consumption of heroin, morphine and cocaine actually increased in Australia in the period leading up to World War II. A second conference in 1931, also in Geneva, called the Conference on the Manufacture of Narcotic Drugs, adopted a Limitation Convention designed to ensure that signatory countries were restricted to manufacturing or importing the controlled drugs identified in 1925 in quantities consistent with their medical and scientific needs. To this end, countries were required to lodge, in advance, their projected annual requirements to a supervisory body that would then set manufacturing and importing limits.[1]

At the time of the Limitation Convention in 1931, the per capita consumption of heroin in Australia was greater than in any other country in the world except New Zealand. We consumed three times as much heroin per capita as the United Kingdom and, for good measure, twice as much cocaine. Within five years we had dislodged New Zealand from its premier position so that by 1936, the year that a third Geneva Convention (for the Suppression of the Illicit Traffic in Dangerous Drugs) was adopted by signatory countries, we were consuming 14 per cent of the world's legally produced morphine and 7.5 per cent of the word's legally produced heroin.[2]

These world record levels of heroin consumption were not a pre-World War II statistical aberration. From 1946 to 1951 our heroin use more than doubled, so that we again had the world's highest levels of consumption. The Permanent Central Opium Board, set up as a supervisory board by the Geneva Convention — no doubt concerned that an illicit market had begun to operate — demanded an explanation. The official explanation was that in some Australian states it was permissible for cough mixtures and some other chemists' preparations to include heroin provided that the amount in total was less than 0.1 per cent. Given that only seven kilograms of the 52 kilograms imported in 1951 were used in proprietary medicines, this explanation was dubious. The real explanation seemed to rest between increased clinical demands and over-prescribing. In any event, the response of the Commonwealth Government was to ban the legal importation of heroin in 1953.[3] But within two decades imports were to resume at levels that both met demand and fuelled it: government bans are an inconvenience, but certainly not an impediment, to illegal heroin use.

The consumption of morphine and heroin in Australia following the 1925 convention was perfectly legal and prescribed by doctors in accordance with the provisions of the relevant international conventions and domestic laws. So too was the consumption of cocaine, although illegal recreational use in Sydney and Melbourne was clearly evident in the 1920s and sensationalised in newspapers as a 'cocaine crisis'.[4] The decrease in the popular use of cocaine from the 1930s coincided with the availability of much cheaper products of similar effect supplied legally by the pharmaceutical industry[5] — amphetamines were consumed throughout the world for more than 30 years before they became controlled substances. They were one of the many products of the pharmaceutical industry that emerged in mid-19th century Germany that Australians managed to consume in greater amounts than most.

Chemistry, drugs and medicine

Antoine Laurent Lavoisier (1743–94) is credited with being the founder of modern chemistry, the discovery of oxygen being one of his more notable achievements. Another was to develop the idea of the living body as 'an elegant piece of chemical machinery'.[6] He also held the government post of farmer-general of taxes in pre-revolutionary France, which, unfortunately for him, meant that his pursuit of chemistry was cut short by a trip to the guillotine.[7] French physician Xavier Bichat (1771–1802), who was opening up corpses and specialising in pathological anatomy, was able to explain anatomy and physiology by deconstructing, as it were, the organs of the body to their elementary tissues. He clearly recognised the resonance of this work with that of Lavoisier: 'chemistry has its simple bodies which form by the various combinations of which they are susceptible composite bodies ... Similarly, anatomy has its simple tissues which ... by their combinations form organs.'[8] Having revolutionised the diagnosis and classification of diseases, these French physicians and their successors now had to turn their minds to therapeutic intervention. If the body and its diseases could be explained in terms of chemistry, it was the curative and prophylactic properties of chemical drugs that had to be investigated next.

This investigation began in university laboratories in the early decades of the 19th century when the baton of scientific medical research passed from France to Germany, although it was in Estonia that the first chair of pharmacology was established, at the University of Dorpat.[9] It was nevertheless filled by a German doctor from Leipzig, Rudolf Buchheim (1820–79). His pupil Oswald Schmiedeberg (1838–1921) succeeded him and later moved to Strassburg, where he trained more than 100 pharmacologists who, in turn, disseminated the science around the world.[10]

The naturally occurring drugs in plants had been used as medicines from the earliest of times, and the knowledge that had been gradually accumulated of the efficacy of specific preparations had long been reduced to writing. These pharmacopoeias — books of drug recipes — had been guiding physicians and apothecaries in Europe for hundreds of years at least, and their range was impressive. The first pharmacopeia issued by the Royal College of Physicians in England in 1618, for example, listed over 2000 preparations.[11] But it was Bichat's successor, François Magendie (1783–1855), who eventually became professor of anatomy at the College de France, who had the clarity of vision to recognise that it was in their 'pure' form that drugs were most reliable. By 1821, research prompted by this insight had led to the isolation of a number of alkaloids, including caffeine, quinine and a strychnine-like alkaloid, brucine.[12] The earlier discovery of basic organic compounds that made these findings possible was the work of an apothecary's assistant from Westphalia, Friedrich Serturner (1783–1841). The specific alkaloid that he discovered, disclosed in experiment results published in the *Journal der Pharmacie* in 1806, was called 'morphium', now known as morphine. Magendie was one of the first people to administer this new drug, and his 1818 paper on the subject contributed to its increased use from the 1820s.[13]

As alkaloids with medicinal properties were isolated in the laboratory, the scientific possibility of synthetic production was opened up. This avoided the need to rely on the expensive and time-consuming extraction of plant matter. But whether natural or synthesised, the widespread availability of these new drugs would depend on the mass production processes of factories just as much as on the technical capacity of laboratories. The German wholesale pharmacist Merck was among the first to realise this, so the company sent some of its employees into the research laboratories to learn the new production methods.[14]

Research chemistry in Germany led to the establishment of the chemical industry, and as it developed it divided into separate branches. The primary chemical industry was concerned with the production of 'heavy' chemicals such as potash, sulphuric acid, soda and fertilisers, while the products of the 'preparations' or 'processing' industry were coal tar chemicals and fine chemicals.[15] Coal tar is a byproduct of the coal gas that was used to provide artificial light for the workplaces and streets of Europe from early in the 19th century. It was regarded as a 'nuisance and embarrassment' until the synthetic compounds that were derived from it found a profitable spot in the marketplace.[16] Paracetamol, phenacetin and aspirin all came to the medical marketplace after being synthesised in German laboratories as byproducts of coal tar distillation.[17] But it was from the artificial dyestuffs industry, that 'triumph of mass chemical synthesis',[18] that pharmaceutical giants such as Hoechst and Bayer were to emanate.

The pharmaceutical industry in Germany emerged, in a roundabout way, thanks to an 18-year-old Englishman with an interest in chemistry who was trying to produce a synthetic drug. The Spanish Jesuits are credited with bringing to Europe, somewhere around 1630, the Peruvian bark from which the anti-fever drug quinine is extracted. It was widely used to treat malaria and was often referred to as 'Jesuits' bark'.[19] The attempt to synthesise quinine by William Henry Perkins (1838–1907) in 1856 proved somewhat ambitious. Its complex structure would take another 90 years to unravel. But in the process he synthesised the first dyestuff, mauveine, whose commercial success was directly responsible for the birth of the artificial dyestuff industry. As the industry developed, in the second half of the 19th century it began to produce new drugs as well as dyes, and its pharmaceutical branch became an industry in its own right.[20]

As the findings from laboratories were transformed into medicinal products in the factories, so too was the relationship between doctor and patient transformed. Diagnosis of disease was still entirely dependent on doctors, but healing now came to rely on the products of the pharmaceutical companies. By 1894, the professor of medicine at Oxford University, Sir William Osler (1849–1919), was able to say 'the physician without physiology and chemistry flounders along in an aimless fashion, never able to gain any accurate conception of disease, practising a sort of popgun pharmacy, hitting now the malady and again the patient, he himself not knowing which'.[21]

Louis Pasteur, Robert Koch and others were still peering into microscopes and making important medical discoveries, but the production and distribution of medicinal drugs became a business whose operating principles were precisely the same as those of the artificial dyestuff industry from which it came. Production was for profit, patients became consumers, and the pharmaceutical companies formed their own research departments. The 1000 production workers in the employ of the German company Bayer in the 1880s were complemented by nearly 30 chemists in the research department.[22]

The chemical industry owes its origins entirely to science. Bernal describes the late 19th century chemist as a 'new kind of scientist, one much more closely tied up with industry than the physical scientist of earlier times', and claims that 'the academic science of the period was ultimately dependent on the success of science in industry'.[23] In the pharmaceutical industry, this new scientist now had an interest in patents and profits.

Patenting healthcare

Controversy concerning the commercial exploitation of patents has proved to be an enduring feature of the pharmaceutical industry, particularly in the United States. The secretion of the adrenal glands, adrenalin, has the useful property of increasing blood pressure, which gives it a number of important medical uses. It was first isolated in the 1890s by a number of scientists, but John Abel (1857–1938), the first professor of pharmacology at Johns Hopkins University in Baltimore, is usually credited with making the most significant contribution.[24] When the pharmaceutical company Parke-Davis applied to patent this new hormone (the name that adrenalin and like substances acquired in 1905), the idea was objected to by some scientists: they thought that the production of drugs was more to do with making people well than realising a profit and that in any event, patenting a substance that occurs in nature ought not to be permissible. The US courts thought otherwise, ruling that once adrenalin had been removed from gland tissue it became an invention, and inventions are patentable. Parke-Davis even managed to secure a US trademark for 'Adrenalin', which meant that in the United States, scientists had to refer to the hormone as 'epinephrine'.[25] It was this sort of commercial practice that opened up a rift between some scientists and drug companies and caused the American Society for Experimental Pharmacology and Therapeutics, which John Abel founded, to exclude industrial pharmacologists from their membership.[26]

Marie and Pierre Curie typified scientists of this era who refused to profit from patents even though the process they created, by which radium is prepared, was widely used in industry.[27] It was a tradition followed by the two Canadians, Frederick Banting (1891–1941) and Charles Best (1899–1978), who initially refused to patent the insulin treatment for diabetes that they discovered at the University of Toronto in 1921. Banting believed that any scientific discovery that had the capacity to improve healthcare should be freely available to all who might derive benefit from it.[28] Only after repeated requests did he and Best patent the process, and only then to prevent others taking out a patent that would restrict Banting and Best's right to make it available to others. Their share of the profits that came from the manufacture of insulin under licence by Eli Lilly in the United States went to the University of Toronto, and it was on the strength of insulin, more than any other single product, that Eli Lilly became one of the largest pharmaceutical companies in the United States.[29]

Perhaps the last of the 'old-fashioned' scientists who believed that the discovery of potentially life-saving drugs was its own reward, were the three who were awarded the 1945 Nobel Prize for the discovery of penicillin: Alexander Fleming (1881–1955), Ernst Chain (1906–79) and the Australian Howard Florey (1898–1968). Florey and Chain had been working on antibacterial agents at Oxford University since 1938, and by 1940 had demonstrated the clinical value of penicillin. The resources of wartime Britain couldn't stretch to its mass production so it was US companies that produced penicillin in the early war years, and thereafter controlled the patents.[30] Florey declined to patent the production process for penicillin because he held the view that a drug with such therapeutic potential should be freely available.[31] The large-scale synthesis of penicillin proved so elusive in the years following World War II that most chemists gave up on the idea. One who didn't was J C Sheehan, who managed to achieve a synthesis in 1957. The fact that it took until 1980 to resolve the resultant disputes tells something about the value placed on patents.[32]

Penicillin proved to be so effective in combating the battlefield infections of World War II that it came to be described as a 'wonder drug'. It was soon followed by streptomycin, one of whose discoverers, Selman A Waksman (1888–1973), is responsible for giving us the term 'antibiotics'.

The infectious diseases that penicillin and other later antibiotics were effective against included the sexually transmitted diseases, syphilis and gonorrhoea. Syphilis, which acquired its name from a Verona physician in 1530, had been a public health problem of some significant concern since Christopher Columbus's crew were thought (not without some controversy) to have brought it back from the 'New World' in 1493.[33] But despite its widespread occurrence, it was a disease surrounded by secrecy and shame, one whose origins were unlikely to be acknowledged at any level. The French called it the Italian disease and the Italians called it the French disease.[34] It was also a disease without a cure, and the effects of the recommended humoral treatment — purging with large doses of mercury — were almost as bad as the disease. An understanding of the chronic illnesses that syphilis can cause (which include blindness, paralysis and insanity) came when the founder of cellular pathology, Rudolf Virchow (1821–1902), was able to show that the infection can be transferred to internal organs through the blood. However, there was still no cure for a disease that early in the 20th century affected something like 10 per cent of the population, including up to one-third of those in mental institutions.[35] Paul Ehrlich proved to be the saviour when he discovered salvarsan, but in doing so he became involved in a controversy the like of which has also proved to be a continuing problem for the pharmaceutical industry.

Ehrlich established a research institute for chemotherapy in Frankfurt in 1899 where he pursued the idea that infectious diseases could be cured by drugs that would replicate the natural production of antibodies and destroy the invading micro-organisms that produced disease, all without damaging the patient.[36] In the course of conducting experiments to determine the causes of disease and test the efficacy of new drugs, scientists of the time often used themselves as guinea pigs. One of the earlier and more heroic examples was the Scottish physiologist and surgeon John Hunter (1728–93). In order to better understand the difference between gonorrhoea and syphilis he reportedly inoculated his own penis with the pus of a gonorrhoea sufferer. The fact that he drew something of a wrong conclusion from the experiment hardly detracts from his stalwart commitment to science.[37] In similar fashion Friedrich Serturner tested the new drug morphine on himself and a number of his friends and was almost killed in the process when he took too large a dose.[38]

When Ehrlich and the Japanese scientist Sahachiro Hata (1873–1938) began testing arsenical compounds on the microbes that cause syphilis, they were well aware of the toxicity of the substances they were experimenting with. After the 606th arsenical that they synthesised showed some promise, it was subject to a rigorous testing procedure that was unusual for the time: it was first tested on animals, then on two volunteer doctors, and then on mental patients suffering from progressive paralysis that would invariably prove fatal. Testing progressed further, so that when Hoechst began production of salvarsan it had been tested on almost 30,000 cases. In a relatively short period of time it proved effective in the treatment of more than one million syphilis sufferers.[39] Nevertheless, the drug that Ehrlich called a 'magic bullet' did have its dangerous side effects, and a significant number of patients suffered from toxic effects on the liver and bone marrow, which led to its critics demanding that the German Imperial Health Office ban the drug.[40] The controversy even led to court proceedings, which completely exonerated the nonetheless distressed and long-suffering Ehrlich; but it was a modified form of the drug, neosalvarsan, that became the main treatment for syphilis until the discovery of penicillin.[41]

When the German Imperial Health Office was established in 1876 it had the unenviable task of regulating the country's drug industry during a period of massive growth, with both the industry and the state resolutely opposed to interference in free trade and in circumstances where legislative authority ultimately rested with individual German states. It was essentially an advisory body, and its powers were, in the main, limited to persuasion. Although it managed to produce several editions of the *Imperial Pharmacopoeia*, which set quality standards for drugs, industry representatives were increasingly able to influence its deliberations. It was unable to control the proprietary medicines market, which was notorious for its false advertising, secret remedies and fraudulent representations, despite the exhortations of groups such as the German Society for Combating Quackery. Its attempt to promote legislation reserving for pharmacists the preparation of a range of products that included ointments, tinctures and essences (known as 'galenicals' in tribute to a long-gone pioneer) failed in the face of industry pressure that was concerned with depriving pharmacists of their monopoly on what had become a booming trade — the preparation of tablets. It was the failure of the Imperial Health Office that led to the industry itself taking over responsibility for drug control; this coincided with a dramatic increase in the manufacture of proprietary medicines.[42]

The 'speciality' or proprietary medicines that German factories were producing amounted to no more than a few dozen in 1870, but by the start of World War I there were more than 10,000 of them.[43] They were imitated in factories in Britain and the United States, exported around the world and consumed in large quantities, but nowhere more so than in Australia.

Marketing pharmaceutical drugs

Hypnotic drugs cause sleep and stupor, and given that the inability to sleep is a common complaint, it is not surprising that the German pharmaceutical industry turned its attention to the commercial application of this class of drugs in the late 1860s. The German chemist Justus von Liebig (1803–73) gave the name chloral to the substance that comes from the reaction of chlorine and alcohol, and in 1832, by adding water to chloral, he first prepared chloral hydrate. Both Rudolf Buchheim in Dorpat and Oscar Liebreich (1839–1908) in Berlin investigated the relationship between chloral hydrate and the anaesthetic chloroform (chloral treated with caustic potash) because of the possibility that chloral might be converted into chloroform in the body, thus providing an effective slow-releasing anaesthetic. Their investigations led to the finding that chloral hydrate produces sleep. Liebreich published an account of this discovery in 1869. The drug was available on the market in a matter of months and came into medical use as one of the earlier and more commercially successful products of the pharmaceutical industry. It held the promise of being able to overcome the difficult medical conditions of insomnia and anxiety, and it proved so effective in inducing sleep in the short term that it became known as a 'mickey finn'.[44] However, besides losing its effectiveness relatively quickly, chloral hydrate, the first synthetic sleep-inducing drug to be marketed, also proved to be habit-forming and began to be used recreationally, by middle-class men in particular. The philosopher Friedrich Nietzsche (1844–1900) and the painter and poet Dante Gabriel Rossetti (1828–82) were two of the more notable men of the time who were debilitated by it.[45] By the 1870s, when the country's manufacturing industry was still in its infancy, chloral hydrate was being manufactured for consumption in Ausralia.[46] It was followed by an even more powerful hypnotic, sulphonal, first produced by the German company Bayer in 1888. It sold well enough to provide the finance for further research on hypnotics; this led to a class of drugs that dominated the sedative-hypnotic market for much of the 20th century — barbiturates.[47]

Barbiturates are derived from barbituric acid, which was first synthesised by the German chemist Adolph von Baeyer (1835–1917) in 1864. It was one of his students, Emil Fisher (1852–1919), working with the physiologist Joseph von Mering

(1849–1908), who produced the first barbiturate to be used clinically. Marketed under the trade name Veronal, it made its first appearance in 1903. Subsequently more than 2500 barbiturates were synthesised, though only about 50 made it to the market, most notably Amytal, first marketed in 1923, and Nembutal and Seconal, first marketed in 1930.[48] Prescribed for epilepsy and high blood pressure as well as insomnia and anxiety, the side effects of barbiturates were immediately apparent: slurred speech and staggered gait, somewhat like the effects of too much alcohol. At doses just five times greater than the amount usually prescribed, barbiturates can cause death from respiratory failure.[49] This led to their association with fatal poisoning, both accidental and deliberate. Virginia Woolf (1882–1941) attempted suicide with Veronal in 1913, and in the same year the sociologist Max Weber (1864–1920) had to take a rest cure due to his dependence on the drug. Veronal was one of the many drugs used by the French novelist Marcel Proust (1871–1922). In more recent times, Marilyn Monroe died in 1962 from an overdose of Nembutal and the US anti-war activist Abbie Hoffman committed suicide in 1989 using a combination of barbiturates and alcohol.[50] Despite the obvious dangers that barbiturates posed, they nevertheless remained on the market. As late as 1965, nine billion barbiturate doses were manufactured around the world,[51] and in Australia 6.5 million prescriptions were still being written for the drug in 1967.[52] It wasn't until 1980 that the Australian Medical Association 'strongly recommended' against the general prescription of barbiturates; however, by then they had been overtaken by a new generation of sedative-hypnotics.[53]

The German company Merck was the first to manufacture cocaine-based preparations. Together with US company Parke-Davis, the company marketed cocaine products in proprietary medicines from the 1880s.[54] The opium-based preparations that were ubiquitous at the time predated the emerging pharmaceutical industry — one of the more popular brands, Godfrey's Cordial, was being distributed by wholesalers around Britain as early as 1731. During the latter half of the 19th century a greater variety of them appeared.[55] Popular brands such as Mrs Winslow's Soothing Syrup (recommended for babies), Bonnington's Irish Moss and Ayers' Sarsaparilla all contained opium in one form or another, and Ayers' Cherry Pectoral was morphine based.[56] Dr Collis Browne's Chlorodyne, which was advertised as a remedy for cancer, cholera, consumption, diphtheria, epilepsy and meningitis, contained equal amounts of morphine and cannabis extract, with a dash of chloroform for good measure. Children were catered for with lollies — available at the corner shop — that contained morphine.[57]

The level of consumption in this period of what are now illicit drugs has drawn latter-day criticism, but it's not difficult to understand why some of the proprietary drugs were so popular. In the first place, drugs containing opiates, cocaine, cannabis extract and the like actually worked in relieving real or perceived pain. The period from the late 19th century to the mid-1920s was still, for many, primarily a time of self-medication, and these were effective drugs that had been used medicinally, in certain parts of the world at least, for thousands of years. They were precisely the same drugs that doctors were prescribing for those who could afford their services.

Not all proprietary medicines contained drugs as powerful as opiates or cocaine, but a significant number of them contained alcohol, often in large amounts. Alcohol has long been thought to have medicinal properties when taken in small doses, so these alcohol-based drugs wouldn't necessarily be harmful, it was thought, provided consumers knew their alcohol content and could control the amount they took. But the contents of all the proprietary medicines were secret, so consumers had no idea if they were swallowing a poison or a placebo. In the case of alcohol this could cause something of a problem for teetotallers if the product was promoted as non-intoxicating. To the discerning consumer, the 'non-intoxicating stimulant' Whisko, which contained 28.2 per cent alcohol, might have offered a clue as to its ingredients in its name, but the catarrh remedy Pe-ru-na, with 28.5 per cent alcohol, or Hostetters Stomach Bitters, with 44.3 per cent, would have been too cryptic for most.[58] However, if you did develop an alcohol problem using these products, the proprietary drug industry happened to have the solution. There was a wide choice of 'cures' for alcoholism, including Eucrasy and Anti-Dipso. Dr Keeley's Biochloride of Gold Cure contained cocaine, not universally known for the treatment of alcoholism despite an editorial in *The Age* newspaper in 1893 attesting to its success in this regard. Dr Tyson's Vegetable Cure for Drunkenness contained so much strychnine that a tablespoon proved fatal in one case, causing it to be removed from the market.

Other products were aimed at promoting the belief that people might have a problem that they weren't aware of … which the inventive industry could obligingly solve, for a small consideration. Fair complexion hardly seems a life-threatening condition, but Dr William's Pink Pills for Pale People sold well enough even though they contained arsenic. From the same alliterative family came Bile Beans for Biliousness, which must have been a serious condition in 1906 given that Australians were consuming three-quarters of a million of them every day when the total population stood at just three million. It's perhaps just as well that their main ingredients were flavoured sugar and vegetable extract.[59] But no matter what they contained, Australians had an appetite for the pills and potions of the pharmaceutical industry that was close to insatiable.

The outrageous claims of the early proprietary drug manufacturers came to the public by way of the established advertising mediums of the day: trade cards and posted bills. The manufacturers were also dependent on advertising in newspapers. Such was the extent of their advertising that newspapers and advertising agencies came in turn to depend on proprietary drug advertisements for a large part of their income. Mass circulation newspapers began to appear in the last decades of the 19th century as a result of improved technology and rising literacy rates. With their bold headlines, pictures and display advertisements, they were visually different from earlier newspapers, which had catered only for an educated middle-class minority.[60] Since the mid-18th century the doctrine of 'caveat emptor', buyer beware, had been a guiding principle of English contract law, and the idea of 'puff' — exaggerated advertising — dates from the same period. David Ricardo (1772–1823), the celebrated political economist whose *Principles of Political Economy and Taxation* Thomas De Quincey credited with saving his reason prior to writing his *Confessions*,[61] even expressed the opinion that 'buyer beware' extended to publicans' right to sell diluted beer if they could get away with it.[62] So advertisers weren't shy in inflating the claims of their products, and to read them is to wonder why there was any ill-health at all at the time. The industry had it all covered, from coughs, colds, cuts and cancer to pimples on the face and boils on the backside. Nostrums were on hand to defeat nervous debility and fever, and a hole in the head could be completely cured, with bleeding staunched, in less than ten minutes. Sexually transmitted diseases took a little longer.[63] In the United States there was a product on the market actually called Snake Oil, alongside Swamproot Compound, Dr Moog's Love Balm and Spanish Fly.[64] None of them managed to compete with Lydia E Pinkham's Vegetable Compound, so celebrated in song, which claimed to cure the worst of female complaints, which apparently included bloating, headaches, depression, indigestion, fainting, flatulence and fallen wombs.[65]

Proprietary drug manufacturers and distributors became the largest single newspaper advertisers in Australia, just as they did in both the United Kingdom and the United States.[66] In the United

States they became the backbone of the business of advertising agencies, some of whom later became part-owners of the drug companies.[67] And it was in the United States that the advertisers had the presence of mind to include in their long-term contracts with newspapers a severance provision in the event of legislative restrictions on their products, thus giving the newspapers good reason to oppose such revenue-threatening measures.[68]

Even though the industry was eventually subject to regulation from the early 20th century, most notably in terms of the elimination of poisons and the limitation on controlled drugs in their products, they managed to resist the disclosure of the 'trade secrets' in their ingredients in Australia until the 1920s.[69]

The popularity of proprietary drugs wasn't entirely due to mass advertising, inflated and improbable claims, doubtful testimonials, or dubious and in some cases addictive ingredients. With the use of anaesthetics during surgery and childbirth and the more general use of morphine by the middle of the 19th century, the idea began to emerge that it was possible to go beyond controlling pain, to eliminating it altogether. The feeling of pain has always been intensely personal, experienced only by the sufferer and verifiable by them alone. The response to pain is equally personal and doctors today have no more idea of how pain is felt by individuals than the physicians in post-revolutionary France who first inquired 'where does it hurt?' Pain is nevertheless experienced in a cultural context, part of the learned experience of coping with the difficult reality of life and the certainty of death. Managing the evident distress that pain causes individuals had long preoccupied earlier societies, even though their understanding of what causes pain was limited by religious or mystical beliefs. Treatments were developed that included the use of available drugs, but from the mid-19th century the subjective experience of individual pain, now stripped of its religious or mystical explanation, was subordinated by the objective opinion of doctors, who not only had a much more informed view of some of the underlying causes of pain but also had the advanced chemical tools to more effectively deal with it. From here it was but a short step for the purveyors of proprietary drugs to market the idea that they had the product that could eliminate pain. It didn't matter where the pain was, and its cause didn't have to be determined by doctors or anyone else; all you had to know was that if you felt pain their drugs could eliminate it. Thus on 7 June 1853 in *La Crosse Democrat* in Wisconsin there appeared an advertisement for Perry Davis' Pain Killer alongside Ayer's Cherry Pectoral. Described as 'any one of the various remedies for abolishing or relieving pain', the expression 'painkiller' had entered the lexicon.[70]

The Perry Davis product was among the first of the proprietary drugs to be manufactured in Australia in the 1870s,[71] and Ayer's Cherry Pectoral was one of the more popular of the imported pain relievers. Eliminating pain was something of a false claim, but indeed most pain can be relieved by drugs. The industry had come up with a powerful marketing idea at a time when the cultural context in which pain was suffered had begun to change. In fact pain no longer had to be suffered; it ceased to be an experience to be learned from and became something that should simply be avoided. The feeling of pain remained a personal experience, but personal responsibility associated with it was limited to procuring the means that the drug industry had developed to alleviate or eliminate it. Sympathy and concern could now be replaced by the provision of a bottle.

Australia's prodigious appetite for drugs (alcohol excepted) dates from the 1870s, and an indication of the size of the Australian market is that it was able to sustain imports from Germany, the United States and Britain and at the same time develop its own industrial production. By 1880, New South Wales alone could boast ten factories manufacturing proprietary medicines.[72] But even though the local German and US firms were doing profitable business, Australia was primarily an Empire market: by 1910 it had become the largest importer in the world of British pharmaceuticals.[73] A decade earlier, Australians had already become the largest per capita consumers in the world of proprietary drugs.[74]

The promise of pain relief remains a prominent feature of over-the-counter medicines to this day, particularly of those that promote themselves as being effective in protecting against coughs, colds, headaches and what the industry calls 'minor ailments'. Headaches seem to have been a problem of some concern for Australians from as early as 1907, when it was estimated that the annual consumption of headache powders was somewhere between five and eight million.[75] The levels of consumption were such a concern to health authorities that restrictions were placed on the sale of headache powders that contained APC (aspirin, phenacetin and caffeine). But in a reversal of the trend to ban drugs, these restrictions were lifted in New South Wales and Victoria following World War II.[76]

The result was that from the 1950s to 1980, when over-the-counter sales of APCs were again prohibited, Australia led the world in the consumption of compound analgesics. As a consequence we also led the world in analgesic-related kidney failure.[77]

Two brands, Bex and Vincents, dominated the Australian APC market. The key ingredient was caffeine, because its addictive nature kept consumers coming back. Taking APCs for headaches meant consuming caffeine, and overconsumption of caffeine led to headaches, for which APCs were recommended. Discontinuing the use of APCs led to caffeine withdrawal and caffeine withdrawal led to headaches, which could be cured by APCs. So taking a Bex then having a cup of tea and a good lie down invariably led to, after a suitable elapse of time, having another Bex, or Vincents, as the case may be. A packet a day (containing 12 powders) wasn't an unusual amount for many people. However, what they mostly didn't realise was that in terms of caffeine alone this was the equivalent of drinking

12 cups of strong black coffee, but in a more concentrated form.[78] And, of course, if the nature of consuming all of this concentrated caffeine wasn't properly appreciated, it was more than likely that APCs would be supplemented with a little more caffeine in the form of tea or coffee.

Around the world, analgesics were among the more popular postwar drugs of addiction, and the doubling of consumption in Australia between 1955 and 1961 had already occurred in countries such as the United States and Denmark.[79] Exactly how many were being consumed in Australia by the mid-to-late 1960s is difficult to accurately determine. According to some industry advertising it was 900 million in 1964 when the total population was some 11 million. According to a Senate Select Committee in 1970, it was closer to three billion.[80]

Countries with high levels of kidney-related problems, such as Sweden and Switzerland, had prohibited the open sale of analgesic compounds by 1963.[81] Of patients with renal failure requiring dialysis or transplants, analgesics were the cause in 7 per cent of cases in the United States and 3 per cent in continental Europe in 1962. In Australia it was 20 per cent, but it took the better part of two decades before APCs became a prescription-only drug.

The level of addiction to caffeine that followed from the massive consumption of APCs meant that symptoms of severe anxiety began to appear in former consumers, the majority of whom were women. Fortunately, a class of drugs able to deal with this worrying condition was already on the market — benzodiazepines.

Together with analgesics, barbiturates and amphetamines, benzodiazepines were the other popular drugs of addiction in the decades that followed World War II.[82] They were all available on prescription following a consultation with your doctor, although prescribed amphetamines were effectively banned from general use in New South Wales in the late 1960s.[83] By 1977, there were

11 million prescriptions issued for tranquillisers, sedatives and antidepressants,[84] with benzodiazepines having by this time replaced barbiturates as the preferred drug of prescription.

Hoffmann-La Roche developed the first of these benzodiazepine drugs in the late 1950s, patenting Librium in 1959. By 1963 they had marketed another 'benzo' that was five times stronger and which would soon become a household name: Valium. It made Hoffman-La Roche a lot of money. This was a good enough reason for the rest of the pharmaceutical industry to produce a few more of them. Ativan, Serepax and Mogadon would all become familiar names to many Australians.

Between 1969 and 1982, Valium — Latin for 'strong and well' — was the most prescribed drug in the United States. At its peak in the 1970s, two billion were being sold each year. It's still a popular drug in Australia, with one million scripts issued for it in 2002, together with another one million for diazepam, its generic name.[85]

In 1988 Prozac came on the market. Often referred to as 'bottled sunshine', the effects of Prozac are similar to, though less intense than, the illicit drug ecstasy.[86] Perhaps this goes some way to explaining why it has been consumed by more than 40 million people throughout the world, including a great number of Australians, making it one of the most successful drugs in history.[87]

The contradictory view that Australians have of the state of their health and wellbeing is clearly evident in the 21st century. The National Health Survey of 2001 showed that 82 per cent of people aged 15 and over considered their overall health to range from good to very good to excellent. Yet 87 per cent reported that they had at least one long-term medical condition. Among other things, more than half have eyesight problems, more than a quarter suffer from either asthma or arthritis, 10 per cent have hypertensive disease, a slightly higher percentage have complete or partial hearing loss and almost one in ten report a long-term mental or behavioural problem.[88]

Over 185 million prescriptions were dispensed through pharmacies in 1998. Almost 36.5 million of these were for drugs affecting the central nervous system, including more than 14 million scripts for analgesics, more than 11 million for tranquillisers, hypnotics, sedatives and anxiolytics (for reducing anxiety) and more than 8.6 million for antidepressants. By 2004 the total number of prescriptions had reached 233.4 million, a 41 per cent increase on the period since 1994.[89]

Australians also have a healthy appetite for illicit drugs. At the end of the 20th century no other country was managing to consume more ecstasy or more amphetamines; only Papua New Guinea, Micronesia and Ghana consumed more cannabis; Australia's heroin consumption ranked seventh in the world after Iran, Laos, Tajikistan, Pakistan, the Russian Federation and Israel; and only in the United States and eight Spanish-speaking countries (the Dominican Republic, Honduras, Spain, Bolivia, Guatemala, Colombia, Ecuador and Peru) was cocaine consumed in greater quantities.[90]

At the beginning of the 20th century Australia was the world's largest importer of British pharmaceuticals as well as the world's leading consumer of proprietary drugs. At the start of the 21st century, the source of Australia's drugs has changed, as has the type of drugs Australians consume, but our appetite for them remains unchanged. It would seem that there are lots of people in pain and lots of places that ache.

Doctors and pharmaceutical companies

By the early years of World War II, the Germans who had shown 'the rest of the world how to make critical raw materials out of a sandbox and pile of coal' — and in the process given birth to the pharmaceutical industry — had been eclipsed.[91] The centre of pharmaceutical innovation shifted across the Atlantic: 60 per cent of the new drugs 'discovered' between

1941 and 1963 came from the United States, and only 6 per cent came from Germany and 8 per cent from Switzerland. Although the extent of this domination didn't last, neither did Germany recover its previous pre-eminent position, because other countries, including Sweden, Italy and Japan, began to play a more prominent role in the global pharmaceutical industry in the 1970s and 1980s.[92] However, as the industry grew both more profitable and more competitive, it proved difficult to shake off the reputation for marketing dangerous drugs without disclosing their composition that had been established by the proprietary drug manufacturers in Germany.

Benzo Junkie is an informed and articulate account of the pharmaceutical industry written by an iatrogenic benzodiazepine addict, Beatrice Faust, who implicates the industry in corrupt practices. The evidence is compelling.[93] Pharmaceutical companies have marketed drugs that were supposedly beneficial in the treatment of various medical conditions but which produced decidedly unpleasant and unwanted side effects. These included hair loss, cataracts and blindness as well as miscarriages, epileptic convulsions, liver and kidney failure and deaths.[94] The thalidomide babies born without limbs are one of the better known examples of the failings of the industry. Ironically, thalidomide was developed as a safe sleeping tablet because of public concern over suicides caused by barbiturate overdose. When it was taken to relieve morning sickness in early pregnancy it led to the birth of thousands of children whose limbs failed to develop.[95]

In any industry, accidents are unavoidable, and unwelcome, but the failings of the pharmaceutical industry are not simply a catalogue of accidents. The companies either knew of the drugs' shortcomings (such as when the trial monkeys died) and tried to cover up, or they should have known via testing procedures that had a little more rigour.[96]

Nor is all of this in the dark and distant past. Research in the United States has shown that slightly more than half of the drugs approved by the Food and Drug Administration have medically serious side effects. Prescription drugs are the fourth commonest cause of death in the United States, and in that country's hospital system alone, there are nearly 2.25 million severe adverse reactions to medication each year.[97] The total number of adverse reactions to medication is conservatively estimated at five million a year.[98]

The United States is the only country where a free market in pharmaceuticals operates — companies can charge what the market will bear and people who can't afford their prices go without or take a bus trip to Canada or Mexico where they can buy the drugs at a much lower price — and it is by far the largest market, accounting for some 40 per cent of global demand. It is also, of course, the most lucrative: it generates nearly 60 per cent of global industry profit.[99] Just under half of all Americans, more than 128 million, take prescription drugs each day[100] — 75 per cent of those over 65 take prescription drugs every day, and some five million in this age group are unable to afford both the medicine that they are prescribed and other basic necessities such as food.[101]

The pharmaceutical industry has consistently been one of the world's most profitable manufacturing industries, and this profitability is shared among an ever-decreasing number of companies. Mergers and takeovers have led to the 20 largest companies controlling 65 per cent of the licit drug market by 2002. That market was then worth about US$430 billion.[102] The global market is, as might be expected, concentrated in those geographical areas of the globe that have the capacity to pay: 88 per cent of the world's medicines are consumed in the United States, Japan and the European Union.[103] Meanwhile, elsewhere, 30,000 children die each day from preventable illnesses.[104]

Big Pharma, as the industry has come to be known, cite research and development costs as the rationale for both their pricing costs and corporate philosophy. Between 2001 and 2003, estimates of the costs associated with bringing a new drug to the marketplace went from US$300 million to US$800 million. By 2006 the costs were said to have climbed to US$2 billion.[105] However, some 80 per cent of R&D money is spent either attempting to replicate drugs that are already successfully marketed by competitors or developing drugs that are only slightly different from their own profitable products in an effort to extend patent protection. New drugs will have new patents, which means they will not be able to be copied by other companies for however long those patents last, where older drugs will be covered by patents that are about to end, which means other companies can then legally copy the drug, sell it more cheaply and so 'steal' the market.[106]

Huge sums are spent on marketing. In the US market, which sets the standard, the money spent on marketing, advertising and administration spending is nearly two-and-a-half times that spent on R&D. Drug promotion directed to doctors and the healthcare industry as a whole cost US$18.5 billion in 2002. Two hundred thousand sales personnel are employed in the United States and Europe to try to influence doctors in their drug prescribing.[107] As an editorial in the *Medical Journal of Australia* in July 2005 noted, the billions of dollars spent each year in promotion by the pharmaceutical industry dwarfs its R&D expenditures — for every dollar spent on R&D, between $2 and $3 is spent on promotion.[108] In Australia, most prescribing of drugs occurs in general practice, where doctors will write a prescription for about two of every three people they consult with.[109] Ninety per cent of the information that these general practitioners receive about drugs comes from the pharmaceutical companies,[110] whose promotional expenditure on doctors is more than $1.5 billion a year.[111]

When drug companies marketed products directly to consumers, the transaction was a relatively straightforward one.

The companies offered their wares to the public by advertising and the consumer had easy access to supply from a variety of convenient outlets. Restricting the supply of drugs to the authority of doctors may have offended free-market principles, and was initially thought by the pharmaceutical industry to be disadvantageous, but readjustment wasn't all that difficult. It simply involved advertising directly to doctors; this could actually have some benefits. A more focused sales and marketing effort, rather than the scattergun approach of mass advertising, held the promise of cost efficiency — the challenge has always been balancing these costs with profitability.

So the drug companies adapted to dealing directly with doctors and sought to make the experience one of mutual benefit. Over time, the interaction was defined by a modus operandi that ultimately rested on the companies' huge financial resources. First, there was the development in the larger markets of a sales force big enough to ensure that a single salesperson had a client base of only about ten doctors, most of whom they could visit somewhere between three and six times a week.[112] And second, there was a marketing budget at their disposal large enough to buy influence through straight-out personal gifts, sumptuous dinners, sponsorship of 'educational' seminars (which could just as well be held in the Bahamas as Brisbane) and free gifts such as tickets to sporting events and travel vouchers.[113]

This selling strategy was certainly successful and indeed still is, although the fine line between the strategy and outright corruption became sufficiently blurred for both the *British Medical Journal* and the *Journal of the American Medical Association* to take notice. Both commented on the nexus between company promotion and doctors' altered prescribing habits and counselled caution on the part of doctors.[114] The rules in Australia — that gifts and hospitality to doctors be related to medical education — were honoured in the breach soon after their introduction.[115]

Spending more on marketing than research suggests that a company's primary emphasis is on sales. Increasing market share is the prime objective, because that's the most effective way to increase profits, and this has led to the extension of advertising beyond the traditional medium of professional journals. Growth means persuading doctors to prescribe more, but how can that growth be generated when direct marketing to doctors has already reached a point beyond which there is the very real risk of engaging in the sort of corruption that invokes use of the criminal code?

Such infractions of the law occur all too frequently. In 2003 AstraZenica pleaded guilty to conspiring to encourage doctors to charge health authorities in the United States for treatment with a prostrate cancer drug that the company provided for free. The civil and criminal charges that followed were settled for US$355 million. TAP Pharmaceutical Products had earlier settled on similar charges for US$875 million.[116] In Italy in early 2003, 37 employees of GlaxoSmithKline and 35 doctors were indicted for corruption and 80 medical visitors were accused of making illegal payments to doctors for prescribing GSK products. A similar scam operated in Germany.[117]

What's left is 'direct to consumer advertising' (DTCA) — a way of getting patients to persuade their doctors to prescribe advertised drugs. DTCA isn't a substitute for existing marketing practices, or an attempt to wind back the clock and eliminate doctors as some unnecessary third party standing in the way of a direct consumer/company relationship. Rather, it complements existing arrangements by bringing additional pressure on doctors to prescribe advertised products. But now the pressure is from consumers, who become the drug company's advocates in the doctor's surgery following company advertisements.

DTCA is presently only permissible in New Zealand and in the United States. It got off to a shaky start in the United States in the early 1980s. It wasn't that the first advertised drug,

Eli Lilly's prescription for ameliorating arthritic pain, didn't have increased sales. It was just that it wasn't quite ready for the market — there were renal failures and deaths among those who took it. DTCA was then banned completely for a couple of years while regulators determined what safeguards and scrutiny should accompany this new form of advertising. DTCA eventually came of age in 1997, when drugs were allowed to be advertised on television.[118]

From this point DTCA really took off. Industry spending went from US$791 million in 1996 to US$3.3 billion in 2003.[119] A 22 per cent increase in visits to doctors in the six months following television advertisements set the trend.[120] Just three years later, half of the US$20.8 billion increase in drug sales came from the near 10,000 drugs subject to little or no DTCA. The other US$10.4 billion came from the 50 most advertised drugs.[121]

DTCA is well suited to the 'lifestyle diseases' prevalent in the affluent world in the 21st century, such as obesity and depression. There are some 1.1 billion obese adults around the globe, and on current trends in the United States, 80 per cent of Americans will be obese by 2040.[122] Australia is currently ranked the fourth fattest nation in the developed world by the OECD,[123] with 51 per cent of Australian adults overweight or obese.[124] Oddly enough, drug companies tell us that the solution doesn't lie in diet or exercise, but with cholesterol-reducing drugs — the top two bestsellers in 2002 had sales of US$13.5 billion. By 2005, Pfizer's cholesterol-reducing drug Lipitor was the bestselling drug in the world, with sales of US$13 billion.[125] Depression is said to be suffered by one million people in Australia and estimated by WHO to become the most prevalent disease in the world by 2020.[126] Again the answer is a little pill, so two antidepressants are already among the world's top ten drugs.[127] And if Viagra works for men, the other half of the population need to know that they are suffering from 'female sexual dysfunction', for which, luckily, treatment is also at hand.[128]

The New Zealand experience of DTCA mirrors that of the United States, and a report by Professors of General Practice from the country's four schools of medicine, with the support of the New Zealand Medical Association, has recommended a ban on such advertising.[129]However, drug companies don't see DTCA as advertising in the generally accepted way in which the term is used. They contend that it's also educational, a valuable community service that alerts the citizenry at large to any previously unknown or unrecognised medical condition that they might have. By happy coincidence, the companies have a recommended course of treatment for such conditions. This is no doubt why Merck spent US$160.8 million advertising their arthritis drug — to let people know that if they happened to have the condition, Merck had an answer in a product called Vioxx. This commendable community activity coincidentally saw sales grow from US$330 million to US$1.5 billion.[130]

Drug companies have even managed to find a way around the bans on DTCA in countries other than the United States and New Zealand: they advertise the disease rather than the drug, and then advise a visit to the doctor. Here they trust that their direct advertising to doctors is sufficient for the connection to be made between the disease and prescribing their drugs. The results show that their trust isn't misplaced, with the European market in prescription drugs expanding at 5 per cent a year (in the absence of DTCA), as opposed to the much more impressive rate of 12 per cent in the United States. Besides being profitable in its own right, this form of advertising also sets up an argument for DTCA in the name of commercial free speech and consumer benefit.[131]

Despite the success of DTCA, doctors continue to be the major focus of drug company money and attention. They will continue to be so as long as they are the gatekeepers between pharmaceutical companies and their consumers. This, in turn, will continue while the right to self-medication is limited to quack remedies on the internet and commodities such as vitamins and herbal products, which are often termed 'alternative' products as if to distinguish them in a pejorative way from the 'mainstream' products of the pharmaceutical industry. All too often, though, the producers of mainstream products inflate their claims about their products and shroud their research in secrecy. They engage in questionable and sometimes fraudulent practices that bear a striking resemblance to those of their earlier, much maligned 19th century predecessors.

Concerns that pharmaceutical companies have altered medical research statistics and concealed negative results have led the International Committee of Medical Journal Editors, representing the world's most influential medical journals, to refuse to publish research unless pharmaceutical companies register all clinical trials before they start them, in order to avoid the later suppression of results.[132] Before this decision, reports showed that drug trials that were financially supported by pharmaceutical companies were up to seven times more likely to report positive results (about the efficacy of the drug being tested) than trials that had no company support.[133]

Presumably, these esteemed journals are anxious to avoid being associated with the events that began to unfold with Merck's arthritis drug Vioxx in 2004. Since its introduction in 1999, Vioxx has been used by between 70 and 80 million people around the world, with sales eventually growing to US$2.5 billion a year. Then a three-year clinical trial showed that it significantly increased the risk of heart attacks or strokes after 18 months of use.[134] It was voluntarily withdrawn from the market in September 2004 amid claims that Merck had attempted to downplay Vioxx's cardiovascular risks for some years.[135] Research then came to light which indicated that between 88,000 and 139,000 people had heart attacks linked to

Vioxx; 30–40 per cent of them were fatal.[136] Pfizer, the world's biggest drug company, worth about US$200 billion, was then asked to withdraw its Bextra arthritis drug because of similar concerns.[137] Less than 12 months earlier, in May 2004, Pfizer had agreed to pay US$430 million to settle allegations that it flouted US federal drug regulations by marketing an epilepsy medicine for conditions that it had not been approved to treat.[138]

Shortly after the Pfizer settlement, in September 2004, US authorities ruled that all antidepressants, including Prozac, must include a warning in the strongest possible terms that they could cause children to harm themselves or commit suicide.[139] The following month Wyeth Australia advised doctors that their antidepressant Efexor, for which 1.5 million scripts were issued in 2003, could increase the risk of suicide, and could harm newborn babies whose mothers had taken the drug during the last trimester of pregnancy.[140] Then, less than 12 months after it was shown that Vioxx users had a 32 per cent higher risk of heart attack, two of the more commonly used painkillers were found to increase the risk of heart attack by 24 per cent and 55 per cent respectively. They are still on the market.[141]

A two-tier market

In the space of some 80 years, drugs that were once freely available have become illicit and new, more powerful drugs are licit, advertised and available following a visit to the doctor. This is despite the fact that, accidental death and injury aside, a significant number of drugs marketed today don't meet the needs of the patients to whom they are prescribed. A senior executive with one of the world's largest pharmaceutical companies, GlaxoSmithKline, is reported as saying that most prescription drugs do not work on half the patients who take them. He is quoted as saying that 'the vast majority of drugs, more than 90 per cent, only work in 30 or 50 per cent of the people' — he is a geneticist who believes that it is possible to develop a genetics test that would predict which medicines work on individual patients.[142]

This perhaps goes some way towards explaining why a two-tier drug market has emerged: the one licit, with supply controlled by drug companies and distributed in the main by pharmacists on the authority of doctors; the other illicit, and dominated by organised crime. They both generate similar sales — more than US$400 billion each year — and they are also in competition with each other. But some of the more dangerous drugs are the more readily available products of drug companies, just as they were in the second half of the 19th century. The truly lifesaving drugs of today's pharmaceutical companies are now disconnected from health, in the first instance by affordability. Many are also disconnected from health because they are a positive danger to it. According to some estimates, 100,000 people die each year in the United States alone from using prescription drugs. Here is history repeating itself both as farce and as tragedy.[143]

3
The food drugs, tobacco and alcohol

Drugs. The word is of Arabic origin reflecting the contribution of Arabic pharmacologists to the history of medicine and acknowledging the number of new drugs they introduced. In 9th century Baghdad it was scholars, led by Hunayn ibn Ishaq (d. 873), who kept the Galenic tradition alive during the Dark Ages by translating his texts from Greek into Arabic. Galen's idea of classifying drugs was carried on and extended by Arabic pharmacologists, who went on to produce drugs in complex combinations designed for the specific problems of individual patients. Such was the influence of Arabic medical scholars that the medical textbook *Canons of Medicine*, written by ibn Sina (Avicenna) (980–1037), was translated into Latin and became the basis of the university medicine that was taught in Europe from 1250 to 1600.[1]

From the late 16th century the market for drugs was large enough to sustain a class of artisans who were skilled in their preparation for medicinal purposes. The retail pharmacists of today can trace their organisational lineage back to the Society of Apothecaries, which was founded in London in 1617 following its formal separation from the Grocers' Company. Its coming of age as a professional organisation dates from the founding of the Pharmaceutical Society of Great Britain in 1841. Its aim was to organise all chemists and druggists around an educational credential in order to enjoy the protection and privileges of a profession, rather than those of a mere trade.[2]

At the beginning of the 20th century druggists were still respectable suppliers of medicinal products called drugs, but by then a change was already under way. Although the expression 'druggist' was a familiar enough term used to describe the purveyors of drugs, its use appears to have been more prevalent in the United States than elsewhere. The common description of druggists' premises as 'drugstores' seems to have been largely limited to the United States, and it was here that the word 'drug' first came to be associated with substance abuse rather than with medicinal products. Following the restrictions on opium smoking and cocaine use, the consumers of these now illicit substances began to be identified in medical journals in the United States as drug addicts from around 1897. By the time the *Harrison Narcotic Act 1914* was passed, the link between the word 'drug' and the word 'abuse' had been firmly established.[3] It was assisted in no small part by the fact that sympathy for iatrogenic addiction to morphine and heroin by middle-class women had, in the public mind, been replaced by fear of and contempt for 'deviant' recreational users who now constituted a criminal class identified in the popular press as 'drug fiends'. The unauthorised use of opiates and cocaine was portrayed as an 'evil' or a 'menace'. By the early 1920s pharmacists in the United States had become so concerned about this misuse of the word 'drug' that they conducted a vigorous campaign against it, which included writing to hundreds of newspapers and magazines. They pointed out that the word embraced a vast range of substances used for medicinal purposes and that prohibited drugs represented but a tiny fraction of these. They urged proprietors, editors and reporters of newspapers and magazines to acknowledge this and to distinguish prohibited drugs in more precise terms. Clearly they met with little success. In the space of just a few years, the word 'drug' had been demonised; it was the description of therapeutic substances as drugs that had to change. These now became medicines.[4]

Today the first association that most have with the word 'drugs' is with illicit substances. Magic mushrooms and cannabis to those working on the counter-hegemonic project. Ecstasy and cocaine to the clubbers and high-income hip young things. Speed and smack to those who are getting seriously wrecked. But the word is not so readily associated with alcohol or tobacco, and these are clearly the most dangerous drugs in common use today. And it is even less readily associated with the food drugs, such as caffeine or sugar, or the vast array of drugs in the medical pharmacopeia. A drug, though, properly defined, is simply a substance whose chemical nature affects the structure and function of living organisms.[5] So there are lots of substances properly called drugs and their chemical properties are unaffected by Acts of Parliament, newspaper headlines or common usage. This chapter looks at some of the more common, less restricted drugs that many of us consume.

Most people seem to want, or need, some type of drug to help them get through the day or night. This is not to say that life is so trying for everyone that some assistance is needed to get through it. It might well be that it's just easier that way. It could also be that some of us have a natural tendency to seek out pleasure-inducing substances. Stuart Walton, in his cultural history of intoxicology, has described how intoxicants in their many forms have been an integral part of the lives of the mass of humanity long before they were ever subject to restriction or prohibition, and have certainly continued to be so since. The exception he notes is the Inuit people, who live in a snow and ice environment and therefore are unable to grow anything. Before their contact with Europeans they were the only known fully formed society to have lived without the use of psychoactive substances. The claim that intoxication plays, or has played, a part in the lives of virtually everybody who has ever lived doesn't seem widely overstated.[6]

Others go even further. The American ethnobotanist Terence McKenna suggests that one drug in particular, the psilocybin mushroom, played a crucial role in the evolution of the human race. Simply put, he claims that the emergence of modern humans from the higher primates, which entailed enormous changes in brain size and behaviour, took place in less than 3 million years. This is contrary to the accepted pattern of evolution in higher animals, which operates over much longer time-spans, often tens of millions of years. What enhanced both brain activity and size, he says, were hallucinogenic compounds such as psilocybin, which was found in the mushrooms that grew in the dung of wild cattle in the African grasslands. At a later point, he continues, these hallucinogens assisted the development of both imagination and language.

We may or may not have eaten ourselves to higher consciousness, 'awareness of awareness', with magic mushrooms, but it is safe to suggest that the ingestion of plants and other simpler substances that required no knowledge of further processing by our primitive ancestors were the start of our drug culture.[7]

There are so many commonly used drugs that to enumerate them would be to produce a pharmacopoeia which would be out of date before it was completed. We live on a planet that is under increasing stress. So too are we. Those who don't have paid work (or enough of it, at least) are forced to worry about their very existence. If they have responsibility for children as well as themselves, that worry is both magnified and projected into the future.

Sociologist Richard Sennett has described what he sees as the resultant condition of those who do have paid work in what he calls the 'new' capitalism, whose dynamics are determined by the demands of 'impatient capital' for increasingly rapid returns. The personal consequence, he says, is the corrosion of character, 'particularly those qualities of character which bind human beings to one another and furnish each a sense of sustainable self'.[8] It's little wonder, then, whether we tend to the hedonism of drugs or not, that we need some help in treating the symptoms of our collective condition.

The drugs that are most frequently used throughout the world are alcohol, tobacco and caffeine. When coffee, cocoa, tea, distilled alcohol and tobacco were first introduced into Europe they were all classified as medicines. Tobacco was regarded as a reliable disinfectant as well as an aphrodisiac, and was thought to be effective in the treatment of a wide variety of ailments, from running sores and rabies to syphilis and insomnia. Cocoa was used for the treatment of diarrhoea, dysentery and catarrh, and tea for the treatment of gout, with as many as ten cups a day regarded by some as a general health requirement. Coffee was described in the manifests of the Dutch ships that carried it as cargo in the 17th century as a medicine, and was sold as a drug. Among other things, it was said to benefit the digestion and be efficacious for the blood, being prescribed for women during menstruation and following childbirth. In some parts of Europe the production and sale of distilled alcohol was a monopoly right of apothecaries, and its medicinal qualities are perhaps best summed up in one of the names given to it: aqua-vita, the water of life.[9]

We now know of course that while excessive consumption of caffeine is not without its health hazards, alcohol and tobacco have the uncomfortable distinction of being major killers. Despite this they are, in most countries, legally available, albeit with some restrictions. They are also an important and enduring source of government revenue. Indeed alcohol and tobacco taxes were once the most important source of government revenue in Australia. In 1830, duties from alcohol and tobacco accounted for 70.9 per cent of all revenue collected in what was then New South Wales, with alcohol constituting 62.5 per cent and tobacco 8.4 per cent. By 1842 this had declined to a more modest 46.9 per cent.[10]

Caffeine and sugar

Caffeine is a mild and reliable stimulant that comes in a variety of forms — coffee, tea, chocolate, soft drinks, and more recently, 'sports' or 'energy' drinks. When taken in the form of coffee or tea it is often mixed with the sweet stimulant sugar.

Coffee originated in Ethiopia and spread from there to Yemen and other parts of the Middle East. It was being drunk in Cairo early in the 16th century and in Istanbul by the middle of that century. Venetian and Armenian traders introduced it to Italy and France in the 17th century and by 1645 the first coffee house in Europe opened, in Venice.

As coffee houses spread, they came to be regarded by those in authority as sites of sedition. As a result they were banned in the Ottoman Empire during the 1660s and in England by King Charles II in 1675. This royal proclamation proved so unpopular that the ban lasted less than ten days; thereafter increased taxation was used as a means of benefiting the Crown from coffee consumption.

Although the first English coffee house was opened in Oxford in 1650, patronised by scholars whose thought processes were no doubt speeded up by the new stimulant, reliable supply — and therefore stable prices — had to wait until the early 18th century. From this time its popularity increased and coffee houses proliferated in London, becoming meeting places for merchants and other men of commerce.[11] Elsewhere they were still meeting places for radicals. It was in a Paris coffee house on 13 July 1789 that the assault on the Bastille was planned, and the preparations for the revolutions that convulsed Europe in 1848 were made in coffee houses in Berlin, Budapest and Venice.[12]

Cacao beans, originally used by Indians in the Amazon, Venezuela and Mexico to make the cocoa drink, were first brought back to Spain by Columbus (1451–1506) in 1493, and later also by Hernando Cortes (1485–1547). Once the Spanish learned how to make the drink they did their best to keep it a secret, perhaps because its medicinal properties were said to be augmented by its qualities as an aphrodisiac. But it couldn't be kept down, and by the 17th century cocoa had spread to other parts of Europe. However, the mass consumption of chocolate bars only began in the 19th century, when a method of combining cocoa butter with chocolate liquor was found by the Dutchman Van Houten in 1828, enabling Joseph Fry and his sons to market the product from 1850 onwards.[13]

The tea bush, another source of caffeine, is native to China, where tea has been drunk from around the 5th century. It arrived in England early in the 17th century — it was supplied by the Dutch, who had opened up the trade route to China. As is often the case with exotic commodities, it was initially the preserve of the upper classes, gaining wider popularity in the following century, when it supplanted coffee as the preferred beverage of mass consumption. Coffee became popular in continental Europe, in part at least because France and Holland had ready supplies from their colonies. The popularity of tea in England similarly rested on Empire economics. The East India Company had by this time established its trade relations with China, and while England's colonies didn't have coffee, they did have sugar plantations. These had been established in the West Indies by 1650. The consumption of Empire sugar more than trebled during the 18th century, by which time it and tea were inextricably linked and sugared tea had replaced beer as a working-class staple. Unlike beer, tea leaves could be re-used.[14]

It would be foolishly romantic to idealise the life led by agricultural labourers and their families in rustic England before the Industrial Revolution, which began in the 1780s. And certainly from 1830, agricultural districts in England had become the 'headquarters of permanent pauperism'. But the regime of the new factory work was different from that of farm work. The rhythms of industry didn't follow the seasons of nature. By any account, working conditions in the factories and mills were incredibly harsh. Likened to the torture of Sisyphus, it so wore men out that 'most of them are unfit for work at forty years, a few hold out to forty-five, almost none to fifty years of age'. For women and children it was, if anything, worse. Wages were meagre, housing conditions miserable, clothing insufficient and food commonly adulterated and sold in short weight. In an already inadequate diet, the proportion of bread and potatoes increased as wages decreased. It was in these wretched conditions that that the energy and stimulation provided by tea and sugar became a necessity. As one contemporary observer had it, 'Tea is regarded in England, and even in Ireland, as quite as indispensable as coffee in Germany, and where no tea is used, the bitterest poverty reigns.'[15]

Tea consumption increased tenfold in the United Kingdom in the 19th century and individual sugar consumption went from an average of just over 20 pounds a year to slightly more than 80 pounds. During the latter half of the century the source of UK tea began to change, from 'foreign' China to the India of Empire. In 1870 China accounted for more than 90 per cent of tea imports, and India less than 7 per cent. By 1903 India and Ceylon between them supplied more than 90 per cent of imports, and China less than 5 per cent. Tea consumption continued to increase during the 20th century until the early 1960s, when it began to decline as coffee became more popular and the consumption of soft drinks became widespread. This trend led to sugar consumption increasing by 25 per cent, from 80 pounds at the beginning of the century to 100 pounds near its end.[16]

The convicts of the First Fleet were deprived not only of

their liberty, but also of their sugar and tea, a habit they had acquired in the mother country. This latter deprivation was later remedied by Governors Hunter and Macquarie, who first replaced butter with a sugar ration and then allowed tea to be exchanged for part of the meat ration. Australians went on to consume sugar and tea in even greater quantities than the British. At the beginning of the 20th century we were already consuming more than an average of 100 pounds each year of sugar — the number of 'Sugarloaf Mountains' dotted around the country today bears testimony to the sugar-refining process first used in Sydney in 1840. The 9 per cent of volunteers rejected in World War I as a result of severe tooth decay and the 46 per cent of dentally unfit Australian soldiers sent to Britain in 1917 are another testament to our consumption of sugar.[17]

Billy tea was to become an icon in Australia and by the late 1920s Australia's tea consumption was reportedly the world's highest. As with Britain, India and Ceylon replaced China as the principal source of tea from the late 19th century: by 1904 they were supplying 84 per cent of Australia's tea and China was supplying just 8 per cent.[18]

Sugar was a different matter. Originally imported from Brazil and later Mauritius, sugar was first planted in Australia at Port Macquarie in the 1820s. But it was not until the 1860s that any sort of industry developed, and it did so in the northern rivers district of New South Wales, near the Queensland border. The Colonial Sugar Refining Company, which was formed in 1855, had, by 1873, established its first sugar mill at Harwood on the mighty Clarence River in northern New South Wales; today the area marks the southern boundary of sugar production.[19]

But Queensland was to become the centre of Australia's sugar industry and sugar was to become central to Queensland's economy. During the 1880s the amount of sugarcane grown along the more tropical Queensland coast increased; the first mill had been established there in 1864. But growing cane is hard work, and in the tropics, to boot, almost by definition too burdensome for white men. This problem cropped up all around the globe where sugar was planted, and slavery was the simple solution. Sugar took 10 million Africans to the Americas and a similar number were either direct or indirect victims of the trade; it took Indians to Fiji, Mauritius, South Africa and the West Indies; and Japanese and Chinese to Hawaii.[20] And from the 1860s it took Pacific Islanders to Queensland. To be more correct, many of them were taken to Queensland against their will by an organised kidnapping racket that was known as 'blackbirding'. The fact that sugar was grown by slaves elsewhere begat the circular argument that Queensland growers couldn't compete without access to cheap 'coloured labour', so tens of thousands of Kanakas, as they were called, came to work in Queensland.

When the *Immigration Restriction Act* — the embodiment of the White Australia Policy — was passed in 1901 these coloured labourers presented something of a problem. A way had to be found to no longer bring them here, and to remove those already here, without damaging the prospects of the sugar industry. The solution was legislation, also introduced in 1901, which phased out Pacific Island labour by prohibiting their entry after March 1904 and deporting all those that remained at the end of 1906. The industry was given time to adjust to the loss of Kanaka labour, and at the same time it was given protection from competition by the *Custom Tariff Act*.[21]

In the year that these Acts were passed, 1901, T A Coghlan, the government statistician, estimated that sugar ate up a hefty 8.4 per cent of the food budget.[22] Tea maintained its popularity throughout the 20th century and was still preferred over coffee until 1979.[23] Figures from 1998/99 show the annual per capita consumption of coffee well ahead of tea: 2.4 kilograms compared with 0.9 kilograms. While the consumption of sugar was by then down to 43.4 kilograms, we were managing to get through 113 litres of soft drinks each year.[24] If you've ever wondered why some young children appear hyperactive after drinking a can of soft drink, it might have something to do with the fact that a 330-millilitre can has the equivalent of 11.7 level teaspoons of sugar.[25]

The patterns of consumption have changed in the last 200 years, but the major change in the consumption of legal stimulants is its increase. Industrialised societies now consume 25 times the amount of sugar they did in the early 18th century.[26]

Tobacco

Tobacco, a plant indigenous to North, Central and South America, is one of those commodities that formed part of the 'Columbian exchange'.[27] The first Europeans to observe the hitherto unknown and decidedly strange sight of tobacco smoking were Christopher Columbus and his crew in 1492.[28] At least one of the crew would come to regret the experience. When Rodrigo de Jerez first lit up on European soil the Spanish Inquisition accused him of sorcery and he was imprisoned for seven years.[29]

Despite this early setback, English, Dutch and Portuguese traders were among those who spread the tobacco habit around the world in the following 150 years. As we've already noted, tobacco was then known for its medicinal properties and was used commercially by apothecaries. But it also had opponents in the 16th and 17th centuries beyond the Inquisitors, and its use was banned in Austria, Russia, Japan, India, the Ottoman Empire and parts of Germany.[30] In England in 1604, King James I published *A Counterblaste to Tobacco*, in which he described smoking as 'A custom loathsome to the eye, hateful to the nose, harmful to the brain, dangerous to the lungs'.[31] Ultimately, though, in a policy tradition that has proved enduring, the opportunities for taxation revenue outweighed all other considerations.[32]

The North American colonies, particularly Virginia, became significant producers and exporters of tobacco from the 17th century, aided by the monopoly that they were granted on imports to England. But the monopoly was no act of charity. One of its provisos was that tobacco crossed the Atlantic in British-flagged ships and English merchants were able to re-export it at a handsome profit.

Virginia tobacco became the preferred variety in both England and America for pipe-smoking, chewing tobacco and snuff. Until the 19th century, tobacco, when it was smoked, was mainly smoked in pipes; the long 'churchwarden' was a particular favourite.

Other modes of consumption were favoured in the Spanish colonies of South and Central America, where cigars and *cigaritos* were popular. By the mid-19th century their popularity had spread to the United States, Europe and beyond. By this time cigars were being manufactured in New York and Philadelphia, and 100 million a year were being imported to the United States from Cuba.

War was to popularise cigarette smoking. In the case of the English it was the Crimean War of 1853–56. The English soldiers' French and Turkish allies introduced them to the habit, which they then took home with them. During the Civil War (1861–65) American soldiers too were to find that cigarette smoking was well suited to battle; consumption doubled in the following decade.

At this time cigarettes were hand rolled, and you mostly did it yourself. 'Tailor-mades' were available, but these too were hand rolled … albeit by workers adept at the process. Nevertheless quality was uneven, production was slow, and when the cost of packaging was taken into account it wasn't easy to convince tobacco consumers to buy the manufactured product.

But this was the start of modernity, and among its most pervasive features were speed and mass production. The steam engine had given rise to railway systems that compressed time and distance; marine engines were replacing sail, bringing continents closer together; the telegraph and submarine cables meant communication at a hitherto unknown speed and reach; canned food could conveniently replace the fresh variety; horses would soon make way for motor vehicles; and electric lighting had already seen day conquer night.

This was an altogether faster world in the faster-developing countries, one well suited to a drug that is both a stimulant and a sedative. The quick cigarette, as opposed to the slow pipe and cigar, seemed an ideal drug for the modern man.

Although England still had its vast Empire and its protected markets, no country was developing faster than the United States, and it was a 21-year-old American, James Albert Bonsack, who in 1880 patented the Bonsack machine that brought mass production to cigarettes. Skilled hand-rollers could make something like 3000 cigarettes in a 12-hour shift but the Bonsack machine installed and perfected at the North Carolina firm of Washington Duke and Sons in 1884 was able to manufacture 120,000 cigarettes in one 10-hour shift.

The cigarette-making business was turned on its head. Instead of supply being the problem, the issue was now an uncertainty of demand. This could only be remedied by advertising, mass marketing and promotion. But increasing demand could only lead to increased competition. The way Washington Duke solved this problem stands as a perfect paradigm for the modern capitalist enterprise.[33]

In 1890 the company joined forces with the other four leading cigarette companies in America to form the American Tobacco Company. By 1910, Duke's Tobacco Trust had 86 per cent of the US cigarette market and dominated the market for all other tobacco products except large cigars. In due course they would buy or absorb some 250 tobacco companies in order to maintain their dominance, despite being twice convicted under anti-trust laws. The convictions merely replaced a monopoly with a well-organised oligopoly, with the result that at the end of the 20th century the four largest firms controlled 98 per cent of the US market.[34]

When the American Tobacco Company launched its assault on the British market and its lucrative Empire business, the end result was the creation of the first global trust. The American company bought Ogden's of Liverpool in September 1901, and the defensive response of the major British companies, led by WD and HO Wills, was to combine and form the Imperial Tobacco Company. Rather than face an expensive and protracted battle, the two combines agreed in 1902 to withdraw from each other's domestic markets and form the British American Tobacco Company to capture the export market.[35]

In Australia, local tobacco companies came to an agreement with the overseas combines, which led to the formation of the British Tobacco Company (Australia) Limited in 1904. The company held a monopoly on the imports of the American and British combines as well as a monopoly on the distribution of Australian producers, the two largest of which, Dixon's and Cameron's, had merged the previous year to form the British Australasian Tobacco Company (BAT).[36]

The English habit of smoking had, naturally enough, been brought to Australia by the English. Indeed, as with hemp, it was thought that the new colony would provide an alternative source of tobacco, in this case to the United States. Although at first Australians were dependent on imports from Brazil, cultivation began at Port Macquarie and the Hunter Valley in the 1820s and proceeded apace during the American Civil War as US supplies became scarce. When US exports resumed at the end of the war, in 1865, these were blended with the homegrown produce. William Cameron established tobacco factories in Sydney, Melbourne, Adelaide and Brisbane between 1873 and 1889.[37]

Males in the colony readily took to smoking (by 1890 Australians smoked twice as much as the British),[38] and they endeavoured to make smoke breaks or 'smoko' a part of the working day. An Englishman working in Victoria in the 1850s observed: 'A curious practice exists in the colony of taking a "smoking time" in the forenoon for a quarter of an hour, and again in the afternoon for a quarter of an hour. All the men leave off work and deliberately sit down and smoke. This, with sundry "nobblers" which they are allowed to take (a nobbler is a small glass of spirits), will count not less than an hour each day for every man, and is equal to a loss of £2,500,000 annually, allowing for only 2 shillings per hour for 80,000, besides the cost of tobacco and spirits.'[39] Smoko at work became both a sign and a site of labour organisation.

Smoke nights, concerts or socials, which in time came also to be known as smokos, were a leisure activity that reinforced smoking as a male activity. In the latter half of the 19th century and early part of the 20th century they were 'evenings marked by drink, smoking, risqué stories, bawdy songs and uninhibited conversation between men only'.[40] In the latter half of the 20th century they were still men-only events — with the exception, of course, of the female strippers not uncommonly supplied for the entertainment of the smoking and drinking males.

In early Australia up to 83 per cent of men smoked. By 1900, 72 per cent of males smoked compared with 3 per cent of females. Male smoking remained fairly constant over the next half-century but the number of females smoking increased dramatically. In 1962 some 57 per cent of males smoked and 29 per cent of females. By 1986 only 33 per cent of males were smoking but the figure for females stood at 29 per cent.[41] This narrowing of the gender divide between smokers continues, with 21.1 per cent of males and 18 per cent of females being reported as daily smokers in 2001. In the important 14–19 age group, however, 16.2 per cent of females were smokers as opposed to 14.1 per cent of males.[42]

Although Wills (Australia) had imported a Bonsack machine and its Capstan cigarettes dominated the cigarette market in the early 20th century, tailor-mades were rather slow to catch on in Australia. Snuff never had a large share of the tobacco market and cigars too had only a minor share, except during the Victorian gold era. Pipe smoking dominated from the early days and still retained almost half the market in the late 1920s. Roll-your-owns were the Australian cigarette of choice. In Britain they were only 2 per cent of the cigarette market, but in Australia two-thirds of cigarettes smoked in 1936 were roll-your-owns, and even in the more prosperous early 1950s rollies were still more popular than manufactured cigarettes. The tide turned in the mid-1950s, though, and by 1974 only 6 per cent of male smokers and 1 per cent of female smokers rolled their own.[43]

As a smoker lights up and takes a deep drag of a cigarette the temperature at the tip rises to about 926°C. This oxidises and releases through the smoke more than 4000 separate compounds.[44] Among other things, there are 43 chemicals in the smoke that are known carcinogens.[45] Cigarettes also contain somewhere between 0.5 and 2.0 milligrams of nicotine, about 20 per cent of which enters the bloodstream and reaches the brain in a matter of seconds, aided by the manufacturers' thoughtful addition of ammonia. Nicotine is a highly toxic substance which is widely used to good effect in pesticides. About 60 milligrams of the pure stuff is a sure-fire remedy for giving up smoking as a consequence of the rather rapid onset of death.[46]

Risk-taking activity will always, of course, be a matter for the risk taker, but when the wherewithal for the activity is legitimately purchased on the open market, knowledge of the risk might seem a fair precondition for any sale. With the use of tobacco, and cigarettes in particular, knowledge of their harmful effects has been around for a long time but was for much of that time largely suppressed.

As far back as 1828 nicotine was isolated in tobacco and its toxicity was known. The number of working-class volunteers for the Boer War (1899–1902) was dependent on the cycle of unemployment, and the numbers accepted depended on their state of health. More than one-third of volunteers were considered unfit, and the large numbers rejected because of 'smoker's heart' (cardiac irregularities caused by heavy smoking) led to concerns about the future adequate defence of the Empire.[47] This, in turn, led to legislation early in the 20th century in both Britain and Australia aimed at prohibiting children from smoking.[48]

From the late 1920s scientific and medical evidence emerged about the toxic nature of the tar found in tobacco.[49] But unfortunately, with tobacco — unlike alcohol, where overindulgence is soon apparent — the deleterious effects are cumulative. So it wasn't until the early 1950s that the link between cigarette smoking and cancer, particularly lung cancer, was definitively made by medical researchers in the United States and England. By the mid-1950s this evidence was confirmed in Australia.[50] And by the early 1960s research conducted by the tobacco industry itself (but not made public) had unearthed numerous cancer-causing compounds in smoke.[51] After the Reports of the British Royal College of Physicians in 1962 and the US Surgeon-General in 1964 there came to be general acceptance, in the medical community at least, of the dangers of smoking.[52]

The response of the cigarette companies in the United States when this bad news began to surface in the 1950s was to fund a new public relations organisation that was larger than the American Cancer Society or the National Academy of Sciences, in financial terms.[53] Protection of profit had clear dominance over public health for these companies, and for the better part of 40 years this strategy worked well. But the bad news kept on coming. In 1988 the US Surgeon-General officially declared nicotine addictive (a fact that the tobacco companies had known since 1963) — it is more addictive than heroin, as it turns out, which is why heroin addicts find it easier to quit than smokers do.[54]

The policy response in Australia to this burgeoning crisis was predictably slow. There was a domestic industry to protect and there were overseas companies to placate. Advertising, mass-marketing and promotion were crucial for the growth of the tobacco industry into the multi-billion dollar worldwide business it had become. Tobacco advertising linked smoking with glamour, independence, sport, and even good health. Actors, sportspeople, even doctors were used to sell the product. Clearly, a curb on advertising, together with warnings to consumers about adverse health consequences, was crucial to any program aimed at discouraging smoking. In this respect Australia was a laggard. In Britain television advertising of cigarettes was banned in 1964. In the United States it was banned in 1966, the same year that health warnings were introduced on cigarette packets. Australia didn't introduce these warnings until 1973 and didn't have a complete television advertising ban until 1976. A national print ban had to wait until 1990 and a prohibition on sponsorship didn't come into force until 1995. Even then mass entertainment events such as the Formula 1 Grand Prix were given very long lead times to get rid of their tobacco sponsorship.[55]

The fact that tobacco companies have for many years engaged in deception and fraud to deadly effect has always been difficult for litigants to prove. Many individuals had tried, but all of them ultimately failed. Big Tobacco was simply too powerful.[56]

The breakthrough came when a number of state authorities in the United States decided to sue the tobacco companies to recover health budget expenditure incurred as a consequence of the companies' activities.

The Master Settlement Agreement that resulted from this legal action in 1998 was seen by many as a turning point that might lead to more responsible behaviour on the part of the industry, more informed choice on the part of smokers and, importantly, fewer young people deciding to smoke — and thus the promise that tobacco smoking might in the future be confined to a small minority. Under the settlement, the industry was to pay the litigant states US$246 billion over 25 years, introduce comprehensive smoking prevention programs, with a particular emphasis on children, and strictly limit advertising.

The results to hand so far are hardly encouraging. In the year immediately following the settlement the industry spent more money than it had ever previously spent on advertising and promotion in the United States: a massive US$8.24 billion. Continuing the grand industry tradition of spin, Philip Morris spent US$100 million advertising the fact that it was an exemplary corporate citizen that gave US$60 million to charity. And of course the settlement only covered the United States. This leaves the tobacco companies free to replicate their reprehensible behaviour in any other country in the world that may have escaped their close attention thus far. Their marketing people are unlikely to have missed the WHO study showing women to be the single largest untapped market for cigarettes.[57]

A product that has a large profit margin and is addictive to consumers is obviously too good a business proposition to let languish. The inconvenient fact that the consumers die prematurely is merely another marketing challenge. And the tobacco companies already know the key to this.

Of those who take up smoking as adults (aged 21 and over), the drop-out rate is more than 90 per cent. The number of those who persist is not sufficient to sustain adequate growth. However, a different pattern emerges with young people: 75

per cent of lifetime smokers are smoking by the time they are 17, and 89 per cent are smoking by the age of 19.[58] Children are indeed the future for the tobacco industry, and in the United States almost 1.2 million become regular smokers each year. In Australia there are more than 250,000 child smokers and some 43,000 start each year. A survey by the University of Michigan in the United States found that more than 40 per cent of 13-year-old students had not only tried smoking, but also thought that smoking a packet or more a day didn't present a great health risk.[59] Which is good news for the cigarette producers, because today's successors to the Bonsack machine which made all this possible can now produce 10,000 cigarettes every minute and capacity under-utilisation simply won't do in the modern capitalist enterprise.

Alcohol

Alcohol, or more precisely ethyl alcohol, the drinkable variety, has been with us for a very long time. Quite how long is difficult to accurately determine, but the basic recipe is easy enough. Simply take any organic material with sugar content, add a little yeast, water and heat, and alcohol is the result. The process can occur naturally without any human intervention, and the four ingredients are said to have been in existence in most parts of the globe for 200 million years.[60] It's not difficult to imagine the pleasurable, intoxicating effect that fermented fruit would have had on our ancestors, and we've been rediscovering the pleasure — and, often enough, the pain as well — ever since.

Mead, an alcoholic drink made from fermented honey, was drunk as long ago as 10,000 years,[61] wine appears to date back to 5400 BCE and beer to around 3700 BCE, when the Egyptians established the first official brewery.[62] With the exception of Oceania and most of North America, tribal peoples of all major parts of the world were familiar with alcoholic drink.[63]

Among the Aztecs it was compulsory, for adults at least, to get drunk at religious festivals so as not to incur the displeasure of the gods.[64] The Bible has some 200 references to wine and vineyards; the ancient Greeks turned wine drinking into something of an art form (the intellectual discussion known as a 'symposium' literally means 'drinking together'); and whatever the truth of the matter, the collapse of the Roman Empire has come to be associated with widespread drunkenness.[65]

If in earlier times, as Roy Porter has said, the production of alcohol made sense as an economical way of dealing with perishable and sometimes surplus produce, so too did its consumption as stored nourishment, a substitute for unreliable water and a social lubricant.[66] Alcohol became associated with festivity, both religious and secular, and it seems that any excuse for a festival would do: births, deaths, marriages, agreements, good harvests — we'll drink to that! But while social drinking was one thing, drunkenness, which is democratic in nature in the sense that all in the community were participating, in time came to be unacceptable, for some. It was acceptable to get 'half-drunk' provided you remained civilised and remembered your place, but getting obnoxious and violent with it was unacceptable, particularly for the lower classes.

It can be argued that the turning point was associated with the production of distilled alcohol, the process by which fermented liquid is boiled with the vapour drawn off into a still and then cooled. The condensed product has an alcohol content of 40 to 50 per cent, as opposed to around 4.5 per cent for beer and 12 per cent for wine. (The alcohol content of spirits is usually described using the term 'proof', which is double the percentage of alcohol: a 100-proof spirit contains 50 per cent alcohol.)[67]

Distilled alcohol is generally thought to have been first produced at the medical school in Salerno, Italy around 1100, by the conversion of wine into brandy. Stuart Walton, however, contends that the process was discovered in the East (probably China) during the first millennium BCE and was known in India around 800 BCE.[68] Distilled spirits had the distinct advantage of being able to be produced from a great variety of organic material. Thus, in time, rum was distilled from sugarcane, whisky from corn and barley malt, vodka from rye, tequila from the juice of the maguey plant, and gin from barley, potato, wheat, corn or rye (and then flavoured with juniper berries).[69]

Franciscus Sylvius, the Professor of Medicine at Leyden in Holland who pioneered clinical medicine, is said (perhaps apocryphally) to have first flavoured distilled spirits with juniper berries around 1650. He was looking for a cure for kidney and stomach disorders. There must have been a lot of such disorders about because the Dutch were exporting 10 million gallons a year of Geneva (from the French for juniper *genievre*) just 35 years later in 1685. At home the Dutch navy was to gain a reputation for its fighting spirit, known as 'Dutch courage', which probably resulted from consumption of the spirit that, in English, came to be known simply as gin.

When the Dutchman William of Orange ascended the English throne in the 'Glorious Revolution' of 1688, he was soon to declare war on France. Among other things, this meant a ban on the importation of French brandy. In order to shore up his support with the English landed gentry, he prevailed on Parliament in 1690 to pass an Act to encourage the distilling of brandy and spirits from corn. 'Brandy' was in those days a generic name given to all spirits, and 'corn' was a reference to any of the four grain crops — wheat, barley, rye and oats. These crops had to be rotated, to make sure the land was continually able to produce and because wheat for bread-making fetched the best price but couldn't be sown in the same field year after year, so 'the economics of 18th century farming only worked if a market could be found for an awful lot of extra barley' (rye and oats were used for oatmeal, oatcakes, flour, and livestock feed). The newly deregulated distilling industry became the market.[70]

Thus did state intervention give birth to the English gin industry. And the English, in turn, became known for public drunkenness on a mass scale. In 1713, 2 million gallons of raw spirit were being produced each year; by 1734 this had risen to 5 million gallons. Although not confined to London, this period of the 18th century became known as the 'London Gin Craze'. It was the time that dram shops (and there were as many as 10,000 gin shops in London alone) advertised, 'Drunk for a penny. Dead drunk for twopence. Straw for nothing.'[71]

Excessive gin drinking was blamed for prostitution, violence and disregard for authority, high infant mortality and, above all, for crime. Unemployment, overcrowding and the wretched conditions of the times apparently had no bearing on the predilection of the poor to drink themselves into oblivion. Clearly, something had to be done. What was done was an attempt at prohibition via the *Gin Act 1736*. This had such salutary effect that by 1743 spirit production had increased to more than 8 million gallons a year, enough gin for every man, woman and child in London to be drinking two pints a week.[72]

Excessive consumption was eventually curtailed by a combination of lower wages, higher taxes, failed harvests and the morals of the emerging middle class.[73] The gin craze subsided (though not the English drinking problem) to the extent that by 1758 production levels had returned to those of 1713: some 2 million gallons a year.[74] It was to be revived again in 1825 when state intervention, this time in the form of free trade in spirits, saw consumption dramatically increase and 'gin palaces' proliferate.[75]

What was more enduring, though, was the notion that only the poor were drunkards and that drunkenness led to criminal activity.[76] And, of course, the criminal activity of the drunken poor that was feared was that which deprived the rich of some of their property. The only thing that was more feared was the possibility of being deprived of all of their property, not to mention their lives, by violent revolution, such as was happening in France in 1789.

The attempt to tax the cheap wine of the workers of Paris played an important part in the events leading up to the storming of the Bastille on 14 July 1789. Earlier that month there were riots among the workers of Faubourg St Antoine, Montmartre and Belleville. They were protesting the building of a new city wall which would enable the authorities to impose taxes on the previously untaxed wine sold on the city outskirts. Drinking and eating places known as *guinguettes* had long been established around the outskirts of Paris. They were frequented by workers because they sold cheap wine; this wine was untaxed, whereas in the city a duty was levied. In 1784 the municipality thought it a good idea to increase its revenue by building a new city wall which would enclose many of the *guinguettes* to the north and east of Paris and subject the cheap wine to tax. Fearing that they would no longer be able to afford a drink, the workers set fire to the half-finished buildings that were to make up the wall in early July 1789. They may have lacked bread and been unable to eat brioche, but they weren't about to be deprived of their wine without a fight; the events at the Bastille soon followed.[77]

The bloodshed of the Paris Commune in May 1871 was also attributed by contemporary writers to excessive alcohol consumption, one going so far as to label the uprising an act of 'alcoholic pyromania'. But while there was plenty of alcohol about, seeking to blame it alone was both a convenient way to downplay — even trivialise — a workers' insurrectionary government and a justification for the repression that followed, when as many as 34,000 were killed and 43,000 were taken prisoner.[78]

After the Paris Commune, the connection between the poor and drunkenness came to be extended to the working class and revolution. Curiously, this seems to have been lost on Lenin who, on coming to power with the Russian Revolution in 1917, banned all known drunks from the Communist Party of the Soviet Union.[79]

Australia was to have its own alcohol-related rebellion in 1808, albeit one concerned with the preservation of a monopoly. From the arrival of the First Fleet in Sydney Cove on 26 January 1788, drunkenness was a not uncommon condition among the populace.[80] The initial naval company sent to keep the peace in the new colony proved somewhat unreliable, so they were replaced in December 1791 by the New South Wales Corps.[81] This fine regiment of non-fighting English soldiers had a monopoly on the import and sale of all goods, including spirits. Rum, the most sought-after import, became the medium of exchange for labour as well as other commodities, and the New South Wales Corps came to be known as the Rum Regiment.

Governors John Hunter and Philip Gidley King were unable to break the monopoly of the regiment so the English Crown sent out Governor William Bligh, formerly in command of the *Bounty*, and charged him with the task of 'upsetting a vicious economic system'.[82] Bligh issued orders prohibiting the use of rum as currency and was rewarded for his efforts by arrest and imprisonment on 26 January 1808. His captors, the New South Wales Corps, celebrated by getting drunk. Though order was soon restored, the new governor, Lachlan Macquarie, was instructed to send the Corps back to England. For good measure he also reduced the number of licensed houses, prohibited them from opening during Sunday service and placed an import duty on spirits.[83]

Drinking and drunkenness were never far from the centre of Australian life during the 19th century. Alcohol was a 'great comforter' to those battling away in the city and the bush. It was there at the Eureka Stockade, at the siege of Glenrowan, at Lambing Flat, on royal visits and during parliamentary debates.

Drunkenness was condemned by parson and press alike, and blamed for nine-tenths of all crime. It also had a devastating effect on the Indigenous population, but it continued despite all of this.[84] The only victory of the temperance movement which began in the 1830s was the prohibition of alcohol sales on Sundays in New South Wales in 1881.[85]

Both England and Australia are indebted to events during World War I for the peculiar licensing laws that prevailed in the 20th century: the closing of English pubs in the early afternoon and their re-opening some hours later, and that bizarre Australian institution, the closing of pubs at six o' clock, which rapidly came to be known as the 'six o'clock swill'.

General Sir John French was the Commander of the British Expeditionary Forces in France in World War I. On 10 March 1915 he staged an attack on German defensive positions at Neuve Chapelle, chiefly to mollify the French, who were concerned that a 'sideshow' in the Dardanelles (at a place called Gallipoli) was diverting troops from France. The Germans were taken by surprise, principally because the British, being short of shells, couldn't proceed with the usual bombardment. For the first and only time in the war, British infantry broke the German line. Perhaps they were more surprised than the Germans: their reluctance to advance until reinforcements arrived gave German reinforcements time to plug the gap. With exemplary timing, the British then attacked. They withdrew three days later, their only achievement being unnecessary loss of life.

Not being one to accept defeat easily, the redoubtable Sir John complained with ferocious audacity that it was shortage of shells that led to his failure. Not to be so upbraided without riposte, the Asquith government in turn laid the blame at the feet of lazy and overpaid workers in the munitions factories who spent their time in alehouses rather than manufacturing munitions. The obvious solution, which was duly implemented, was to restrict the opening hours of pubs and impose an afternoon closing time. At the end of 1915 French was recalled. Asquith lost the prime ministership the following year and his parliamentary seat in 1918, but afternoon closing remained until near the end of the 20th century.[86]

In 1916 soldiers at the training camps at Casula and Liverpool in western Sydney rioted and broke into hotels in the city. In the drunken revelry that followed, military pickets shot seven soldiers, killing one of them, at Central Station. Several states imposed 6 o' clock closing and the federal government banned alcohol in military camps.[87] The early closing of pubs was supposed to be a temporary measure, but it lasted until 1955 in New South Wales and 1967 in South Australia. It no doubt gave heart to the prohibitionists, who were able to bring enough pressure to bear to force referendums in several states. Prohibition referendums were held in Queensland in 1920, New South Wales in 1928, Victoria in 1930 and Western Australia in 1950.[88] None succeeded, so we were able to avoid the disastrous prohibition period of 1920–33 in the United States, which proved such a boon to organised crime.

We didn't escape such consequences entirely, though. Restricting alcohol sales simply led to sly grog-selling. This, together with the criminalisation of SP (starting price) bookmaking, prostitution and drugs, created by the 1920s an illicit market serviced by a professional criminal class.[89] This criminal class was in turn able to corrupt police, politicians and, in time, members of the judiciary. The illegal selling of alcohol was an important source of revenue for Australia's criminals until the mid-1950s, when more rational licensing laws began to be enacted.[90]

Today more than 80 per cent of Australians aged 14 and over consume alcohol with varying degrees of regularity and only about 10 per cent have never indulged. In the financial year 2000/01 our per capita consumption of pure ethanol (this is a way in which researchers collect and compare alcohol consumption) was 9.32 litres per annum, which ranked us 23 in the world, and each year we spend more than $14 billion on various forms of alcohol.[91] In the halcyon days at the beginning of the 19th century our total annual consumption of alcohol was enough for more than 26 litres of spirits and 12 litres of wine for every man, woman and child in the colony.[92]

If the worry is that alcohol might fuel revolution, young females and males from an early age are in the vanguard. The very word 'drinking' is, in English, synonymous with drinking alcohol and by 2003, 70 per cent of Australian women aged between 18 and 23 were doing enough of it to be categorised as binge drinkers (consuming five or more drinks in one session). As to young males, a survey of school students at Waverley College in Sydney's exclusive eastern suburbs, following a drunken rampage that caused $80,000 worth of damage in Bondi, revealed that the average age at which these young men had had their first full alcoholic drink was 11.8 years. More than one-third had their alcohol supplied by their parents.[93]

Although the legal age of 18 for drinking alcohol in Australia is arbitrary, it does appear to have general support. The idea that children and adolescents need to be protected from exposure to these sorts of activities is both instinctive and appropriate. However, imposing a moral code by legislative fiat will almost always give rise to controversy of some sort. No doubt there are many who would contend that teaching children to consume alcohol responsibly is a part of responsible parenting and that this necessarily involves imbibing in a controlled environment before the age of 18.

Alcohol is clearly a dangerous drug when more than a moderate amount is consumed (that is, more than one or two drinks per day for adults), and the danger increases with increased consumption. The same thing can be said, although to a somewhat lesser degree, for caffeine and sugar. Prolonged smoking of tobacco is simply deadly. It is a decidedly odd public policy, then — though one that has stood internationally for 80 years — that leads most members of the public to condemn illicit drugs yet largely ignore the equal, if not greater, dangers of some licit drugs.

Of the total drug-related deaths throughout the world in 2000, tobacco was responsible for 71 per cent (4.9 million deaths); alcohol for 26 per cent (1.8 million deaths); and illicit drugs 3 per cent — (223,000 deaths).[94] In Australia tobacco accounts for 80 per cent of drug-related deaths (around 19,000 deaths each year) and alcohol accounts for 16 per cent.[95]

There are also social costs of drug abuse and misuse in Australia: labour costs (absenteeism and lost productivity) and the costs of healthcare, crime and road accidents (including ambulances and fire costs). These costs came to $34 billion in 1998–99. In rounded terms, tobacco was responsible for 60 per cent of these costs ($21 billion), alcohol for 22 per cent ($7.6 billion) and illicit drugs for 19 per cent ($6.1 billion). They are borne by individuals, business and government. However, governments bore just one-third of the social costs of illicit drugs, slightly less than one-quarter of the alcohol-related costs and a mere 11 per cent of the costs associated with tobacco. During the same period, government revenue from alcohol exceeded costs by $1.7 billion; tobacco revenue exceeded costs by $2.8 billion.[96] Total government revenue associated with tobacco products was more than $8 billion in 1998–99 and the federal government, which collects more than $5 billion from tobacco excise, until recently spent just $2 million a year encouraging people to give up smoking through its national anti-smoking campaign.[97]

4
Stimulants for work and pleasure: Cocaine and amphetamines

The early hunter-gathering people of Peru were probably chewing coca leaves as long ago as 15,000 years,[1] and the cultivation of the leaf has certainly been an important aspect of Andean cultures for the last 5000 years.[2] The use of cocaine, the active ingredient of the coca plant, however, is much more recent. It owes its origins to mid-19th century German chemistry and its popularity, starting from that period, to the medical profession, to the emerging pharmaceutical industry, and, in the United States at least, to employers who were quick to recognise its value as a boon to labour productivity.

There are something like 250 species of the coca plant native to the tropical slopes of northern South America, but the two most widely cultivated for their cocaine content are *Erythroxylum coca* and *Erythroxylum novogranatense*.[3]

Andean cultures used the coca plant for various social, mystical, religious and medicinal purposes and, more than 3000 years ago, had worked out that separation of the alkaloid cocaine was best achieved by chewing the coca leaves together with lime-rich material. Its use as an anaesthetic helped Peruvians develop unprecedented knowledge of surgical techniques — including amputations, excisions and a form of skull surgery known as trephining. Coca is the most powerful natural stimulant known, so it was, and indeed still is, used for endurance and to ward off hunger and thirst. Particularly beneficial at high altitudes, it was elevated to divine status during the Inca period.[4]

Then, in the early 16th century, the conquistadors arrived. They came to serve their god and their king ... and to get rich. As Hernando Cortes explained, he and his men 'suffered from a disease of the heart which is only cured by gold'.[5] At first they disapproved of the natives' consumption of coca and endeavoured to prevent its use. However, when they noted that productivity in the gold and silver mines was trending downwards, they were quick to allow consumption to resume.

The South American invasion and occupation resulted in what some historians call the Columbian Exchange. Europeans got potatoes, pineapples, dahlias, sunflowers, magnolias, maize, chillies, chocolate, turkeys, tomatoes and tobacco. The Spanish, in particular, got massive wealth in the form of plundered gold, silver and emeralds. The indigenous people throughout the Americas got widespread death from introduced diseases such as smallpox, malaria and measles; the diseases so devastated the population that the African slave trade was begun to provide a replacement workforce.[6]

One commodity that didn't travel well from the new world to the old was coca leaves. By the time they reached Europe much of their potency was lost; early experiments proved disappointing. Hermann Boerhaave is credited with reviving interest in the plant with his *Institutiones Medicae* in 1708, but the important breakthrough was still 150 years away.[7]

It wasn't until Albert Niemann, a chemist at Gottingen University in Germany, isolated the alkaloid cocaine from coca leaves in 1860 that the drug came into popular use. Early demand focused on alcoholic drinks. The combination of cocaine and alcohol produces a particularly intoxicating metabolite called cocaethlyene, which has an elimination half-life three to five times longer than that of cocaine.[8] This helps explain why Vin Mariani, a mixture of Bordeaux wine and extracts of coca leaves developed by the Corsican pharmacist Angelo Mariani, became such a successful product in 1863.

Vin Mariani was promoted as a tonic-stimulant for the fatigued and overworked body and brain. As an added bonus it prevented 'malaria, influenza and wasting diseases'. Early tipplers included the writers Henrik Ibsen, Alexandre Dumas, Jules Verne, H G Wells and Emile Zola. The royalty of Europe who enjoyed a drop included Queen Victoria, the kings of Spain, Serbia, Greece, Norway and Sweden, the Prince of Monaco, the Prince and Princess of Wales and the Czar of Russia. The Shah of Persia and US presidents Ulysses S Grant and William McKinley also imbibed, as did the sculptor Rodin and the actress Sarah Bernhardt. American inventor Thomas Alva Edison, who gave us the gramophone and the incandescent light bulb among a thousand other inventions, had early in life acquired the habit of going for long periods with little sleep, and his consumption of Vin Mariani must have assisted him in maintaining the habit in later life.[9] Frederic Auguste Bartholdi, creator of the Statue of Liberty, claimed that he would have designed the statue three times larger if he had been drinking Vin Mariani then.[10] Pope Pius X indulged, as did Pope Leo XIII, who was so impressed by the drink that he awarded Mariano a special gold medal.[11]

Vin Mariani enjoyed continuing success until the end of the 19th century, but it was a drink invented by Civil War veteran John Pemberton, a druggist from Atlanta, Georgia, that was to become an icon of American capitalism. Bankrupt and addicted to morphine, Pemberton promoted his French Wine Coca (made from wine, kola nuts and coca leaves) as a general cure-all, and as a specific cure for morphine and opium addiction. In 1886 he pre-empted the prohibition of alcohol in Atlanta by removing the wine and renaming the product Coca-Cola. By 1902 Coca-Cola had also beaten the prohibition of cocaine in Georgia by taking out the 'coke' as well,[12] although the company was still being prosecuted seven years later for violations of the *Pure Food and Drug Act 1906*.[13] A product called 'decocainized flavour essence', which involves the use of 175,000 kilograms of coca leaves each year, is probably still used in Coca-Cola today,[14] but acknowledging the coke in Coke, much less its original appeal, has never been a company strongpoint.[15]

By the mid-1880s cocaine consumption began to increase rapidly, and two of the more notable works of fiction that featured cocaine use were published around this time. *The Adventures of Sherlock Holmes*, serialised in 1891, owes something to the amount of time Dr Arthur Conan Doyle had on his hands as a result of the slow business he was doing in what was then an 'overcrowded' medical profession,[16] but Robert Louis Stevenson rather entered into the spirit of things when he wrote *The Strange Case of Dr Jekyll and Mr Hyde* in 1886 during a six-day period of cocaine consumption.[17]

As might be expected, the German pharmaceutical companies were among the leading manufacturers of cocaine, with the output of Merck rising from less than half a kilogram in 1883 to more than 83,000 kilograms just two years later.[18] By 1884, German companies had begun to set up facilities in Lima, closer to the source of supply. Towards the end of the decade the British were sourcing their supply from Ceylon and considering setting up coca plantations in one of their other colonies, Australia. Some years later the Dutch established plantations in their colony of Java.[19]

The other pharmaceutical company that had the presence of mind in 1884 to send a representative to South America, in this case Bolivia, to source coca leaf was the American company Parke-Davis.[20] This initiative would have a profound effect on the way in which cocaine was marketed in the United States, which in turn would influence US authorities in their eventual prohibition of the drug.

In the mid-1880s, Europe was still the centre of the world and Great Britain still its most influential country. But this was also the time that the United States was taking the 'giant steps' that would see it become the world's largest economy within 30 years. Already the most populated country in the world outside Russia and China, and attracting by far the largest number of migrants, it could also boast more than twice the number of universities as the rest of the world combined.[21] The United States had learned the lesson from Europe (and Germany in particular) of the link between scientific research and industrial development and production. But unlike Europe, where research laboratories were linked to the universities, it was in America that the first private industrial research laboratory had been set up: in Newark, New Jersey in 1876. Thomas Alva Edison financed the operation from the proceeds of the sale of the ticker-tape automatic repeater for stock exchange prices that he invented in 1871.[22] Like the Parke-Davis challenge to the German pharmaceutical industry in the production and distribution of cocaine, it was a sign of things to come.

Parke-Davis was able to take advantage of the advertising industry that had been pioneered in the United States 20 years earlier, and promote cocaine in a way that created demand instead of being subject to it.[23] By 1885 the company had developed coca leaf cigars and cigarettes and its sales pitch boasted that cocaine would 'make the coward brave, the silent eloquent, free the victims of alcohol and opium habit from their bondage, and, as an anaesthetic render the sufferer insensitive to pain'. As well as marketing their own cocaine products, they also supplied the proprietary medicine manufacturers in the United States — and by the end of the century these numbered in the thousands.[24]

Cocaine was marketed in the form of lozenges for the relief of sore throats, as toothache drops and most notably, from the mid-1890s, in sprays and snuffs as a cure for asthma, hay fever, colds and catarrh.[25] It was the cheaper and more easily administered snuff that led to sniffing becoming the most common form of taking cocaine; the catarrh cures became an easy and cheap way of using cocaine whether you had catarrh or not.

And if you were using cocaine for recreational purposes there was a particular brand that had obvious appeal. In most preparations the cocaine content rarely exceeded 5 per cent, but Ryno's Hay Fever and Catarrh Remedy weighed in at a hefty 99.95 per cent. It came with a recommendation that it should be used 'two to ten times a day, or oftener if really necessary' for the relief of blocked-up nasal passages.[26] Prolonged use at this dose would have quite likely relieved users of their nasal septum, if nothing else.

One of the consequences of the massive industrial expansion in the United States in the late 19th century was a level of personal stress that led to the neurasthenia George Beard had discovered in 1869, and which was now spreading downwards from the middle-class 'brain' or white-collar workers. Although he thought that the beneficial effect of coca was exaggerated, Beard had noted in 1880 that 'it has, without doubt, a special and most interesting sustaining and tonic power. It relieves the pain and uneasiness that follows overexertion, and the peculiar distress that comes from sleepless nights, for which purpose, I may say, caffeine may also be used'.[27] So for those unable to afford the rest cure of Silas Weir Mitchell in those stressful times, the alternatives were caffeine and cocaine.

Although industrial expansion was increasingly dependent on the technical innovations of science, such as the Bessemer converter and the Siemens-Martin open-hearth furnace,[28] it nevertheless continued to also rely on work processes that were physically demanding. These labour processes themselves became subject to what was called 'scientific scrutiny' by a discipline that came to be known as 'scientific management', pioneered by Frederick Winslow Taylor (1856–1915). 'Speedy' Taylor turned his mind to increasing the efficiency of labour in the late 1880s when he was chief engineer at the Midvale steelworks in Philadelphia.[29] The science involved consisted of a time-and-motion study that systematically broke down the components of a given task and assigned to each an optimum completion time. The rest was close supervision to ensure that the tasks were properly completed, and payment by results. This obsession with speed was later parodied by Charlie Chaplin in the film *Modern Times* and Taylor himself was said to have succumbed to nightmares in which he was beset by machinery. Following a nervous breakdown, he died while compulsively winding his watch in the early hours of the morning.[30]

With or without Taylorist production techniques, hard physical work certainly lent itself to the consumption of a powerful stimulant like cocaine. In November 1902 an article appeared in the *British Medical Journal*, sourced in part from the *New York Medical News*, entitled 'The Cocaine Habit Among Negroes'. According to this article, the habit of consuming cocaine was said to have its origins among waterfront labourers in New Orleans and to have spread from there to other workers, including those on cotton plantations where employers issued regular rations of the drug as they had previously done with whisky. On the New Orleans waterfront, the article explained, the drug enabled workers 'to perform more easily the extraordinary severe work of loading and unloading steamboats, at which, perhaps for seventy hours at a stretch, they have to work without sleep or rest, in rain, in cold and in heat'. Cocaine seemed, the article said, to be the only stimulant that could make such arduous work possible: 'Under its influence the strength and vigour of the labourer are temporarily increased, and he becomes indifferent to the extremes of heat and cold.' Picking cotton was apparently not as arduous as waterfront work, but it required 'extraordinary long hours' as a consequence of labour shortages. Cocaine use was encouraged by plantation owners because it enabled field hands 'to put in a big day's work'.[31]

Just as the Spanish had discovered with coca leaves nearly 400 years earlier, employers in the United States in the 1890s found that cocaine was well suited to their labour productivity requirements. Wherever there was hard work, the workers doing it were likely to be using cocaine that they either bought themselves or had supplied to them. Cocaine became a part of the wage deal: employers provided it to their workers up and down the country, from the cotton plantations and road and levee construction sites in the south to the textile and silk mills in the north.[32] In the hard-rock mines of the west, miners worked a minimum 84-hour week — at least 12 hours a day, seven days a week. Those who worked at smelting the ore had a similarly punishing schedule, except that they also worked a solid 24 hours every second Sunday.[33] According to 'Big Bill' Haywood, secretary of the Western Federation of Miners from 1900 and a founding member of the Industrial Workers of the World, cocaine and morphine (and later on heroin) were sold at every company store in his work environment.[34] Haywood had worked in the mining industry since he started in 1884 as a 15-year-old.

The increase in supply of cocaine and the manipulation of demand for it was the province of drug companies, but without its use and promotion by the medical profession widespread consumption was unlikely to have occurred. With the increased levels of consumption that came from self-medication and the recommended dosage of doctors who prescribed cocaine as a general tonic for nervousness, sinus ailments, asthma, and opiate and alcohol addiction, dependency began to surface as a problem. Doctors began to prescribe cocaine by injection, as they did with morphine, and, as with morphine, this led to addiction among the middle class. With cocaine, however, it was professional middle-class males rather than females who acquired the habit, with doctors prominent among them. By the end of the 19th century doctors were estimated to have made up some 30 per cent of problematic users.[35] Perhaps the most prominent of them was William Stewart Halsted (1852–1922), who became the first Professor of Surgery at Johns Hopkins University Medical School. Halsted was the first surgeon to introduce the wearing of rubber gloves during surgical operations, and that was principally because his operating room nurse, who also happened to be his fiancée, was allergic to the antiseptic then in use.[36] He was also the first to use cocaine for nerve-block anaesthesia and his experiments with the drug led to a ruinous level of dependence. It took a slow trip on a sailing ship to the Windward Islands in the company of a caring friend to overcome his cocaine dependency. But even then it was replaced by a morphine dependency that he carried with him to the grave.[37]

Combating cocaine dependency with morphine went very much against the trend at the time, which was to promote cocaine as a cure for opiate addiction. Pemberton's French Wine Coca was advertised as God's best gift to medicine and an infallible cure for a wide range of complaints, from nerve trouble and neuralgia to constipation, headaches and all chronic and wasting diseases. As an added bonus it invigorated the sexual organs,[38] and was a 'great blessing' to those unfortunates addicted to morphine or opium.

The idea that cocaine could cure morphine addiction was totally false. It was most likely to result in one addiction being replaced with another that was as bad, if not worse, and it was just as likely to lead to dependence on both drugs. The first reference to its use in curing opiate addiction appears to be an account by W H Bentley, an American doctor who in 1880 reported in the Detroit *Therapeutic Gazette* that he had successfully treated opium addicts and alcoholics with a coca preparation prepared and supplied by Parke-Davis.[39]

This report was picked up four years later by an ambitious young man with a medical degree, Sigmund Freud (1856–1939), who had swapped research work on the nervous system of lower vertebrates at a laboratory in Vienna for practical experience at the city's General Hospital. Freud's father lost his capital in the downturn of 1873 and with it the capacity to support his large family. To make matters worse, the impecunious young Freud had fallen in love and was desperate to marry as soon as financial circumstances would permit. This meant earning a living as a physician, but Freud had qualified in medicine without ever seeing a patient in bed, let alone examining one. His residency at the hospital, which began in July 1882, was designed to remedy this deficiency, but it merely confirmed his earlier instinct that he wasn't suited to general practice, and in May 1883 he transferred to the hospital's psychiatric department.[40]

In the spring of 1884 he had been separated from his fiancée Martha Bernays for two years (she lived in Germany with her family) and his immediate prospects were not particularly bright. He needed to come up with some noteworthy medical discovery that would establish his name and fortune. After reading a paper by a German army doctor on the subject, the discovery that he hoped to demonstrate to the rest of the medical world was the therapeutic application of cocaine. In April he wrote to his fiancée of his intention of procuring the drug and trying it:

> with cases of heart disease and also of nervous exhaustion, particularly in the miserable condition of nervous exhaustion after the withdrawal of morphium (Dr Fleischl). Perhaps others are working on it; perhaps nothing will come of it. But I shall certainly try it, and you know when one perseveres, sooner or later

one succeeds. We do not need more than one such lucky hit to think of setting up house.[41]

The Dr Fleischl mentioned in the letter was Ernst von Fleischl-Marxow, a research colleague and friend of Freud's who had become dependent on morphine while using it for the relief of pain following several operations.

Freud duly set to work on his cocaine project after obtaining a supply of the drug from Merck at a price that he initially feared might prove prohibitive to further research.[42] In the heroic tradition of self-experimenting, Freud took the drug for the first time on 30 April and at the same time offered it to Fleischl-Marxow as well. By the end of the first week of May Fleischl-Marxow was using the drug continually; by 19 June Freud's celebrated paper on cocaine had been written and in the following month 'On Coca' (*Uber Coca*) was published.[43] Freud's cocaine use offers an explanation for why the project was completed with such speed, although it hardly compares with Robert Louis Stevenson's subsequent effort. 'On Coca' certainly made a name for Freud, but not quite in the way that he had sought. His views on the therapeutic value of cocaine were widely circulated in Europe and the United States and used to popularise the use of the drug in medical practice for a range of complaints that, importantly, included morphine addiction.[44]

For such an influential work, 'On Coca' contains little that wasn't already known at the time. Freud's survey of the literature on the drug relies heavily on the Index Catalogue of the Surgeon-General's Office, United States Army, 1883. Original research is limited to Freud's account of his own cocaine experience and his observations of others. Clearly 'On Coca' owes a debt of some magnitude to the *Therapeutic Gazette*. Of the 35 references to the therapeutic uses of coca, which appear in 27 separate notations, 23 are sourced from the *Therapeutic Gazette*. For good measure the *Gazette* is referenced in the text in a footnote which also mentions the manufacturer Parke-Davis and Co.[45] The critical reference that Freud relies on, that of W H Bentley in the *Gazette* of September 1880, also makes mention of 'the well-known house of Parke-Davis and Co.' and reads like a testimonial for a quack nostrum.[46]

According to its September 1880 edition, the *Gazette* was 'a monthly journal devoted to therapeutics and the introduction of new therapeutic agents'. Coincidentally, its self-styled 'medical publisher' was George S Davis of Parke-Davis and Company. The company had the foresight in the 1870s to set up a publishing enterprise, with George Davis at the helm, whose basic aim was to sell the company's products to the medical profession by providing them with 'positive medical research'. The *Gazette* belonged to a stable of company publications that included the *Medical Age*, *New Preparations* and the *Bulletin of Pharmacy*. In the 1880s the product they were promoting to the profession was the new therapeutic cocaine[47] that Freud had referred to as an 'antidote' to morphine.[48]

Despite Freud's report in 'On Coca' that it had cured Fleischl-Marxow's morphine dependency with such alacrity that he was able to dispense with the treatment after a mere 10 days, cocaine was an antidote that wasn't doing Fleischl-Marxow much good at all.[49] Just 12 months after he had first taken cocaine, he was consuming it in quantities that were described by E M Thornton, author of *The Freudian Fallacy*, as 'enormous' — a gram each day during one 3-month period in early 1885. He had also resumed his consumption of morphine: he was 'speedballing', as it later came to be known. Notwithstanding Freud's first-hand knowledge of Fleischl-Marxow's condition, and regardless of the fact that he warned his own fiancée, whom he supplied with cocaine, against dependency, Freud again championed cocaine as a cure for morphine addiction in a paper delivered in March 1885 and published in August of that year.[50] In the same month, an account appeared of Freud's evaluation of Parke-Davis's cocaine compared with that of Merck. It concluded that 'this preparation should have a very great future'.[51]

Parke-Davis's 'innovative business practices', first evident with the promotion of cocaine in the late 19th century, were to set the pattern for the drug business in the next century and beyond.[52] Freud, though, was headed for trouble. As reports of cocaine dependency began to surface in the years immediately following the publication of 'On Coca', he was accused by the psychiatrist Albrecht Erlenmeyer of 'unleashing on the world the third scourge of humanity', the other two being alcohol and morphine.[53] Freud's defence against this accusation, and others, was published in 1887, and has been rather gently described as 'somewhat tendentious'.[54] Disingenuous and mendacious might be more accurate. His behaviour at the time has been more aptly described as that of a charlatan.[55] For all his enthusiasm for cocaine use in medical practice, Freud had missed its most important property, that of a local anaesthetic, which was discovered by a colleague, Dr Carl Koller. For all his professed love of his fiancée, he implicated her in this failure, which caused him to miss out on the attendant early fame, although he later conceded that he bore her no grudge.[56]

By 1891 Fleischl-Marxow was dead. Freud wrote no more of cocaine after 1887.[57] There is some evidence, though, that Freud resumed his use of cocaine in 1892 and may have continued using the drug until around 1912. The direct outcome of this drug use is said to be those new theories which would eventually coalesce into the therapy that finally did make him famous: psychoanalysis.[58] Both inside and outside the medical profession, views on the therapeutic value of Freudian psychoanalysis have waxed and waned. If, however, there is anything to the opinion expressed by neurologist Macdonald Critchley that psychoanalysis is 'the treatment of the id by the odd',[59] the explanation for the odd might well lie in Freud's cocaine use.

In medical practice the use of cocaine was phased out when organic chemists developed a less hazardous synthetic compound, Novocain, in 1899,[60] but its use in other areas continued. The German army doctor whose paper first caught the attention of Freud was Theodor Aschenbrandt, who published his observations on the recuperative powers that cocaine had on the exhausted troops of a Bavarian artillery company that was under his medical care during manoeuvres in 1883. The lesson seems to have been very well learned but much less well acknowledged. Cocaine was certainly administered to combatants in France during World War I, including to Australian troops, who were also given cocaine at Gallipoli. The extent to which it was used will probably remain unknown. It is known, though, that by 1919 some returned soldiers in Melbourne were demanding cocaine from chemists without a prescription, contrary to the regulations about the sale of the drug. And more importantly for them, no doubt, they were being given it. Its use among soldiers in Sydney had been evident some years earlier.[61] Cocaine use by allied troops, predominantly Canadians, in London in 1916 was largely responsible for its stricter control by regulation in Britain under the *Defence of the Realm Act* in that year.[62]

As medical use began to decline, recreational use increased. This was spectacularly evident in the United States where, in the 13-year period from 1890, cocaine consumption increased fivefold.[63] The sympathy that had previously existed for middle-class medical addicts was now replaced by fear of 'crazed cocaine fiends' as cocaine became a working-class drug. This fear was exacerbated by the fact that cocaine was now associated with a particularly sordid type of user — that of the petty criminal class. Cocaine became the drug of choice not just for the proletariat but for the lumpen proletariat.[64] Prostitutes started to become significant cocaine users in the early 20th century, and with them came pimps, petty thieves, gamblers and other assorted undesirables. In the United States cocaine also came to be associated with African-Americans. In the South, 'cocaine-crazed negroes' with their 'increased and perverted sexual desires and nearly superhuman strength' were held to represent an urgent and growing danger to the white community.

The police chief of Asheville, North Carolina, is said to have exchanged the firearm he was issued with for one of a higher calibre after shooting a 'cocainised nigger' twice with so little effect that he had to finish him off with a club.[65] The fact that this danger was contemporaneous with an epidemic of lynchings, legal segregation and the introduction of discriminatory voting laws was, it seems, entirely coincidental.[66]

By the end of World War I, cocaine was well on the way to becoming a prohibited drug in those countries where it hadn't already been banned. The drug companies had seen the writing on the wall and were content to realise their profits from other synthetic drugs.[67] But making the use and possession of cocaine a criminal activity when a large group of users were already criminals was hardly the epitome of deterrence. Those who continued to use the drug simply turned to illicit suppliers as the dynamics of the market changed. Cocaine leaked out of the manufacturing plants of Amsterdam and Hamburg, and was smuggled by seafarers and supplied illicitly by dentists and pharmacists.

Much of Australia's illicit supply came from Chinese seamen who bought cocaine in those Asian ports where it was not yet prohibited and smuggled it into Sydney's Chinatown, from where it found its way to east Sydney prostitutes via the infamous Tilly Devine and Kate Leigh.[68] The market for illicit cocaine in Australia in the 1920s wasn't a particularly large one, though. Sydney's notorious 'razor gang wars' of the late 1920s may well have been a struggle for the cocaine trade, but it was a small trade, largely confined to prostitutes and their associates. In 1926 an estimated 15 women regularly took cocaine in Sydney and there was just one prosecution for a cocaine offence. By 1929 prosecutions had risen to 34, but two years later they had dropped back to five, and in 1933 there was again just one prosecution.[69]

By the late 1920s, with cocaine eliminated from proprietary medicines, superseded as a local anaesthetic and strictly controlled in its now limited application in medical practice, its continued consumption was dependent on its popularity as a recreational drug and as a stimulant that aided productivity in the workplace. The worldwide depression that began when the stock exchange on Wall Street crashed on 29 October 1929 had the obvious effect of dampening demand in the workplace as industrial production fell by something like a third, with employment levels not far behind, in its immediate aftermath. By the early 1930s, well before production and employment levels had recovered, the pharmaceutical industry had provided a substitute for cocaine that could be used both recreationally and in the workplace as well as providing relief for the tired troops and others who would become involved in the conflict that was to begin in 1939. Amphetamines would be as readily available in the coming decades as cocaine had been in the previous ones.

Cocaine was to make a comeback in the United States in the 1970s: demand for it increased as the supply of amphetamines decreased as a consequence of legislative restrictions.[70] Ironically, it was the legislative initiatives of the presidential 'drug wars', beginning with Richard Nixon in 1969, that opened up the supply lines of cocaine from Colombia.

For Nixon, marijuana was a drug of mass disobedience. Those who smoked it were unpatriotic, law-breaking hippies and worse who opposed the Vietnam War and many of his other policies. By concentrating on its suppression, he diverted the illicit drug traffic to cocaine. After engineering the downfall and murder of Salvador Allende in Chile, the dictator Augusto Pinochet was only too happy to please his benefactor Nixon by delivering Chilean drug traffickers up to the United States. Those who were left took themselves and their considerable expertise off to Colombia, and Pinochet himself would eventually stand accused of being involved in the trafficking of cocaine to both the United States and Europe. As an increasing supply of Colombian cocaine was entering the United States through Florida, Nixon's successor, Gerald Ford, was concentrating on heroin from Mexico. The administration of Ronald Reagan, president from 1981 to 1989, also concentrated on suppressing the subversive marijuana while illegally supporting the Nicaraguan Contras, who returned the favour by saturating American cities with cocaine.[71]

And so it continues. The Clinton–Bush 'Plan Colombia', which began in 2000 and is as much about eliminating Marxist and grassroots democratic movements as cocaine, cost American taxpayers more than US$3 billion in its first year of operation.[72] Despite saturating large parts of the country with glyphosates — to the considerable benefit of US chemical companies — the 'spectacular success' that it could report three years later was to have increased the area of Colombian coca cultivation by 25 per cent between 2000 and 2001.[73] In mid-2005, satellite imagery showed that the total area of coca under cultivation in Colombia was much the same as it was in 2003. Of the 12,000 subsistence farmers deprived of their land, livestock and livelihood as a consequence of the fumigation program, only 12 had received any sort of compensation. The program nevertheless continues, despite the fact that plantations successfully poisoned are simply replaced by new ones in Colombia and neighbouring Bolivia and Peru.[74]

As cocaine began its resurgence in the United States in the 1970s, its demand was initially evident among the middle class rather than the lower-class labourers it had been associated with earlier in the century, and who had contributed so much to its prohibition. Recreational users were now found among those with a talent for music, art, designing fashion and showing it off, as well as among their unfortunate hangers-on waiting for that Warhol moment. Some even sported silver coke-spoons around their necks. The cocaine experience would be incorporated into their art and music, and be appreciated vicariously by a large audience. And what of the labouring classes? Well, the concept of a post-industrial society had already emerged in the United States as early as 1962 and the old industrial working class was in evident decline soon after.[75] The options and futures markets had emerged in Chicago in the early 1970s and the Eurodollar market, the safe haven that Soviet-held US dollars took refuge in and which would soon lead to the global dominance of finance capital, had begun its spectacular rise.[76] Cocaine suited this new class of brain worker: it gave them the 'edge' they needed while transferring millions of dollars or deutschemarks or contracts for pork belly futures across cyberspace in search of short-term profit. As if to confirm its status among high-income earners, it was often snorted (this expression had now replaced sniffing) using high-denomination banknotes.

But markets need to grow. Millionaires may have dominated the cocaine market in the early 1970s, but cocaine, at least according to alienated young men in the 1890s, could also make the dispossessed feel like millionaires.[77] Expanding the market to include these potential new customers meant that the price of the drug would have to be lowered. It was the preserve of the middle class only because the working class couldn't afford it, but a simple chemical process solved this problem in the early 1980s.

In its white crystalline powder form, cocaine hydrochloride is a water-soluble salt that can be injected or snorted. Removing the hydrochloride results in a cocaine that can be smoked (called freebase). This means it gets to the brain faster; it also has a more intense effect. Early attempts at freebasing in the late 1970s involved ether, which has the unfortunate tendency to explode at light-up time. A more reliable method was discovered in the early 1980s: treatment with baking soda that produces small rocks which emit a cracking noise when smoked.[78] Crack cocaine could now be sold in small amounts that the urban proletariat could afford. The market expanded dramatically. In 1977 it was estimated that something like 10 per cent of young Americans (18 to 25-year-olds) used cocaine. By the mid-1980s it was one-third.[79] From a marketing perspective, crack was a goldmine because its effect lasts for a mere 15 minutes, after which the consumers were queuing up for more. The net result came to be described as an epidemic, which reignited the debate about whether or not cocaine was addictive in the same way that heroin was held to be. Cocaine, like many other drugs, can lead to psychological dependence, but it is not physiologically addictive.[80] It's understandable that it might appear to be, though, as crack users come back for more and more, with an appetite for the drug that seems almost unquenchable.

If the various methods of using cocaine in the 1980s reflected a class divide in much the same way as its use a century earlier had, when the middle class were injecting and the working class sniffing, so did the legislative response. Cocaine powder was snorted by predominantly white consumers, and although white crack smokers outnumbered African-Americans and Hispanics, crack was much more likely to be the way in which consumers in these minority groups used the drug. In 1986 laws were enacted in the United States that provided for mandatory minimum custodial sentences for cocaine possession. With crack cocaine a 10-year sentence is triggered for violations that involve 50 grams, but with powdered cocaine the same sentencing doesn't come into effect unless the amount involved is 5 kilograms. In other words, people who were found with cocaine that could be injected or snorted (and these were mostly white Americans) could have 100 times the amount of smokeable cocaine a person could be found with (and these were more commonly African-Americans) before attracting the same penalty.[81]

Before the 1986 drug laws were introduced the average sentence for federal drug law violations among African-Americans was more than 10 per cent higher than for whites. By 1990 it was closer to 50 per cent. Seven years later, official reports showed that 90 per cent of those convicted in federal courts for crack cocaine distribution were African-Americans; a little ironic, perhaps, as the majority of users were white.[82] At the time, something like 21 per cent of prison inmates were incarcerated for drug offences — 8 per cent for possession, 13 per cent for trafficking (which includes dealing in small amounts) — and 90 per cent of those were African-Americans. Whichever way you look at it, it is hard to escape the conclusion of the British drug charity Release, that this resembles 'a war on black ghetto youth'. In 2002 the United States had the highest rate of incarceration in the world, with a prison population of more than 2 million that included almost 12 per cent of all African-Americans males aged between 20 and 34.[83] Included in the 2 million were 1.3 per cent of all males in the country and 4.8 per cent of all African-American men: this means African-American males are more than three and a half times more likely to be imprisoned than white males. This sentencing disparity crossed the gender divide, with African-American women eight times more likely to be incarcerated than white women, and Hispanic women four times more likely.[84]

The consequences of this continuing deep-seated racism go beyond those felt by the victims and their families. In some states in the United States, those with criminal records are denied the right to vote. Florida, the state that decided the presidential election for George W Bush by 537 votes in November 2000, is one such state. African-Americans in Florida vote 90 per cent Democrat, yet 31 per cent of African-

American men in Florida are denied the vote because they have a felony conviction. The disenfranchising of these men, and many other African-Americans, cost the Democrat candidate Al Gore the presidency, a result which may have profoundly influenced the course of world history.[85]

Cocaine consumption seems to have stabilised in the United States since the high usage rates recorded in the mid-1980s, but millions of Americans still regularly use the drug. The large Colombian cartels that have been broken up have merely been replaced by hundreds of new trafficking organisations, ensuring that supply is ever ready to meet demand.[86]

A simple, coherent explanation for the high level of drug consumption in the United States has so far proven somewhat elusive. The introduction of smokeable crack provides a reason for the market growth of cocaine, for example, but not for underlying demand. Perhaps those looking for a simple solution are always going to be disappointed. There are, though, some features of US society that can help us understand the trickle-down effect of cocaine consumption once it was established as a preferred drug among the celebrities of the middle class. The United States has a greater disparity between rich and poor than any other developed country, with just 1 per cent of the community owning one-third of the country's wealth. Yet 19 per cent of the adult population claim to be part of that richest 1 per cent and a further 20 per cent believe they'll be part of it in their lifetime.[87] So even if the potential market for cocaine in the United States is limited to those who are up there, those who think they're up there and those who think they'll be up there soon, that's already an impressive 40 per cent of the adult population.

The cocaine industry generates sales around the world in excess of US$70 billion and has a consumer base of at least 15 million people.[88] Outside the United States, cocaine consumption in the advanced economies seems to be slowly but steadily rising, led by the Spanish, whose per capita consumption levels in 2005 were the world's highest. A study of British consumption patterns among 15 to 24-year-olds in 2004 concluded that the drug was used at levels similar to those in the United States, and in the London area alone there are said to be some 50,000 crack cocaine addicts.[89] Innovative scientific testing in Italy in 2005 revealed that consumption levels were almost three times higher than what the official figures showed.[90] In Germany in 2003, 90 per cent of all Euro banknotes were found to have traces of cocaine within seven months of the new currency being circulated. Testing in the European Parliament building in 2005 (in the toilet areas, not surprisingly) found evidence of significant levels of cocaine use.[91]

In Australia, cocaine has long been known as the preferred drug of Sydney and Melbourne's high-income set, and as in Europe its consumption has been steadily increasing since the late 1980s. Following an alleged case of horse-doping with the drug in Sydney in mid-2005, press reports confirmed that cocaine is as much a part of the big race day scene as champagne and chatter about eastern suburbs property prices.[92] Although crack doesn't seem to have caught on, Sydney and Melbourne consumers still manage to get through something like 3 tonnes of cocaine a year, with the decadent Sydneysiders consuming some 87 per cent of it. Intravenous users account for almost half of all the cocaine used in Australia, which may indicate a shift in drug use from some of those who previously used heroin. As for the rest, cocaine is now being snorted by consumers who are as likely to be chefs and waiters as stockbrokers. This widening of the consumer base has been assisted by the drug being packaged in smaller, more affordable caps — 0.1 gram — that sell for about $50 each.[93] But price is still a significant factor with cocaine consumption. Those tiny caps don't go far, and even a gram is easily consumed among friends on a big night out. At prices that range from $200 a gram (60 per cent pure) to $350 a gram (85 per cent pure), cocaine is likely to remain an occasional luxury for most, particularly given the competition from 'the poor people's coke', amphetamines.

Amphetamines

German chemists were experimenting with thousands of chemical compounds in the late 19th century. Naturally, not all of them found their way to the marketplace. Some of those that did were quickly withdrawn when the ill effects on those that they were administered to became obvious.[94] Others never made it beyond the laboratory, being left on the shelf for want of some profitable purpose. Such was the fate of the drug that came to be called amphetamine, which was first synthesised by the German pharmacologist L Edeleano in 1887,[95] the same year the Japanese chemist Nagayoshi Nagai (1845–1929), who spent 14 years studying chemistry in Berlin, isolated the alkaloid ephedrine from the Chinese medicinal herb *ma huang*.[96]

Ma huang, derived from ephedra plants, has been known in Chinese medicine for 5000 years. It is recorded in the earliest Chinese pharmacopoeia, *Shen Nung Ben Cao Chien* or *The Herbal Classic of the Divine Plowman*. Around 2800 BCE the Divine Plowman, Shen Nung, reputedly tested and recommended 365 herbs, one for each day of the year. They were divided into three categories. The upper category herbs sustained life, the middle category herbs smoothed the mental state and the lower category herbs cured illness. Ma huang was classified in the middle category and came to be used for the treatment of colds, asthma and low blood pressure.[97]

Despite its lineage, or perhaps because of it, ephedrine was little used in commercial practice. It was only in 1926 that it was approved as a drug by the Council of Pharmacy and Chemistry of the American Medical Association, following clinical investigation at the University of Pennsylvania and the Mayo

Clinic. It was used in the treatment of asthma. Its commercial exploitation followed so quickly that one manufacturer attempted to monopolise the supply of ephedra plants from China. This in turn prompted research on a synthetic substitute. One was developed by the chemist Gordon Alles and tested in the pharmacology department of the University of California at San Francisco in 1927 and 1928. These research results were passed on to the laboratories of the pharmaceutical company Smith Kline and French in Philadelphia; they had been conducting similar research, looking for a nasal decongestant. The new drug was given the name 'amphetamine', and in 1932 Smith Kline and French marketed its freebase, an oily liquid, in the form of an inhaler called Benzedrine that was recommended for the treatment of asthma and nasal decongestion.[98] Speed was out of the blocks.

By 1937 amphetamines were available in pill form, soon known as bennies or pep pills. Together with related stimulants, they were marketed as useful for a wide range of medical conditions, including depression, epilepsy, schizophrenia, bed-wetting, obesity, Parkinsonism, narcolepsy, and drug and alcohol addiction.[99] Methamphetamine hydrochloride was marketed in Germany around the same time.[100] So amphetamine, methamphetamine and analogous drugs were being marketed by pharmaceutical companies throughout the world from the 1930s on.[101] The bewildering number of amphetamine-related stimulants on the market led to some confusion with terminology but it's now generally accepted that 'amphetamines' (plural) refers to amphetamine, methamphetamine and dexamphetamine.[102] In the Australian vernacular it's usually called 'speed' or 'goey'.

Not long after amphetamines were released into the marketplace, the world was convulsed, from 1939, by a conflict much bloodier than the one that had ended just 21 years previously. It was truly a world war, one that engulfed 60 countries, left 55 million dead and set new standards in cruelty and oppression. Most of the major combatants put the new drug to good use among their armed forces. British intelligence was aware of the use of amphetamines among German troops, in the Bavarian tradition (see Theodor Aschenbrandt's observation of cocaine consumption by Bavarian troops in 1883), and Britain distributed some 72 million pills among their own fighting men. American forces, who entered the war following the Japanese invasion of Pearl Harbour in December 1941, managed to get through 200 million pills in less than four years. The drug was well suited to kamikaze pilots — the extent of Japanese consumption became apparent immediately after the war's end.[103]

Amphetamines increase heart rate and breathing rate, and raise blood pressure.[104] This helps boost energy levels and alertness, thus making amphetamines ideal for those fighting in the field as well as those back at headquarters directing the action. From his position at the rear, Adolf Hitler was in the habit of taking Vitumultin tablets, which consisted of amphetamines combined with a vitamin preparation. After the fall of Stalingrad in early 1943, he was said to have aged rapidly, and to have then received amphetamine injections on a regular basis.[105] British Prime Minister Sir Anthony Eden (1897–1977), found the drug particularly useful in helping to keep a stiff upper lip during the Suez crisis of 1956, and US President John F Kennedy (1917–63) also found it helpful during stressful periods in the early 1960s. Indeed both he and his wife were reported to be 'strongly addicted' to amphetamines, which they took on medical advice during his presidency.[106] The use of amphetamines by US forces continued during the Korean War, and in the Vietnam War they were said to have consumed more amphetamines than the US and British troops did between them during the whole of World War II.[107] However, in Vietnam, the amphetamines seem to have been counteracted by the equally large quantities of cannabis, opium, heroin and LSD that the US troops were consuming. Amphetamines were apparently still being handed out during both the first Gulf war in Iraq and the conflict in Afghanistan: in early 2003 the lawyer representing two US Air Force pilots involved in a 'friendly fire' incident that killed four Canadian soldiers and injured eight others in Afghanistan blamed the use of amphetamines issued by the air force and known as 'go pills' for the pilots' impaired judgment.[108]

As well as their use as an aid-to-combat and in medical practice, amphetamines, almost as soon as they were introduced, were used recreationally and as self-medication. They were particularly associated with the prominent American beat generation writers of the 1950s and 60s, William Burroughs (1914–97) and Jack Kerouac (1922–69). Kerouac's most famous work, *On the Road*, published in 1957, was written on a single scroll of paper more than 36 metres long in the highly suggestive speed of three weeks.[109] They had an illustrious predecessor in Graham Greene (1904–91), who wrote many acclaimed works: in the 1950s alone he wrote *The Quiet American*, *The Third Man* and *Our Man in Havana*. In 1938, with the aid of a bennie for breakfast and another at lunchtime, he was able to complete a spy novel in a mere six weeks, although *The Confidential Agent* isn't among his better known works.[110] The 'poet of the thirties', W H Auden (1907–73), began taking bennies when he migrated from England to the United States just before World War II to take up an associate professorship at Michigan University, and he was still taking them when he was appointed Professor of Poetry at Oxford University in 1956. His period of amphetamine use, which lasted from 1939 until 1957, has been held by some to coincide with his best poetry.[111]

While the beats were seen by many as a bit 'out there', anti-establishment, hedonistic and willing to experiment with any number of drugs, a significant number of people around the world shared their taste for speed from the mid-1940s. Amphetamines assisted many of those who were trying to cope with the traumatic effects of war, and the difficult period of postwar reconstruction. Yet it was in Sweden, a country that had managed to escape direct involvement in World War II, that widespread amphetamine use in civil society first emerged as a problem. What's more, it became evident during the war: in 1943, 200,000 Swedes, around 3 per cent of the total population, were using the drug regularly, but the number of 'problematic' users (the term used by researchers) was estimated to be no more than a few hundred.[112]

There has been some speculation that the availability of amphetamines in Sweden during the war was related to the use of the drug as an appetite suppressant, as obesity was a problem for the prosperous Swedes even then, at a time when most of the rest of Europe had slimmed down because of meagre wartime rations.[113] This may well have been so, but a drug which in low doses increases energy and alertness, enhances self-image and induces a state of euphoria has some fairly obvious attractions. Unfortunately, though, repeated use builds up tolerance, so that more of the drug is needed to produce the same effect, and excessive use can lead to a condition known as amphetamine psychosis. Apparently indistinguishable from the endogenous illness (literally growing or proceeding from within — in this case a psychosis that occurs as a consequence of a more 'natural' process rather than through amphetamine use), the condition is characterised by delusions of persecution, auditory or visual hallucinations and feelings of omnipotence.[114] It is also said to mimic schizophrenia, one of the conditions for which it was first recommended as a treatment.[115] By 1954, 55,000 people in Japan were estimated to be suffering from methamphetamine-induced psychosis as military stocks of the drug came onto the black market and were supplemented by over-the-counter sales.[116] The number of Japanese injecting methamphetamines at this time has been estimated at between 550,000 and 1.5 million.[117]

From the 1950s, amphetamine use in several countries around the world occurred in what have been described as epidemics that seemed to last nearly a decade. Epidemics occurred in Sweden in the 1950s and 1960s, in the United Kingdom in the late 1950s and 1960s and in the United States in the late 1960s and early 1970s. The Australian epidemics in the middle and late 1960s were said to be less severe than in other countries.[118] The one thing they all had in common was that they were largely iatrogenic. In Sweden, amphetamines pills had been a prescription-only drug since 1939; in the United Kingdom this had been the case since 1954 and in the United States since 1951.[119] The Australian epidemics were accompanied by a large increase in the prescription of amphetamines by GPs.[120] And while the doctors were busy scribbling, the pharmaceutical companies were just as busy cranking up production. In the United States alone, the number of tablets manufactured went from 3.5 billion in 1958 to 8 billion in 1966 and 10 billion four years later.[121]

The growth of the illicit market, clearly evident from the early 1950s, was just as impressive. The consumer profile of amphetamine users bore a striking resemblance to that of morphine and heroin users years earlier. Middle-aged middle-class women were prescribed amphetamines by their doctors, and 'deviant' young males were injecting amphetamines sourced from the illicit market.[122] As early as 1952, the WHO began to express concerns about the patterns of amphetamine consumption, but it wasn't until 1971 that international restrictions were imposed by the Convention on Psychotropic Substances. The convention, which came into effect in 1976, covered 32 psychotropic substances, including hallucinogens and hypnotics as well as amphetamines. Within 20 years, the number of controlled psychotropic drugs would increase beyond 100.[123] But by 1971, the illicit market in amphetamines was so well established that the attempts at control — restricting the prescription of amphetamines to two medical conditions: narcolepsy and attention-deficit hyperactivity disorder (ADHD) — were unsuccessful; it continued to operate, and eventually expanded.

The illicit market benefited from the increased production of the drug companies — it is said that somewhere between one-half and two-thirds of the pills produced in the United States before 1971 were distributed through illegal networks.[124] The injecting use of amphetamines that was so widespread in postwar Japan had also been recorded in Sweden as early as 1949[125] and by the mid-1950s it was also occurring in the United States. The Beat poet Allen Ginsberg was living in San Francisco when his first book, *Howl and Other Poems*, was published in 1956, but by the late 1950s the San Francisco beats were on the way to being succeeded by the slightly more respectable beatniks. Injecting liquid amphetamines with heroin was a feature of the beats' drug use that was shared by various groups of African-Americans in the city, with the amphetamines sourced from two drug company products: Desoxyn and Methedrine.[126] When these two drugs were withdrawn in 1962 and 1963, demand for a powdered form of water-soluble speed was sufficiently great to open up a new market in supply that has been evident in one form or another ever since.

Bathtub crank made its debut in San Francisco in late 1962. As the name implies, the first batch of illicit methamphetamine was made in a bathtub which was located, appropriately enough for San Francisco, in a flower shop. However, an immediate problem surfaced with the production of homemade speed — the smell. All those chemicals bubbling away gave rise to a distinct odour that neighbours or passers-by were unlikely to miss, and the assault on the olfactory senses was such that it could have easily provoked complaints to the authorities.

The problem was solved in the first instance by resorting to the methods that Chinese opium smokers had developed after opium was first prohibited in San Francisco in 1875: windows and doors were covered with wet blankets to contain the obnoxious fumes.[127]

Homemade crank, which could be injected or snorted, soon developed a consumer base beyond bohemians and African-Americans, but it had a special appeal to one group in particular — bikie gangs. It didn't take them long to work out that they could just as easily make it themselves as pay someone else to do so. Within a few years bikie gangs, through the adroit application of violence and intimidation, controlled the production, distribution and much of the sale of speed in California. In time, they would dominate the trade in other parts of the country and in other parts of the world.

Bikie control of the speed market and its association with violence led to a change in both consumption patterns and the consumer base during the 1960s. The beats and their successors began to show a preference for major hallucinogens such as LSD, and the minor hallucinogen cannabis. Middle-class occasional users moved away from speed and embraced the different drug experience of the legally available Valium. Injecting and otherwise heavy use of speed became associated with marginalised working-class youth, thus establishing its reputation as a redneck drug. The aggressive and violent presence of these 'speed freaks', as they were known in San Francisco, shattered the 1960s' promise of love and peace made by those on a different drug trip: the hippies.

It is the chemical composition of drugs like speed that illustrates the impossibility of enforcing their total prohibition. As the early amateur chemists in San Francisco discovered, speed isn't difficult to make. It isn't quite as easy as cultivating cannabis in the backyard, and care needs to be taken during the cooking process, but it isn't necessary to have a chemistry degree to interpret the instructions of a basic recipe; nor is access to sophisticated industrial capacity required to produce profitable amounts of the drug. For the past 40 years, the larger producers have dominated the market, as they tend to do with most commodities, but it is the illicit status of speed, with its concomitant high profitability, that justifies the risks associated with production. This helps explain why a cottage industry of small entrepreneurs has grown up around the world. These people produce speed at home … and in premises rented for the purpose, motel rooms and mobile labs. The response of law enforcement authorities has been to restrict the availability of the otherwise quite legally purchased chemicals necessary to produce speed. Not surprisingly, this has led to both the development of an illicit market in these chemicals and new manufacturing techniques. In Australia, prior to the introduction of a ban on over-the-counter sales of cold and flu medications containing pseudoephedrine in 2006 it was easy enough to buy these preparations, which could then be processed to remove buffers and produce ephedrine. A packet containing just 30 tablets was enough to produce 20 street deals of speed, which could then be sold for a total of $2000.[128] When the ban was introduced, the then justice minister, Chris Ellison, said that as much as 90 per cent of the pseudoephedrine used in illegal drugs came from community pharmacies. Two years after the ban came into effect customs officials reported a 'significant' increase in the amounts of ephedrine and pseudoephedrine smuggled into the country, particularly by outlaw motorcycle gangs.[129]

The market for speed has expanded in the more advanced economies since the 1970s, partly because the number of users from among the socially marginalised has grown (together with their overall numbers) and partly as a result of increased consumption by recreational users determined to extract the maximum amount of pleasure from weekend activities without being bothered by the inconvenience of sleep. The latest amphetamine epidemic to emerge is centred on the use of crystal meth or ice, which is a smokeable form of methamphetamine. Initially imported from Asia, its use first surfaced as a problem in the United States in Hawaii in the late 1980s following the successful eradication of the local cannabis product known as 'pakalolo'.[130] By 2003 somewhere between 10 per cent and 15 per cent of Hawaii's population were estimated to be using the drug.[131] In 2005 the homemade product was fuelling an epidemic among predominantly white users in rural areas of states such as Iowa, Tennessee and Missouri. The increase in violence and crime associated with ice has led to a remarkable result in Arkansas: the racial majority of the prison population has changed from African-Americans to whites.[132] The ice high lasts for 24 hours, with some users reporting that the effects can still be felt after two or three days. In the United States it sells for US$50 a gram but some dealers in Australia are reported to be asking ten times this amount, $500 a gram. Despite this hefty price tag, the drug is increasing in popularity.

The global market for amphetamine-type stimulants in 2005 consisted of at least 26 million consumers, with almost two-thirds of them in Asia.[133] Cambodia, Indonesia, Laos, Taiwan, Malaysia, South Korea, the Philippines, Thailand and China (although reluctant to admit it) all have significant numbers of users, and North Korea does an impressive export line.[134] In Japan, where the industry is largely controlled by the Yakuza (organised crime syndicates),[135] there are more than two million regular methamphetamine users, and in 2003 there were said to be some 600,000 addicted to the drug.[136]

In Australia in 2001, nearly 1.5 million people said they had sampled speed at some point in their lives. The number of those addicted to methamphetamines is reportedly as high as 73,000, more than twice the number said to be dependent on heroin in 2005.[137] After cannabis, it is the country's second most commonly used illicit drug, and control of large parts of the industry rests with those groups who can trace fraternal ties back to the bikie gangs in 1960s San Francisco. According to the Australian Crime Commission, Queensland bikie gangs are the largest producers of amphetamines in Australia and the Queensland Crime and Misconduct Commission reported that 162 speed laboratories were found in the state in 2002. In New South Wales, 72 laboratories were uncovered in the period from the beginning of 2002 to mid-2003, and in Western Australia, in the first six months of 2003, police reported a 35 per cent increase on the number of laboratories uncovered in 2002.[138] The number of speed laboratories detected around the country increased from 137 in 1999 to 346 in the year ending in September 2004. Some 60 per cent of these were uncovered by accident — through phone-ins, neighbours and when police visited houses for traffic incidents or with other warrants.[139]

While Queensland might lay claim to being the centre of speed production in Australia, it is in Melbourne where control of the industry is most contested. In the five years to 2003 there were 18 unsolved underworld murders in Melbourne, and between April 2003 and June of the following year, known criminals were being murdered at the rate of almost one a month. All the killings were said to be linked to control of the amphetamine market. According to former Melbourne drug squad sources, the criminals moved into the trade when police shut down the illegal gambling industry they had been running in the inner-city suburb of Carlton in 1994 — that was done to increase the profitability of the legal industry emerging on the Yarra in the shape of the Crown Casino. This coincided with the shutting down of bikie-controlled speed laboratories in the northern and western suburbs of Melbourne. Seeing a market vacuum, the ex-illegal gambler criminals moved into the amphetamine industry ... and have been squabbling over its control ever since.[140]

Besides bikies, self-employed cooks and a well-established criminal group, the other source of amphetamines is the pharmaceutical industry. The controls that were placed on the drug following the 1971 convention essentially restricted its medical use to the treatment of two conditions, as noted above. The first is the rare syndrome of narcolepsy: uncontrolled fits of sleep. It seems reasonable enough to use this drug, which keeps its users awake, for this syndrome. The second is much more controversial: ADHD in children. On the face of it, it does seem rather odd that a drug that is prohibited for adults because it is considered too dangerous is regarded as safe for children. And the logic of prescribing a drug that increases activity to those who are already overactive isn't immediately apparent. Yet those doctors who prescribe the drug say that its benefits are plain enough to see in those children taking it. Those in the medical profession who advocate non-drug treatments, and who contend that ADHD is in any event over-diagnosed, are themselves criticised by colleagues who believe that something like 10 per cent of all children could benefit from taking amphetamine or amphetamine-related drugs.[141]

The discovery that amphetamines can have a beneficial effect on children with behavioural problems was made by accident at a residential home for children with severe behavioural disorders in Rhode Island in the United States in 1937. The director of the institution, Dr Charles Bradley, prescribed Benzedrine for some of the children to raise their blood pressure in an effort to cure the headaches they were suffering from. It didn't do much for the headaches, but it did improve their behaviour and scholastic performance. Among the children, bennies became known as 'arithmetic pills' as a consequence of their effect on performance in that subject. From the 1950s, methylphenidate (an amphetamine derivative) was marketed under the brand name Ritalin. Together with dexamphetamine, it became a common treatment for ADHD sufferers by the 1970s.[142]

Sometimes referred to as 'kiddies' cocaine', dexamphetamine and Ritalin were being used by millions of US children — about 5 per cent of boys and 2 per cent of girls — in the mid-1990s. A decade later six million school-aged children were diagnosed as suffering from ADHD.[143] In Australia, nearly 20 million Ritalin tablets and almost 40 million dexamphetamine pills were prescribed to children with ADHD in 2001.[144] Australia and New Zealand rank third-equal in the world after the United States and Canada in the prescription of these drugs.[145] For reasons that are not entirely clear, Western Australian children are prescribed the drugs at a much greater rate than children in any other state. The population of New South Wales is almost four times higher than that of Western Australia, yet the prescription of ADHD speed is four times higher in Western Australia than in New South Wales.[146] In early 2003 it was reported that 18,000 children in Western Australia were managing to get through two million Ritalin tablets and 13 million dexamphetamine tablets each year.[147] One of the by-products of this level of prescribing is a thriving black market. Prescribed 'dexies' are on-sold at around $1 a pill to fellow students and adult recreational users, and in 2002 it was claimed that 20 per cent of 16- and 17-year-old boys and 17 per cent of girls of the same age in Western Australia use dexamphetamine recreationally.[148] Truly the State of Excitement, dependent only on your schoolyard supplier.

It also seems that childhood ADHD isn't something you grow out of very easily in Australia, as half of those diagnosed with the condition as children are still presenting with the problem as adults. Naturally, there are more adults with ADHD in Western Australia than anywhere else in the country; the incidence of the condition in Western Australia, at least according to the measurement of prescribed dexamphetamine, is ten times higher than in some other states. And it's a growth area for drug companies, with the 40,000 prescriptions for dexamphetamine issued to adults in Western Australia in the financial year 2003–04 representing a 15 per cent increase on the previous year.[149] This reflects the overall growth rates of dexamphetamine prescriptions — they rose almost sixfold in a decade, from 46,000 in 1994 to nearly 250,000 ten years later. When the other ADHD drug, Ritalin, became available through the Pharmaceutical Benefits Scheme (a federal government system that subsidises the cost to consumers of various drugs) in August 2005, reducing its cost from $49 to $29.50 or $4.70 for concession cardholders, the number of prescriptions being written for the drug increased tenfold in just five months.[150]

There are also side benefits for the drug companies, via some of the side effects of prescribed speed — anxiety and insomnia. These are treated with antidepressants and sleeping pills. As more children are diagnosed with ADHD and carry the condition through to adulthood, there will be a growing number of lifelong consumers of speed-related medication. Not quite a return to the halcyon days of the late 1960s for the drug companies, but nevertheless encouraging signs for their bottom line. And there is certainly scope for growth in the adult market. The typical signs of adult ADHD are said to include risk-taking behaviour, consistent under-achievement, lack of social skills and having extra-marital affairs.[151] All of which could indicate that the condition is indeed under-diagnosed. Assuming that this is rectified, more pills will be prescribed, and therefore more will find their way to the illicit market in the future.

In the workplace, Ritalin has made inroads into the cocaine market in the financial services sector in Manhattan,[152] and a positive test for speed in workplaces that use this kind of employee surveillance can now be excused by a doctor's prescription. If visiting the doctor is too bothersome, caffeine — now available in industrial strength packets at pharmacists — will have to suffice as the substitute stimulant.

5
Hallucinogenic dreaming: Cannabis, LSD and ecstasy

Two other medicinal herbs that appeared alongside ma huang in the first Chinese pharmacopoeia were huo ma ren and chu ma. Huo ma ren is the name for the seeds of a plant that was recommended as a mild laxative; the female variety of the plant, chu ma, had a wider application, which included the treatment of gout, rheumatism, menstrual problems, beri-beri, malaria and, oddly enough, absentmindedness.[1] The more familiar name of the plant is cannabis, classified as *Cannabis sativa* in 1753 by the Swedish doctor and naturalist Carolus Linnaeus (1707–78), who was sufficiently interested in studying the plant to grow it on his windowsill.[2]

Native to Central Asia, cannabis was probably first cultivated as long ago as 10,000 years, and from that time on the hardy weed has established a presence in most parts of the globe.[3] For a plant that has been around for so long it is surprising that there is still disagreement as to whether there are three distinct species (*Cannabis sativa, C. indica* and *C. ruderalis*) or simply one species, *C. sativa*, and two subspecies.[4] Controversy as to its correct botanical classification to one side, it's certainly possible to discern a variety of distinct uses of the cannabis plant throughout its long history. Its seeds have been used as a food source, and the oil contained in them has been used for lighting and in the production of soap, varnish and paints. The plant fibre, commonly called hemp, is used in rope, cloth, canvas and paper-making, and its leaves, seeds and oil are used as a medicine and intoxicant.[5]

It was hemp rope and canvas that powered the sailing fleets of the ancient Phoenician, Greek and Roman civilisations. The larger sailing ships of the 17th century used between 50 and 100 tonnes of hemp fibre, and it needed replacing at least every two years, so large tracts of land had to be set aside for the cultivation of cannabis.[6] This level of demand for hemp led to its production being declared mandatory in a number of countries; in the early days of the American colonies it was even used as legal tender.[7] The Gutenberg Bible was printed on hemp paper, as were the American Declaration of Independence and the first drafts of the American Constitution. Until the last decades of the 19th century, being in the paper-making business meant being in the hemp business.[8]

As a medicine, cannabis has long been used in most of the continents of the world. In Africa it was used as a cure for dysentery and malaria and in India it was also used for dysentery as well as a general cure-all to treat headaches and venereal disease, to induce sleep and to increase appetite. In Arab medicine hashish (cannabis resin) and benj (cannabis leaves) were used as an analgesic and in the treatment of asthma, diarrhoea and venereal disease. Galen was writing of its medicinal properties more than 1800 years ago, and in comparatively more recent times the English clergyman Robert Burton (1577–1640) advocated its use for depression in his *Anatomy of Melancholy* (first published in 1621). Some years later the English physician Nicholas Culpeper (1616–54) attempted to provide a comprehensive list of the uses of cannabis in the two important medical texts that he published in 1649 and 1653.[9]

In India, the use of various cannabis preparations as intoxicants has been known for thousands of years. The Hindu god Shiva was known as the lord of bhang, the name for a cannabis drink made of ground leaves, seeds and stems. Ganja, some two or three times stronger, is made from the flowers of female plants, and charas is the name given to the even stronger pure cannabis resin.[10] For several hundred years at least, the ubiquitous weed has been used as a recreational drug in Egypt, North Africa and the Middle East.[11]

However, despite the fact that hemp had been grown in Europe for more than 1000 years,[12] it was only following Napoleon's occupation of Egypt — from 1798 to 1801 — and the French invasion of Algeria in 1830 that cannabis for recreational use came to be widely known in Europe.[13] For although cannabis grown for its fibre content contains the psychoactive chemical delta-9-tetrahydrocannabinol (THC), the source of the cannabis 'high', it is present only in small amounts. In Egypt and Algeria large numbers of the invading French were exposed to cannabis that was specifically cultivated for its high THC content and they readily took to the experience.

From the 1840s on, hashish parties were popular among the literati of Paris. The more prominent of those who took part were Honoré de Balzac, Gustave Flaubert, Charles Baudelaire, Alexandre Dumas and Victor Hugo.[14] This was also the time when cannabis came into prominent use in European medical practice, thanks largely to the efforts of a young Irish doctor, William O'Shaughnessy. Born in Limerick in 1809, O'Shaughnessy received his medical education in Edinburgh and then sought to establish a practice in London, but his inability to obtain a licence (the profession's solution to overcrowding) from the Royal College of Physicians meant that he was prohibited from doing so within seven miles (11 kilometres) of the city. After a brief period in the provinces, he went to India in 1833 to work with the Bengal Medical Service of the East India Company, and eventually became Professor of Chemistry at the Medical College in Calcutta. From his studies and experiments with cannabis in India he was able to show that it was a particularly valuable drug in the relief of pain, and that it also acted as a muscle relaxant and anti-convulsant in the treatment of tetanus and rabies.[15] The publication and dissemination of these findings in 1842 attracted the interest of the medical community in Europe, and in that year he brought a supply of cannabis back to England; it was marketed by the London pharmacist Peter Squires as Squires Extract. Three years earlier, on the other side of the Atlantic, cannabis had been introduced into homeopathic medicine.[16]

The period from 1840 to 1900 stands as the high point of cannabis use in western medicine. More than 100 major papers were published in the medical literature, recommending its use for a wide range of illnesses and disorders,[17] including the treatment of asthma, coughs, insomnia, opium withdrawal and menstrual cramps.[18] It was for this last condition that Queen Victoria was prescribed the drug.[19]

The pharmaceutical companies were quick to add cannabis preparations to their list of proprietary medicines, and around 30 different products were available over the counter well into the 20th century. At the tobacconists', cannabis cigarettes were marketed as a remedy for asthma. The leading US companies that had cannabis-based medicines on the market included Squibb, Eli Lilly and Parke-Davis.[20] In 1887 the *Therapeutic Gazette* carried an article by H A Hare on the value of cannabis in treating migraines, and Parke-Davis later entered into a joint venture with Eli Lilly and developed their own potent strain of cannabis, Cannabis Americana.[21]

By the end of the 19th century, however, the medical use of cannabis was in decline. From the perspective of doctors administering the drug, it had a number of shortcomings. The potency of the available preparations was too variable and there didn't seem much prospect of standardised doses becoming available. This meant that the effect on individual patients was a hit-and-miss affair that doctors had no control over. Cannabis was taken orally, which meant that it could take an hour or longer to become effective. Doctors would have to spend this time twiddling their stethoscopes until the patient's reaction could be observed. Cannabis is also insoluble in water, so it couldn't be administered by injection and provide the immediate relief that injected morphine could. Perhaps the final nail in its coffin was the increased availability of synthetic hypnotics and analgesics such as chloral hydrate, barbiturates and aspirin, all of which turned out to be much more dangerous to health than cannabis could ever be.[22]

At the beginning of the 20th century cannabis was still readily available in the Western countries where it had been introduced the century before, and once again it was in the United States that its recreational use first became evident. Going back to the beginning, cannabis was introduced to Latin America and the Caribbean from the early 15th century by African slaves. Much later, in the early decades of the 19th century until World War I, close to half a million Indian labourers were brought to the Caribbean and surrounding areas of the colonised northeast coast of South America to work on the sugar plantations. They brought their ganja with them.[23] So by the early years of the 20th century the recreational use of cannabis had spread from the Caribbean to the US Gulf Coast ports of Houston, Galveston and New Orleans. Then half a million Mexicans migrated to the United States between 1915 and 1930, and they too came with a custom of consuming cannabis, which they were happy to spread among the locals, some of whom began to develop a taste for it.[24] Marijuana, a Spanish-Mexican word initially used to describe tobacco, became a familiar term for cannabis in the Americas and beyond.[25] In the 1920s, as Mexican labourers and African-American jazz musicians from New Orleans travelled north to cities such as Chicago and Detroit, marijuana travelled with them, but it was thanks to the prohibition of alcohol that it travelled further and the market for its consumption expanded considerably.[26] Just as opium had its illicit dens and alcohol its speakeasies, so too did marijuana come to have its secretive places of consumption. They were called 'tea-pads', and during Prohibition several hundred of them 'sprang up like weeds' in New York City alone.[27]

At the dawn of alcohol prohibition in 1920, the open sale and possession of marijuana had already been banned for six years in the cities of New York and El Paso, and in the years that followed an increasing number of states — at least 12 by 1923 and 18 by 1933 — passed laws against marijuana.[28] As deliberations got underway at the International Opium Conference in Geneva in November 1924, the Egyptian delegation argued that hashish was more dangerous than opium and pressed the case for its prohibition on the ground that the vast bulk of those declared insane and incarcerated in their country's lunatic asylums were users of the drug (this was not true).[29] The United States was willing to support the proposal on an expedient quid pro quo basis alone, but the delegation would also have been aware of the growing desire among US state lawmakers to ban the drug. Cannabis now joined cocaine, opium, morphine and heroin as a drug subject to international control and condemnation.

In the United States, marijuana was demonised in much the same way that opium and cocaine had previously been. It was portrayed in some sections of the press as a 'sex drug', and as a drug that drove its users mad. In New Orleans, a year after the Geneva Conference had concluded, marijuana was confidently claimed by city officials to be responsible for a crime wave; they said the human derelicts who used it were so depraved as to be corrupting school children with the drug. The usual suspects were rounded up: African-Americans, low-class whites, those addicted to other drugs, and criminals of any and every description. Jazz musicians could now be added to the list, as well as that low breed of Mexican who used 'loco weed' not only to become intoxicated but also to treat the venereal diseases that his base habits disposed him to.[30]

The bureaucratic apparatus responsible for enforcing alcohol prohibition in the United States was set up by the Bureau of Internal Revenue. It established a Prohibition Unit that from 1920 had a separate Narcotics Division, headed by Colonel Levi Nutt. But Nutt's organisation became corrupted by the gangsters who controlled the illicit market for opiates and cocaine; it was disbanded in 1930 and replaced by the Federal Bureau of Narcotics (FBN).[31] The FBN had a slow start, but soon its commissioner, Harry Anslinger (1892–1975), began to exert what was to be a profound and enduring influence on the policy approach taken to cannabis in the United States, and in most of the rest of the world. But right from the start he had a little help from his friends.

The FBN was set up under the aegis of the United States Treasury Department and Anslinger, who had been employed in the consular service before transferring to the Prohibition Bureau, had the good fortune to be married to the niece of the Secretary of the Treasury, the prominent banker Andrew Mellon. He was appointed commissioner despite someone else already having been nominated for the job.[32] Anslinger was a racist who had decidedly odd opinions about drug addiction.[33] In his view it had to be suppressed by criminal sanctions because it was not a treatable medical condition. Once incarcerated, a person could stop taking drugs simply because they were (supposedly) no longer available, but upon release the mental problem of addiction remained. It could only be overcome, he believed, by the addicted persons themselves — by which means doesn't appear to have been specified.[34]

When Anslinger first took office, marijuana wasn't high on

his list of drugs to be suppressed. Opiates and cocaine were his prime targets and his modus operandi was the same as that of his rival at the Federal Bureau of Investigation (FBI), J Edgar Hoover: they both relied on paid informers and double agents. Given the superior strength in the United States of organised crime groups that used similar methods, this meant they were only able to secure convictions against street users (addicts, as Anslinger would classify them) and those suppliers considered expendable by their superiors.[35] But this was the era of the Great Depression, and restraint in government spending meant budget cuts at the FBN which severely restricted the capacity of the organisation to purchase both information and the full-time services of informers. Corruption became evident, just as it had with the FBN's predecessor organisation. Mellon had departed from the Treasury in 1932 to take up the post of ambassador to the United Kingdom, and by 1936 Anslinger, who had suffered a nervous breakdown the year before, was facing pressure from the head of Treasury over his organisation's deteriorating performance. His survival, and that of his organisation, came to depend on a campaign against the evils of marijuana.[36]

Despite its popularity among some groups, the problems caused by marijuana use were relatively insignificant compared with those associated with other drugs in the United States in the 1930s. But its users were mainly members of minority groups that could be easily marginalised on race grounds alone. Just as importantly, the marijuana market wasn't controlled by the organised crime figures whose power and influence had increased considerably during Prohibition. Neither Anslinger at the FBN nor Hoover at the FBI could seriously challenge the dominance of organised crime. Associates of America's pre-eminent gangster, Meyer Lansky, would even claim that he blackmailed Hoover by procuring photographs of his acts of sexual congress — which, unfortunately for Hoover in the circumstances, were with someone of the same sex.[37]

Anslinger's survival strategy was to inflate the dangers of marijuana use with propaganda material that bore little if any relationship to known facts and to stigmatise the drug by associating it with Mexican and African-American consumers. In 1936 the film *Reefer Madness* was released. Its plotline had two high school students entice other students to use the drug, with the predictable result that all their lives were ruined. The following year an article in *American Magazine* headed 'Marijuana: Assassin of Youth' blamed marijuana for the violent death of a young girl in Chicago. Marijuana had by now become a narcotic that was 'as dangerous as a coiled rattlesnake'.[38] Anslinger was assisted in his demonising of marijuana by newspaper magnate William Randolph Hearst (1863–1951), whose sensational brand of journalism led to his publications being given the sobriquet 'yellow press'. Hearst was also a racist, with a particular hatred for Mexicans said to stem from the loss of 800,000 acres (about 324,000 hectares) of valuable forestry timber to the Mexican bandit turned revolutionary, Pancho Villa.[39]

Hearst's newspapers had previously carried articles about cocaine-crazed African-Americans who raped white women. The same newspapers were now able to switch the drug to marijuana and run similar stories. His newspapers described marijuana-smoking Mexicans as violent and degenerate. Paradoxically, they were also both lazy and responsible for depriving law-abiding Americans of their jobs during the Depression. In Hearst's *Washington Herald* in April 1937 Anslinger claimed that 'if the monster Frankenstein came face to face with the monster marijuana, he would drop dead of fright'.[40] According to Anslinger, marijuana had a particular effect on African-Americans and Mexicans, causing them to 'have perpetrated some of the most bizarre and fantastic offences and sex crimes known to police annals'.[41] All these stories had one small defect: they weren't true. What, on the other hand, was true but not acknowledged was that cannabis had been one of the more important agricultural crops in America since colonial times. Beyond its wide commercial use, it had been quietly smoked for recreational purposes over generations. Six earlier US presidents, including George Washington, had smoked the drug both at home and abroad but, curiously enough, the habits of these heads of state weren't mentioned.[42]

In 1937 the federal legislation on marijuana that Anslinger had initially resisted was passed into law — in the absence of any scientific material supporting its provisions and over the objections of pharmacists and the American Medical Association. *The Marijuana Tax Act* made it compulsory for anyone who grew, transported, prescribed or sold marijuana to register and pay taxes. Failure to comply was an offence, but it was virtually impossible to comply given that marijuana use (except for medical purposes) was an offence against state laws. Anyone failing to register for the tax was liable to prosecution for a federal offence, but federal registration brought with it the liability to be prosecuted under state laws. The Act was also unconstitutional, violating the Fifth Amendment provisions on self-incrimination by requiring a person to pay a tax in order to possess an illegal substance.[43] Nevertheless the Act, together with FBN regulations, put an end to the medical use of cannabis, and save for one notable exception, it also halted research on the drug for the better part of 30 years. In 1941 cannabis was removed from the US Pharmacopoeia and National Formulary, reportedly at the request of Anslinger, who had long held that cannabis had no therapeutic value. Clearly unaware of the circumstances in which Robert Louis Stevenson's book was written, he testified before a congressional committee: 'Opium has all of the good of Dr Jekyll and all the evil of Mr Hyde. This drug [marijuana] is entirely the monster Hyde, the harmful effects of which cannot be measured.'[44] Under the provisions of the *Marijuana Tax Act* thousands were arrested, many were jailed and tens of thousands of tonnes of the drug were destroyed. The one thing it didn't do was stop people using the drug for recreational purposes. There was a clear demand for mild hallucinogens and the market expanded in the years to come.

The other notable achievement of the *Marijuana Tax Act* was to destroy the American hemp industry; there is still controversy over whether this was an unintended consequence — unavoidable collateral damage in the war on marijuana use — or a chief part of its unstated but intended purpose. The case for the latter centres on the threat that a resurgent hemp industry posed to the interests of the Du Pont company, William Randolph Hearst and Andrew Mellon, and is most persuasively made by Jack Herer in his book *The Emperor Wears No Clothes*. Simply put, technical advances in the harvesting and processing of hemp led to increased productivity and availability and a dramatic drop in price. By the mid-1930s hemp was emerging as a serious competitor to wood pulp and hydrocarbons. The Ford Motor Company was advancing plans to use hemp as a primary source for both building and fuelling vehicles.[45] This development threatened the profitability of Hearst's operations, which was dependent on his forestry holdings. It similarly threatened Du Pont, which dominated the petrochemical industry and owned Ford's rival vehicle company, General Motors. Mellon's problems stemmed from the fact that he financed Du Pont's acquisition of General Motors and owned Gulf Oil.[46]

These interests came together in various ways to block the advance of hemp's industrial applications, but none was more obvious than Du Pont's lobbying of the Treasury Department for cannabis prohibition and an assurance that the company's synthetic petrochemicals could fill the void left by the elimination of hemp-seed oil from the market.[47] Their efforts were immediately rewarded, as in 1935 Treasury commenced the secret drafting of the Bill that would become law two years later.[48] Coincidentally, other companies had by now joined Ford to present a broader challenge to Du Pont and Mellon by promising to replace petroleum hydrocarbons with cannabis carbohydrates.

Herer certainly makes a convincing case and it's plain that the interests of Du Pont, Hearst and Mellon were well served by the passing of the *Marijuana Tax Act* and the concomitant destruction of the American hemp industry. The other commercial interest that was threatened by the demise of the hemp industry, the canary birdseed trade, was placated by being allowed to import hemp seed, provided that it was first sterilised.[49]

In 1942, with the United States at war and important sources of hemp controlled by Japan, the US Department of Agriculture sponsored a revival of the hemp industry by initially requesting some 20,000 farmers to plant 36,000 acres of hemp seed; there were plans to increase this to 300,000 acres and to build 71 processing mills. Hemp was necessary for the war effort, particularly for the US Navy: hemp rope was used by all US naval and commercial ships. As part of the promotional effort a film called *Hemp for Victory* was made in 1942. When Herer went looking for a copy nearly 40 years after the war ended, no record of it could be found in the archives and he was told it didn't exist. He eventually managed to track it down, thanks to persistence and an element of good luck, but this affair did rather make his point about a cover-up.[50]

While *Hemp for Victory* was being screened and US farmers were being exhorted to do their patriotic duty and start growing cannabis again, Anslinger was busy updating his files on African-American jazz musicians and others in the entertainment world whom he suspected of smoking it. Louis Armstrong was kept under surveillance, given that he had already transgressed — in 1931 he had spent 10 days in jail for marijuana possession, followed by a six-month suspended sentence. The legendary drummer Gene Krupa fared even worse, doing time in San Quentin prison for possession of marijuana. Count Basie, Duke Ellington, Cab Calloway, Dizzy Gillespie and Lionel Hampton were among the more prominent musicians Anslinger kept files on, and the actor Robert Mitchum became familiar with prison life from the inside when he was convicted on marijuana charges in 1949.[51]

Another activity that Anslinger was engaged in during the early 1940s, in collaboration with the Office of Strategic Services, the predecessor organisation to the Central Intelligence Agency, was the search for a drug that would act as a 'truth serum'. He was able to learn firsthand of the effect on people's veracity levels of a particularly potent form of marijuana. The most obvious effect of high-grade marijuana on those being tested was uncontrollable laughter. Others got paranoid and all got hungry. It was a finding that he declined to share with the American public.[52]

In the 1950s, despite heroin being again a major problem in the United States thanks to supply from Meyer Lansky's French Connection in Marseilles, Anslinger was still concentrating on marijuana. During congressional hearings on the *Marijuana Tax Act* in 1937 Anslinger had testified that marijuana users didn't graduate to heroin, opium or cocaine, but now he had come up with the politically expedient proposition that cannabis was a 'gateway' drug that led to heroin use. On the basis of this newfound threat he worked with the Democrat politician Hale Boggs to ensure the passage into law of the first mandatory minimum sentences for drug possession. Marijuana, cocaine and opiates were all treated the same: a first conviction for possession attracted a two-year sentence, a second conviction 5–10 years, and a third 10–20 years.[53] When asked about the heroin coming into the United States, the connection that Anslinger made was with 'Red China', which he falsely accused of exporting the drug; in fact they were already making significant headway in cleaning up the legacy of the widespread opiate use and addiction bequeathed them by the British.

Jumping aboard the anti-communist bandwagon, Anslinger joined his good friend in Washington, Senator Joe McCarthy (1909–57). McCarthy was a circuit judge in the state of Wisconsin who was unconstitutionally elected to the Senate in 1945 and showed his contempt for the law by taking his seat in defiance of a Supreme Court ruling. From 1953 onwards McCarthy demonstrated his disregard for the rights of others from his position as chairman of the Senate Permanent Subcommittee on Investigations. Together with the chairman of the House Un-American Activities Committee (HUAC), he exploited the new medium of television, broadcasting live hearings of the bullying and smearing by innuendo of witnesses summoned to appear before them. The presumption of innocence was replaced by guilt by association, and the lives and careers of many Americans, a number of them in the entertainment business, were destroyed. McCarthy eventually brought himself undone by accusing the US Army, the State Department, the Democratic Party in general and the Truman Administration (1945–52) in particular of treason and being 'soft on communism'. Truman's response was to label him a 'pathological character assassin', and 'McCarthyism' entered the lexicon, defined as the public accusation of disloyalty unsupported by facts.[54]

Anslinger and McCarthy had more in common than friendship. They were both fervent believers in an ideology called Americanism, in which citizenship was defined neither by birth nor residence but by what a person believed in, and thought.[55] The United States was built on individualism and free (i.e. private) enterprise, and they were what people should believe in. It was 'un-American', according to these two, to believe otherwise. When the idea that the US Congress should establish an Un-American Activities Committee was first proposed in 1934, the un-American activity that was to be investigated was the racist propaganda of fascist Germany that was being spread by organisations such as the Ku Klux Klan. This threat from the right was quickly forgotten as HUAC was turned into an anti-communist crusade by conservative opponents of the New Deal of President Franklin Delano Roosevelt (1882–1945).[56] The notion that the business community, through taxation measures, should accept some responsibility for general welfare, not to mention the dangerously radical idea of public ownership, was clearly un-American for some.

What was un-American for Anslinger was taking drugs, although this rather depended on who was consuming them; McCarthy was a morphine addict and it was Anslinger who supplied him with the drug.[57] Anslinger remained in office for 32 years. He didn't survive the presidency of J F Kennedy (1917–63), but he did survive the president, who was assassinated on 22 November 1963. Kennedy's assassin, Lee Harvey Oswald, was shot and killed two days later by Jack Ruby, a petty gangster from Chicago who had run errands for Al Capone as a child and had been recruited as a double agent by the FBN in 1946.[58]

The most striking feature of Anslinger's reign as America's first 'drugs czar' was the increased use of illicit drugs and the institutionalising of their supply. World War II certainly interrupted the supply of opiates everywhere, but US troops landing at Normandy on D-day could still find dealers to supply them with illicit morphine.[59] The publicity that Anslinger's policy approach gave to marijuana actually helped popularise the drug, and the experience of those who tried it as a result led to a disregard, if not a contempt, for official government pronouncements on the deleterious effects of drugs. Categorising marijuana with heroin and cocaine led to some street-level suppliers favouring distribution of the more dangerous drugs. If the penalty for dealing in any of the three was the same, it made perfect sense to deal in the less bulky, more easily concealed and more profitable drugs. This may have ultimately led to an increase in their consumption.

Anslinger refused to even acknowledge these lessons, let alone learn from them. He set the pattern for successive drug czars, and they followed dutifully. In the years immediately following his departure from the FBN there was a massive increase in drug consumption in the United States, with marijuana leading the way.

In the 1960s the Vietnam War met the coming of age of the post-World War II generation. This was a combustible mix in the United States, and it saw a questioning of authority and political direction. Marijuana use, partly because it was forbidden, became a symbol of youth rebelling against the prevailing conservative wisdom. Popularised by counterculture figures such as Alan Ginsberg, it crossed the divide between the marginalised and the middle class, and became popular in the suburbs and on college campuses across the nation. Large numbers of the conscripts sent to Vietnam clearly didn't want to be there, and they consumed large quantities of cannabis in order to temporarily transport themselves somewhere else. Between 1965 and 1967, the number of arrests for use and possession of marijuana by US military personnel in Vietnam increased by more than 2500 per cent.[60] After the Vietnamese National Liberation Front and the North Vietnamese Army's Tet offensive in 1968, during which 67,000 troops attacked 102 towns and villages in South Vietnam, including the capital, Saigon,[61] the US military chiefs intensified their efforts at suppression by ordering the military police to cut off supply lines. The troops turned to heroin instead.[62]

In the United States in 1969, 4 per cent of the total population had used marijuana, but among college students the figure was 22 per cent; five years later the figure among college students was more than 50 per cent.[63] Across all 18 to 25-year-olds, more than one-quarter were regular users of marijuana in 1972 and more than one-third were five years later. A massive 60 per cent of this age group had tried the drug at least once. In the even younger 12 to 17-year-old group, the 7 per cent of regular users in 1972 had increased to 17 per cent five years later.[64] With so much pot being smoked by so many people, the laws that purported to prohibit its use became unworkable. Despite the threat that such mass disobedience posed in the conservative mind, it was, if nothing else, logistically impossible to jail one in every five 12–17-year-olds and six out of every ten 18–25-year-olds in the country, together with all those over the age of 26 who were using the drug. Sheer weight of numbers seriously compromised the law at this point. The other important factor was middle-class consumption. Jailing African-Americans and Hispanics was one thing, but jailing the cream of America's overwhelmingly white middle-class youth was quite another.

The policy response to this massive increase in marijuana consumption was to relax the punitive laws. From the mid-1960s to the mid-1970s, 11 US states decriminalised marijuana use, and in most other states possession was downgraded from a felony (generally a crime for which more than a year's jail time is a possible punishment) to a misdemeanour (generally a crime for which punishment does not exceed one year in jail).[65] In 1977, US President Jimmy Carter even went as far as supporting legislation decriminalising the possession of up to one ounce of marijuana.[66] Congress, however, was against him, and under his successor, Ronald Reagan, the campaign against marijuana use was again taken up as a conservative cause. It was continued during the presidencies of George Bush, Bill Clinton and George W Bush, with punishment for a first offence now ranging from probation to the death penalty.[67] More than 10 million Americans have been arrested for marijuana offences in the past 20 years, with the rates of arrest steadily increasing. In

1998, 695,000 were arrested, in 2001 it was more than 720,000 and in 2006 it was 830,000.[68]

None of this has had much of an effect on consumption. In the last full year of Reagan's presidency, 1988, the number of marijuana users in the United States was estimated to be between 20 and 25 million.[69] Today about one-third of Americans (around 90 million people) have smoked marijuana at least once and the number of regular smokers is variously estimated at between 20 and 50 million, with more than two million lighting up every day.[70] The value of the outdoor-grown crop alone was estimated at up to US$25 billion in 2001, easily surpassing the US$19 billion value of the largest legally grown crop, corn.[71] The value of the indoor-grown hydroponic crop can only be guessed at.[72]

Another way to look at the extent of marijuana consumption in the United States since the 1960s is by looking at the habits of the country's presidents and their immediate families from that time. President J F Kennedy was by all accounts the first president to smoke marijuana in the White House, in 1962. He used it for relief from the chronic back pain he suffered, and smoked the drug both before and during his presidential term. Lyndon Baines Johnson, president from 1963 to 1968, didn't follow his example. Richard Milhous Nixon, a prominent member of the House Committee on Un-American Activities who occupied the White House from 1969 until 1974, when he resigned in disgrace over the Watergate scandal, restricted his drug intake to alcohol, sleeping pills and the anti-convulsant Dilantin.[73] Sons of Presidents Ford and Carter admitted to smoking dope in the White House during their fathers' terms, between 1974 and 1980. The next occupants to stay on Pennsylvania Avenue, Ronald and Nancy Reagan, were there from 1980 to 1988 and didn't sully the premises with the smell of weed … but they both smoked marijuana, and got the giggles, when Reagan was governor of California, from 1966 to 1974.[74] George Bush, who was president from 1988 to 1992, didn't smoke dope no matter where he was, but his vice president, Dan Quayle, was known to smoke pot, among other drugs, at college.[75] Bill Clinton, who succeeded Bush at the White House and stayed until 2000, did, on his own admission, smoke marijuana, but not on American soil. He neither inhaled nor had sexual relations with Monica Lewinsky. His vice president, Al Gore, a less complicated man, simply admitted to having tried marijuana.[76] President George W Bush has been remarkably evasive on the subject of his illicit drug use, but some members of his family and former friends haven't. He is reported by them to have used both marijuana and cocaine during the 1960s and early 1970s. On the account of his former sister-in-law, he snorted cocaine on more than one occasion at Camp David during his father's presidency.[77] Illicit drug use, and smoking marijuana in particular, seems on the evidence to be a very common American activity. It's the punishment for it that's selective.

Cannabis in Australia

Cannabis arrived in Australia with the First Fleet in January 1788 thanks to the English botanist Sir Joseph Banks (1744–1820), who was considered by some at least to be 'the Father and Founder of the Australian colonies'.[78] Banks had accompanied James Cook on his expedition round the world on the *Endeavour* between 1768 and 1771 and was one of the few in England who had some firsthand knowledge of the place that Cook had named New South Wales. He also had considerable influence within the British government and with its monarch, George III. It was his evidence before the House of Commons committee on transportation in 1779 that sparked interest in the idea that Australia could be a useful place for a penal colony, given that America, which had been obliged to take 40,000 British convicts from 1717 had, on 4 July 1776, declared independence and would be taking no more convicts.[79]

Besides being a repository for sections of the British criminal class, Australia, like all other Empire possessions, was expected to play its proper role as a source of raw materials for the mother country. There were two such raw materials Britain was thought to be particularly lacking in at the time. In Banks' view, she was dangerously dependent on Russia for hemp supplies and on Spain for fine wool, and it was to Empire that he looked for a remedy. Five years before the arrival of the First Fleet it had been proposed that colonising Australia might lead to the development of a hemp industry that would make Britain self-sufficient in the commodity; the cannabis seeds that Captain Arthur Phillip brought with him in 1788 (supplied by Banks) were intended for this purpose.[80] The other possibilities canvassed for developing a hemp industry for the Empire at the time were Ireland and India.

India was, of course, long familiar with cannabis cultivation, so it's no surprise that Governor King of New South Wales was able to notify Banks in 1804 that the 10 acres (2.5 hectares) of cannabis he had planted in Sydney with seeds sent from India in 1802 were coming along very nicely (though it may have been a particularly psychoactive type of hemp).[81] Seed was again imported from India in 1803 and a flourishing plantation of 500 acres (just over 200 hectares) was established on the Hawkesbury by a settler. Two looms were making sailcloth from Hawkesbury hemp in 1804, and in 1807 the *Buffalo* was fitted with homegrown hemp sails. But demand for the local industry was contingent upon Sydney becoming an extensive whaling port, so the practical suspension of whaling in 1810 saw the hemp industry gradually disappear.[82] India instead became the source of hemp for the Empire and Australia the source of its fine merino wool.

So the cannabis that was used in Australian medical practice in the 19th century had to be imported. By the 1860s Australia had its own literary celebrity writing about the drug. Marcus Andrew Hislop Clarke (1846–81) had attended the same private school in England as De Quincey, Coleridge and Keats before migrating to Melbourne in 1863, at the tender age of 17. Best known for his novel *For the Term of his Natural Life* (1874), Clarke had read De Quincey and, like him, was an opium smoker who was also fond of a drink.[83] The plainly titled 'Cannabis Indica', which appeared in the February 1868 edition of the *Colonial Monthly* was, on his account, something of a psychological experiment.

A number of writers, most famously De Quincey, had previously written accounts of their drug-taking experiences with opium and 'haschich' after the effects of the drug had worn off. Marcus Clarke wanted to give the world a story composed while still under the effects of hashish (*Cannabis indica*), which he described as a narcotic more powerful than opium. Relying on De Quincey's account of the effects of opium (under its influence the powers of reason are in abeyance) and the French physician Moreau's account of the hashish experience, he declared that the cannabis effect was different. With cannabis, according to Clarke, the reasoning faculties are in full play and the user not only remains articulate but is able to work out the 'most subtle chains of reasoning'. What was in fact different about Clarke's experiment was that he dictated his cannabis-induced story to a doctor who, as well as administering the drug, also recorded his own objective account of Clarke's behaviour during the experiment.

The cannabis that Clarke took, at 7 pm one night, consisted of two pills, each containing about three-fifths of a grain. He washed them down with a warm cup of tea. It must have been particularly potent because at first he fell into a stupor. He was able to start dictating his story at 10.30 pm, and he continued until 3.15 the following morning, after which he fell into a long sleep.[84] It would be generous to say that the story itself is unremarkable, and it didn't apparently do much for the circulation of the *Colonial Monthly*. Clarke became its editor the month after the story appeared but had to extricate himself from the financial disaster of the enterprise in September of the following year.[85]

Clarke's writings on cannabis also appeared in other publications. In the month that followed the publication of 'Cannabis Indica' he was again writing of opium and 'hatchis' in the conservative Melbourne daily the *Argus*, asserting that opium, when smoked, rarely induces visions of extraordinary beauty; as with hatchis, it is opium when eaten that has this effect.[86] In his 'Peripatetic Philosopher' column, which appeared in the *Argus*'s weekend magazine *The Australasian* from late 1867 to the middle of 1870, he made reference to the Yorick Club that he and other writers and journalists established in 1868 for the purpose of discussing literary matters while getting pleasantly intoxicated. Somewhat tongue-in-cheek, he refuted the allegation that he and other club members sat around smoking 'green tea'. The green tea was cannabis.[87] The medical doctor who assisted Clarke in his cannabis experiment was not named in the 'Cannabis Indica' article, perhaps for reasons connected to professional ethics. However, the name that a playful Clarke gave to the fictitious medical practitioner who appeared in a later series of articles for *The Australasian* was Dr Cannabis.[88]

Unlike Marcus Clarke, most Australians took their cannabis in the form of proprietary medicines. Dr J Collis Browne's Chlorodyne sold particularly well, perhaps because the six grams of cannabis extract that it contained (together with morphine and chloroform) was in the form of black Nepalese hash.[89] Surprisingly, perhaps, in view of later developments, some of the cannabis proprietary remedies sold in the 19th century were still available in the 1940s and 1950s. Cannabis cigarettes aptly named Cigares De Joy were advertised as a cure for asthma and bronchitis in the 19th century, particularly suited to ladies and children, and they were still available after World War II. Those who had an authority to purchase Dangerous Drugs could still buy cannabis in bulk in 1947 at prices that ranged from 1s 6d an ounce to 9s 6d a pound. Dr Poppy's Wonder Elixir, which had cannabis extract in it, at 2s 6d for a 15-ounce bottle, came recommended as an early morning drink to see you through the day — it was still on the market in the 1950s.[90]

The one group of migrants who brought their cannabis seeds with them and grew, ate and smoked the drug within their communities were the Afghan cameleers who opened up the Australian outback from the time they first arrived for the Burke and Wills expedition in 1860.[91] The number of cameleers who came to Australia isn't known with any precision, but it's been estimated that there may have been as many as 1500 living in the camel camps that came to be known as Ghantowns.[92] There were about 20 of these settlements scattered around Australia; the outskirts of railhead towns and ports in South Australia, Queensland, Western Australia and New South Wales. Port Augusta, Oodnadatta, Fremantle, Port Hedland, Cloncurry, Townsville, Bourke and Broken Hill all had their Ghantowns. The cannabis that the cameleers grew was a variety of some potency that was baked into cakes called 'marjoms' and smoked in bongs known as 'narghiles'.[93] As late as the 1960s, descendants of these earlier cameleers in Broken Hill were given to wondering why the miners preferred to get intoxicated and belligerent drinking beer when there was plenty of 'happy weed' to be smoked.[94]

Despite the fact that by then cannabis had been consumed without any fuss in Australia for the better part of 100 years, *Smith's Weekly* was able to tell readers, in its 23 April 1938 issue, of a warning from America that marihuana [sic], a 'Mexican drug that drives men and women to the wildest sexual excesses', had suddenly made its first appearance here. The 11 June issue was further able to reveal that marihuana cigarettes, the ones that make you 'behave like a raving sex maniac', had been sneaked into the country and smoked at a Sydney party. The reliable informant for these stories turned out to be none other than the FBN's man in Hawaii, who was anxious to let us know that 'if prompt action is not taken, marihuana will flood Australia and New Zealand'. According to the April article, it already had. It was growing wild all along the Queensland coast.[95]

Anslinger's propaganda had arrived in Australia barely six months after the *Marijuana Tax Act* had come into effect in the United States. The *Smith's Weekly* articles were a part of his attempt to ensure that the use of marijuana (the term had never before been used in Australia) was sensationally publicised and just as sensationally prohibited in all the countries where he could bring his influence to bear. Inconvenient facts that might impede his proselytising mission were simply ignored. Crude as the strategy was, it certainly managed to get the attention of those in high places. Prime Minister Joe Lyons' department dispatched memoranda to the director-general of health and the Queensland premier suggesting that some sort of investigation of the *Smith's Weekly* claims might be in order. Queensland police were sent north from Brisbane searching for the sex drug. They had no success. The NSW Parliament was moved to declare *Cannabis sativa* a noxious weed and the Queensland government, ever anxious to keep up, followed suit. The Director-General of Health told the prime minister's department that on his advice Indian hemp had been cultivated for its fibre in Australia for more than 50 years, had probably grown wild in Queensland, and in any event contained little resin.[96] Nobody in authority seems to have been advised that cannabis cigarettes were on open sale.

As in the United States and other advanced economies, cannabis use became popular in Australia again in the decade that became known as the swinging sixties. In 1960, in Australia's premier hedonist state, New South Wales, the authorities first reported the use of Indian hemp among a small group in what was described as the 'theatrical world'. The Greek migrant in Queensland who, three years earlier, was the first person to be convicted of growing an illegal crop, was slightly ahead of the times.[97]

Consumption increased rapidly along the east coast of Australia from the mid-1960s thanks initially to the pioneer settlers in the Upper Hunter Valley, who had scattered some seeds about in the early 1820s — by 1846 cannabis was recorded as growing wild on the banks of the Hunter River near Singleton. When it was rediscovered in November of 1964 it stretched along the river for tens of kilometres, from Singleton to East Maitland, and some of the plants were as high as two metres. It took the NSW Department of Agriculture five years to eradicate the newfound crop. They had considerable assistance, often at night and on weekends, from the many dedicated young people who travelled to the area and stuffed sleeping bags, sacks and pillowcases with as much of the noxious weed as they could carry and were conscientious enough to take it home with them before disposing of it. By all accounts it was a good smoke.[98]

Just as the local cannabis was beginning to run out, US troops on rest-and-recreation leave from Vietnam arrived in Sydney with a smoke that was much stronger (sometimes dipped in opium). They were happy to pass it around or sell it. Not long after they had stopped coming, the counterculture communes found that the high-grade cannabis they grew had a ready market. Backyards, balconies and quiet spots in the bush were pressed into service to meet growing demand; despite all this effort, locally grown cannabis still had to be supplemented by imports. Cannabis from many parts of the world found its way to Australia: hashish from Lebanon and buddha sticks from Thailand were the most common imports.

Cannabis was a young person's drug, and its widespread use made the older generation of politicians and others in authority uneasy. The mere fact that it was illegal meant that those who smoked it had no respect for the law. Their other activities confirmed that they didn't have much respect for anything else either, beyond a personal liberty that was threateningly permissive. These dope smokers were taking to the streets demanding an end to Australia's involvement in the Vietnam War and encouraging others to resist conscription. They were university students, subsidised by taxpayers, who were trying to take over the universities to participate in demonstrations when they should have been studying. They were promiscuous, still in bed in the afternoon, and didn't go to church, even on Sundays. What's more, they were supported by the Communist Party of Australia, which demanded that the drug be made legal. Women's liberation, gay liberation — it was all too much for some. In the country's parliaments politicians fell over themselves to condemn cannabis.

It had by now gone from a sex drug that induced violence to a drug that was tearing at the moral fabric of society by making its users indolent and depriving them of motivation.[99] Surfers were a prime example. They smoked the drug as they travelled up and down the coast searching for waves in cars that they unashamedly called 'shaggin' wagons'. As for hippies, it was enough to draw attention to their lack of personal hygiene.

While tougher penalties were being called for, something far more sinister was occurring with cannabis supply in the early 1970s. It was being taken over by organised criminal groups. There had always been cannabis entrepreneurs — those who earned all or a large part of their income from cannabis — but it was very much a small-business venture. Illegality and increasing demand made it profitable enough for organised crime groups to invest in huge plantations and large-scale imports. The crackdown on these activities following the murder of Griffith anti-drug campaigner Donald Mackay in 1977 led to a cannabis drought that was accompanied by an increase in the availability of heroin (see Chapter 9). Suffice it to say that criminal groups were able to exert considerable influence over the supply of cannabis until the advent of hydroponics, which allowed small entrepreneurs to capture a significant share of the market with a superior product at lower prices.

The response to illicit drug use in Australia has, since the 1960s, centred on cannabis. Given that no drug is completely safe for all people in all circumstances, it is obvious enough that cannabis can and will create problems for some. But as drugs go it's more harmless than most others, licit or illicit. This is hardly reflected in the statistics that inform us of the use of criminal sanctions. The scores of people who were arrested for cannabis offences each year in the mid-1960s had increased to thousands in the 1970s and tens of thousands in the 1980s, rising to 78,948 in 1995–96. Despite something of a relaxation of the laws prohibiting its use in a number of states since the late 1980s, the number of arrests for cannabis offences since 1972 has consistently represented between 70 per cent and 80 per cent of all drug arrests. In 2002–03, 74,973 people were arrested for drug offences throughout Australia. Just over 8000 were arrested for amphetamine-type stimulants and nearly 4000 for heroin and other opioids. The 55,689 arrested for cannabis were 74 per cent of the total. In 1974 it was 72.52 per cent, in 1981 it was 83 per cent and in 1994 it was 85 per cent.[100] It seems that the link made between cannabis use and civil disobedience in the 1960s is a strong and continuing one in the mind of officialdom.

Proving once again that prohibition will never succeed, high rates of arrest and incarceration were accompanied by increased consumption and increased numbers of consumers. In 1973, when our population was around 13 million, 500,000 marijuana users were smoking their way through 40 tonnes of the drug. By 1984 (population now around 16 million), 1,175,000 users were consuming 94 tonnes, and in 1998 (population around 19 million), 2,700,000 were managing to get through 210 tonnes.[101]

In 2004, close to half of all Australians over the age of 14 said they had tried the drug at least once.[102]

Although they continue to represent the majority of consumers, cannabis use is no longer the primary preserve of the young. More than five million Australians aged 14 and over have used cannabis, but the numbers of regular users over the age of 40 now outnumber those in the 14–19 age group.[103] Clearly a significant number have continued to use the drug into middle age, but some of those aged 50 and over who never turned on in the 1960s and 1970s are now turning to cannabis for strictly medical rather than recreational purposes. A study conducted by the University of New South Wales and reported in October 2005 showed that older Australians were regularly using cannabis in preference to prescribed medication for the relief of pain associated with arthritis and multiple sclerosis, as well as for depression and nausea. One of the participants in the study took up smoking cannabis at the age of 70 and had been using the drug for two years because it was far superior to the painkillers she had been prescribed.[104]

The lack of research into the medical use of cannabis is one of the major tragedies of its prohibition. The research that has been done, particularly since the 1990s, shows that there is scientific evidence of sufficient rigour to support the therapeutic use of cannabis to treat both nausea and vomiting associated with cancer chemotherapy and loss of appetite and wasting syndrome in AIDS. There is further evidence, both scientific and anecdotal, to indicate the therapeutic potential of cannabis for the general relief of pain and in the treatment of multiple sclerosis, spasticity, spinal cord injury, glaucoma, migraine and epilepsy.[105] The argument that the pharmaceutical industry already produces THC products that can satisfy these areas of medical need is unconvincing. The two THC products that the industry has developed, dronabinol (THC in a sesame oil suspension) and nabilone (synthetic THC) are in capsule form and, according to patients, not as effective as smoked cannabis.[106] This in itself, given the lung problems associated with the smoking of any substance, points to the pressing need for research on more efficient and effective delivery methods. Saying that the pharmaceutical industry has developed products that can treat all the conditions for which cannabis is or could be useful is no more reason to prohibit cannabis than the efficacy of cannabis is reason to prohibit the pharmaceutical products.

In contrast to the lack of medical research, there have been a significant number of inquiries into the recreational use of cannabis, starting with the Indian Hemp Drugs Commission in 1893, which was prompted by concern in Britain about the effects that consumption might have 'on the social and moral condition' of the peoples of India. Among the more prominent of the inquiries that followed were the La Guardia Report of 1944, commissioned by the mayor of New York, the Wootton Report in England in 1968, the La Dain Report in Canada in 1970 and the Shafer Commission Report in the United States in 1972.

The Indian Hemp Commission found that the use of bhang was almost universally harmless, and was in some cases beneficial when taken in moderation. Even when abused it was less harmful than alcohol. The La Guardia Report found that prolonged use of marijuana didn't lead to 'physical, mental or moral degeneration'. The Wootton Report concluded that the dangers of the drug were overstated and recommended a relaxation of the laws covering personal use. Both the Shafer and La Dain Reports came to the view that there were no grounds to justify prohibition of cannabis for personal use. With the exception of India, where the status quo on cannabis use was maintained, the findings of all these inquiries were pilloried by parliamentarians and press alike. Hysteria and political self-interest easily trumped science. When, in late 1995, the British medical journal *The Lancet* declared in an editorial that 'the smoking of cannabis, even long term, is not harmful to health', it too was largely ignored.[107]

Australia's contribution to the inquiry process was a Senate Standing Committee Report in 1977 called 'Drug problems in Australia — an intoxicated society?'. The committee reviewed the international studies on cannabis as well as three Australian studies. It noted that a senate select committee in 1971 had recommended that the Australian government should initiate action at the international level to transfer cannabis and its derivates from the narcotics schedule of the 1961 Single Convention on Narcotic Drugs to a more appropriate schedule in the Convention on Psychotropic Substances, and further recommended that this initiative be pursued as a matter of urgency. After observing that 'supply will always match demand, as the history of all attempts at prohibition plainly illustrates', it concluded that cannabis possession and cultivation should not be defined in law as a crime, but should be discouraged by the imposition of a fine. In the year following the report more than 14,000 people were charged with cannabis offences; three years later the number had almost doubled.

Opponents of cannabis often point to the deleterious effect that the drug is supposed to have on mental health, and cite the Swedish study of Andreasson and others that appeared in *The Lancet* in 1987. It's an old claim, one that was used to justify the international prohibition of cannabis in 1925. It was also made in India where, in 1893, the asylums in that country were said to be full of lunatics who owed their condition to the consumption of cannabis. The Indian Hemp Drugs Commission went to every asylum in India and examined the medical records of every inmate who it was claimed was suffering from a cannabis-induced illness and were able to find almost no patients in these institutions whose condition could be said to have been caused by the use of cannabis: 'In the few genuine cases of cannabis-induced psychosis the illness proved to be short-lived and reversible on stopping the use of the drug.'[108] The Swedish study examined the drug-taking habits of 45,570 Swedish army conscripts and tracked their health progress over 15 years. Of the 246 who presented with schizophrenic illness, a disproportionate number were cannabis users, which led to the conclusion that cannabis was an independent risk factor for schizophrenia. However, more than half the cannabis users who developed schizophrenia had also taken amphetamines, drugs of some popularity in Sweden, with links to schizophrenia that have been long known. Other schizophrenia risk factors, such as deprived social backgrounds, were also evident in the cannabis-using group. Importantly, the Swedish study did not prove any cause-and-effect relationship between cannabis use and schizophrenia; such a relationship seemed highly unlikely to most people, according to a detailed review of the epidemiological evidence.[109]

The number of people around the world who have smoked cannabis in the last 40 years is in the hundreds of millions at least. The 2005 World Drug Report put the number of current users at 160 million, so it would be reasonable to expect the epidemiological evidence to show a sharp increase in schizophrenia if its use was linked to cannabis. Reviews have shown that this is not the case,[110] although the results of a study reported in April 2005 linked teenage cannabis smokers and their genetic profile to increased risk of schizophrenia. The study, by the Institute of Psychiatry at King's College London, involved 803 people in Dunedin, New Zealand. It found that of those who inherited a particular variant of a gene known as COMT (about a quarter of the population), up to 15 per cent were likely to develop psychotic conditions if exposed to cannabis in early life. However, neither the drug nor the gene raised the risk of psychosis by itself.

In December 2005 scientists at Melbourne's Monash University reported that a compound in cannabis, cannabidiol, may actually be protective against psychosis. In early 2006, the Mental Health Foundation in the United Kingdom reported the results of scientific studies that linked a number of mental illnesses, including attention-deficit disorder, depression, Alzheimer's disease and schizophrenia, to junk food and the absence of essential fats, vitamins and minerals in people's dietary intake.[111] Taken as a whole, these various studies seem to indicate that anyone diagnosed with or predisposed to psychotic illness might do well to avoid cannabis, along with junk food, amphetamines, cocaine and a whole range of other drugs, both licit and illicit.

Given the encouragement that it deserves, research into the medical use of cannabis has some hopeful prospects following the Canadian decision in 2001 to legalise the drug for medical use and authorise its cultivation for that purpose. The fledgling enterprise has something of a headstart thanks to 20 years of breeding by the illicit growers, who have managed to make cannabis Canada's most valuable agricultural product.[112] However, the Dutch position on self-medication, which dates back to the 1970s and is still often enough referred to as an 'experiment', has taken some time to be respected for its honesty and followed for its effectiveness. In the Netherlands more than 1000 Coffee Shops are licensed to sell small quantities of cannabis, which can either be consumed on the premises or sold as takeaway. Needless to say they do a brisk trade, despite the fact that the consumption of cannabis has never been made legal. Dutch authorities quite deliberately choose not to enforce the law, preferring a process of regulation that is pragmatic rather than punitive. The result, measured simply in terms of consumption, is a lower rate of use than that in the United States.[113]

This more pragmatic approach was followed by Italy and Spain in the 1990s, when the possession of cannabis for personal use was decriminalised. Belgium and Switzerland adopted similar policies in 2001, the year Portugal took the heroic decision to decriminalise the possession of all drugs.[114] A more rational approach to cannabis use is slowly emerging around the globe — almost 70 years after Anslinger launched his 'reefer madness' campaign.

Lysergic acid diethylamide (LSD)

LSD (lysergic acid diethylamide), the much more powerful hallucinogen that, like cannabis, came of age in the 1960s as a recreational drug, owes its origins to the pharmaceutical industry in Switzerland. There in 1918 in the Sandoz laboratory in Basle, Dr Arthur Stoll isolated the alkaloid ergotamine from the cereal fungus ergot.[115]

The acute toxicity of ergot has been known for thousands of years. The hallucinogenic associated with the Eleusinian mysteries of ancient greece is thought to have been made from ergot-infected barley, and the disease which wiped out more than a third of the population of Athens during the Peloponnesian War (431–404 BCE) is also thought to have been ergotism. Poisoning from ergot-infected rye bread killed around 40,000 people in France towards the end of the first millennium. First known as 'holy fire' after the sensation caused by inadequate blood flow, ergotism came to be associated with St Anthony in the 11th century and thereafter was commonly called St Anthony's Fire. It is thought to have been responsible for low fertility and high death rates in Europe between the 14th and 18th centuries, and as recently as 1951 an outbreak of the disease in France killed several people.[116] In medicine, ergot use has been known from the 16th century to induce uterine contractions and control bleeding after childbirth.[117] In 1938, in the course of investigating other possible medical uses of ergotamine, a protégé of Stoll's working in the Basle laboratory, Dr Albert Hoffman, synthesised a number of compounds based on the alkaloid. The twenty-fifth in a series he was working on, labelled lysergic acid diethylamide-25, was duly catalogued and filed after some limited laboratory tests on animals failed to reveal anything of immediate promise.

Five years later, on 16 April 1943, Hoffman was again working on LSD-25 when he felt a little queasy, knocked off early and took himself home to bed. What happened next is the first account of an 'acid' experience: 'As I lay in a dazed condition with eyes closed there surged up from me a succession of fantastic, rapidly changing imagery of a striking reality and depth, alternating with a vivid, kaleidoscopic play of colours. This condition gradually passed off after about three hours.'[118]

When he recovered from his discombobulated state, Hoffmann realised that he had come across a drug of powerful proportions. He had accidentally absorbed the tiniest amount through his fingertips and life suddenly presented itself in technicolour. So in the heroic tradition of self-experimentation, he decided that the only thing to do was to draw a deep breath and repeat the experience. This he dutifully did three days later, when he took a careful dose of 250 micrograms, just 250 millionths of a gram. The result was a full-on trip that thankfully went from bad to better and included an out-of-body experience.[119]

Such a mind-altering substance clearly had potential in neurological research and psychiatry. It was the son of Arthur Stoll, Dr Werner Stoll, who first alerted the wider scientific and medical community to LSD, with papers that were published in the Swiss Archives of Neurology in 1947 and 1949. Sandoz marketed LSD under the brand name Delysid, and was initially prepared to make it freely available to researchers around the world on the condition that they in turn made all their research material available to Sandoz.[120]

By now World War II had given way to the Cold War, and one organisation anxious to take up the Sandoz offer without fulfilling the obligation that went with it was the

United States' Central Intelligence Agency (CIA). In a 1950 internal memorandum headed 'An Analysis of Confessions in Russian Trials', CIA analysts contended that the confessions of Stalin's purge trials in the 1930s and that of Cardinal Mindszenty in Hungary in 1949 were inexplicable unless the minds of the confessees had been reorganised and reoriented by methods other than physical torture. The newer or more subtle techniques that they considered might have led to the confessions included: various methods of psychoanalysis, some of which involved drugs; psychosurgery which separated the frontal lobes of the brain; electric shocks; and the use of drugs including cannabis, insulin and cocaine.[121] This analysis — that the Soviet Union was likely to be using mind-controlling drugs — led to the obvious conclusion that the United States had to establish a research program that would give them the same capacity, then allow them to counteract the Soviet drug program and eventually gain superiority in this new area of psychological warfare. What's more, the need for such research was pressing. The Soviets too were aware of this new drug LSD, and throughout the late 1940s and early 1950s they were reportedly attempting to both buy up the entire Sandoz supply and establish their own production capacity.[122]

The US effort came together in a CIA project known as MK-ULTRA. It was authorised by the director of the CIA, Allen Dulles, in April 1953 and would eventually embrace 149 sub-projects in behavioural modification, toxins and drugs.[123] Some of the research was decidedly amateurish, with CIA officials responsible for the program testing the drug on themselves and then on other agency members without their knowledge. Trials were carried out on predominantly African-American inmates at Lexington prison hospital, and in one case a group of seven men were given LSD continuously for 11 weeks.[124] In order to test the drug on unsuspecting members of the public, the CIA turned to the FBN agent who had organised similar trials with cannabis under Harry Anslinger's instructions in the 1940s. With Anslinger's blessing, George Hunter White now turned his attention to LSD.

Setting up shop in Greenwich Village in New York, White's strategy was to invite people back to his flat, slip them a mickey finn of LSD, take notes about their reaction and send the results back to HQ. In 1955 the operation was transferred to San Francisco, where it became decidedly more voyeuristic. Drug-addicted San Francisco prostitutes were paid by the CIA to bring their clients back to a brothel that the CIA had set up. When the unsuspecting clients were relaxed and comfortable they were surreptitiously given drinks laced with LSD and had their subsequent performance appraised by White, who would watch from behind the safety and anonymity of a two-way mirror, sitting on a portable toilet sipping martinis. Displaying a sense of humour, the code name of this project was Operation Midnight Climax. White continued his FBN work chasing illicit drug users during the day while partying at night with fellow CIA agents on hashish and LSD until 1963, and as he himself would say, 'Where else could a red-blooded American boy lie, kill, cheat, steal, rape and pillage with the sanction of the All-Highest?'

Certainly not in the US Army Chemical Corps, although they were good enough to assist with their own modest contribution to the CIA's acid research, managing to find 1500 army volunteers glad of the opportunity to serve in such a noble cause. It was these army scientists who were the first to use the word 'trip' to describe the LSD experience.[125]

Soon after MK-ULTRA began it became obvious that there were problems with supply. Sandoz had a monopoly on LSD production and they manufactured the drug in milligram quantities. The fact that they agreed to keep the CIA informed of production levels, the identity of buyers and any intelligence that they were receiving from the Soviet side couldn't disguise the equally important fact that they were, after all, a foreign company. The patriotic solution was to get an American company, Eli Lilly, to produce it instead, setting a precedent with patent and intellectual property rights that others would not be encouraged to follow. By the middle of 1954, Eli Lilly had the capacity to manufacture LSD, and they advised the CIA that they would shortly be able to supply the drug by the ton rather than the milligram.[126]

Outside of the CIA and the US military, the broader medical profession was also keen to explore the possibilities of this new drug. Psychiatrists developed two methods of LSD therapy, one on each side of the Atlantic. In England and parts of Europe, low-dose or psycholytic (mind-loosening) therapy was used in conjunction with more traditional forms of treatment such as psychoanalysis. In the United States and Canada, high-dose psychedelic therapy was a sort of chemical shock treatment aimed at inducing a mystical or conversion experience. The state of altered consciousness that these high doses of LSD brought about was thought to assist the healing process of patients with deep-seated psychological problems.[127]

The therapeutic value of LSD is a contentious issue. Hoffmann tends to the view that the adverse reaction to its widespread recreational use meant that it was never really given the chance it deserved. Its indiscriminate use in high doses didn't help either, and while it undoubtedly helped some patients, the celebrities Cary Grant, Jack Nicholson, James Coburn and Andre Previn prominent among them, an unacceptable number had 'bad trips'. The high number of patients who became psychotic as a result of being prescribed the drug justified its withdrawal so that a more sober and considered approach could be taken to any further clinical trials.[128] But it wasn't the adverse reactions of patients that led to its withdrawal, and Hoffmann was certainly correct about the adverse reaction by authorities to its recreational use.

In California in the mid-1950s, a small and privileged group of scientists and writers, including Aldous Huxley, were using LSD recreationally. Huxley was introduced to LSD by the original acid guru, Captain Alfred M Hubbard. Colourful is a very inadequate description of Hubbard. An officer in the OSS, the intelligence organisation that was the forerunner to the CIA, he made his name, and lots of top-level friends, with swashbuckling exploits in World War II. He then made a fortune in the uranium business, settling in Vancouver, where he became head of the Vancouver Uranium Corporation. Turned on to acid in 1951, he thought it a mystical experience and spent the rest of his life, and a large amount of his money, trying to convert everyone else. He claimed to have bought 6000 bottles of LSD and then to have given them away to thousands of people the world over.[129]

Aldous Huxley took mescaline, another hallucinogen, under the supervision of Dr Humphry Osmond, a psychiatrist working with mescaline and LSD in Canada, and wrote about the experience in his book *The Doors of Perception* (1954), which takes its title from *The Marriage of Heaven and Hell* by the English poet and mystic William Blake (1757–1827).[130] He later took LSD in the company of Hubbard and again wrote about the experience in *Heaven and Hell* (1956). Thereafter both he and Osmond thought that a new name should be given to the unique LSD experience. Huxley proposed 'phanerothyme' but Osmond's 'psychedelic' (mind-manifesting) was preferred.[131]

Harvard academics Timothy Leary and Richard Alpert were also acid pioneers from the early 1960s, although Alpert is little remembered and Leary's legacy is likely to rest on the phrase 'turn on, tune in, and drop out'. There is no doubt, though, that Leary in particular was hounded by the establishment. He was sentenced to a total of 20 years' imprisonment for cannabis possession and another five years for escaping, although he only served about two years before being paroled for good behaviour after collaborating with the FBI. Perhaps Leary was singled out because he was such an establishment figure doing such an anti-establishment thing. He was hardly 'the most dangerous man in America', as President Nixon called him, although he did manage to do some considerable harm to those who helped him escape from prison when he informed on them.[132]

Early acid advocates Ken Kesey and Alan Ginsberg were much more dangerous to the established order. Both took LSD for the first time courtesy of government research programs. Kesey was paid US$75 a day to take acid at the Menlo Park Veterans' Hospital in 1960 as part of the MK-ULTRA program. Thereafter he worked in the hospital's psychiatric ward where he got the material for his first novel, *One Flew Over the Cuckoo's Nest*. Ginsberg was given LSD in an experiment conducted at the Mental Research Institute in Palo Alto, California in 1959.[133] Kesey went on to tour the United States in a psychedelic bus with his band of Merry Pranksters, inviting people to take the 'Acid Test'. Ginsberg went on to become one of the leading organisers of radical anti-Vietnam War protests. Both were in-your-face, anarchic challengers of authority.

By any measure there was certainly a lot going on in the United States in the 1960s. President J F Kennedy was assassinated. His brother Robert became the favourite to move into the White House just a few years later, but he too was assassinated. Martin Luther King Jnr met the same fate, and so did Malcolm X. Forty-six people were killed and more than 20,000 were arrested across hundreds of American cities in the riots that followed King's assassination and it took 55,000 troops and National Guards to restore order. There were riots and clashes on university campuses and massive, violent street protests against the Vietnam War, which eventually led to the political demise of President L B Johnson. There were sit-ins, be-ins and love-ins, plus a distinctive style of music and a distinctive style of dress. It was very much a young person's decade: *Time* magazine's Man of the Year in 1967 was 'anyone under twenty-five'.[134]

This social upheaval wasn't confined to the United States. Paris erupted in 1968, and so did Prague. Sixties music influenced by acid (as well as cannabis) politicised young people all over the world. There were anti-Vietnam War demonstrations in London, and in Australia there were the beginnings of what would shortly be the biggest mass protest movement the country had ever seen. But events in the United States were really at the forefront. The protest movement there was led by those associated with the hippie counterculture and the 'new left', and it was acid and cannabis that brought them together. Marxism was by now 'the opiate of the unstoned classes', and if smoking cannabis was joining the revolution, dropping acid was making it. It's estimated that four million people turned on to LSD in the United States in the 1960s; 70 per cent of them were of high school or college age and many had at least some involvement in radical politics — during the early months of 1969, one-third of the country's students were involved in demonstrations across some 300 colleges and universities. [135] Acid anarchists were everywhere: the San Francisco Diggers; the Up Against the Wall Motherfucker Collective, with their acid-armed consciousness manifesto; the Weathermen, who were responsible for Timothy Leary's escape from prison; the Yippies (Youth International Party); the Jesse James Gang; and the White Panthers. Nothing was sacred. Psychedelic religions were established, such as the Neo-American Boohoo Church, whose members used LSD as a sacrament. The Students for a Democratic Society radicalised students across the nation, the Gay Liberation Front was established, and although it was still very much a male-dominated world, the women's liberation movement was taking shape.

Some images of the era are enduring: the crowd of 75,000 anti-war demonstrators that surrounded the Pentagon in

October 1967, sticking daisies down the gun barrels of guarding soldiers and proclaiming that 'Che lives'; the indiscriminate violence meted out to both protesters and onlookers alike at the Democratic National Convention in Chicago in August 1968; the Monterey and Woodstock music festivals. But perhaps the most symbolic gathering was the Human Be-In at Golden Gate Park, San Francisco on 14 January 1967, where 25,000 people celebrated peace and love and LSD and looked forward to the coming summer of love. Unfortunately it all started to turn sour in that Haight-Ashbury summer. There were too many people, too many amphetamines, too much harassment and too much exploitation. By the time the cannabis drought and abundant speed supply had helped ruin the summer, LSD had already been banned in California — in October 1966.[136]

More than anything else, it was the Vietnam War that brought hippies and the left together. Napalming children in Southeast Asia couldn't possibly represent the future. It was unjustified, unconscionable, and it had to be opposed; everyone had to oppose it. And large numbers did, in a grand coalition where LSD was synonymous with peace. But the coalition was over before the war was.

The hippie movement that was such an important part of the coalition came from the San Francisco beats who had moved to the Haight-Ashbury district in the early 1960s. They were now pejoratively called 'beatniks' — a breed of youth that was more middle class and less degenerate than the original beats and whose drug of choice was cannabis — by the press, which considered them subversive, and as threatening as Soviet sputniks. 'Hip', a slang word from the days of opium smoking, was also used to describe African-Americans who were wise enough to abandon the cotton fields of the south for the cities of the north. In beat parlance, to be in the know was to be 'hip', which was turned pejoratively into 'hippie' by Herb Caen, a journalist at the *San Francisco Chronicle*.[137] After the Haight-

Ashbury summer, the revolutionary version of the new world order didn't seem very different from the existing order as far as the hippies were concerned. They eventually left to construct an alternative on the periphery, where cannabis was easier to grow.

One group in 1960s America that didn't take to LSD in a big way was African-Americans. In ways that we now forget unless reminded by a hurricane, America in the 1960s was strictly racially segregated. And it was in the 1960s that African-American resistance confronted white oppression in a series of violent clashes. In the Watts district of Los Angeles in August 1965, African-American resentment over poor housing and education opportunities, police violence and unemployment finally erupted. In the riots that followed, 34 were killed, more than 1000 were injured and nearly 4000 were arrested. It took 16,000 police and National Guards to restore an uneasy peace. Ronald Reagan was elected Governor of California the following year by an electorate that blamed the increased civil rights of African-Americans for the violence.

Six months before the Watts riots, Malcolm X, the 'black shining prince of African-American manhood' was shot dead in Harlem. His body was riddled with more than 20 bullets, just to make sure. Malcolm X was the first prominent African-American leader to speak out against the Vietnam War. He highlighted the fact that it was a war waged by white America but fought by African-Americans. In 1965–66 the casualty rate for African-Americans was double that of whites, and in 1967, while 64 per cent of eligible African-Americans were drafted into the war, only 31 per cent of eligible whites were.[138] It was much easier for whites to avoid the draft by being at college and then joining the reserve. George W Bush did exactly that. He avoided Vietnam: family influence allowed him to leapfrog into the Texas Air National Guard.[139]

In 1967, just four months before the Human Be-In at the Golden Gate Park, it took 12,000 Californian National

Guards to quell the riots in the African-American areas of San Francisco. A curfew was imposed, more than 350 were arrested and 51 were injured. African-Americans didn't live in Haight-Ashbury because residential racial segregation confined them to the Bayview-Hunter's Point neighbourhood and the Fillmore district. What was for some intended as a summer of peace and love was for others a long year of violent confrontation: there were African-American uprisings in 128 US cities in the first nine months of 1967.

Martin Luther King Jnr, in what was surely one of the most moving speeches ever given in English, 'had a dream' that one day his four little children would be judged by the content of their character and not the colour of their skin. In September 1963, less than three weeks after he delivered that speech, four young girls were murdered when the Sixteenth Street Baptist Church in Birmingham, Alabama where they were worshipping was blown up by white supremacists. It wasn't until May 2002 that the last surviving perpetrator of that bombing was brought to justice. The answer to this massive and escalating assault wasn't to be found in LSD or flower power; it was to be found in an organisation set up in October 1966 by Huey P Newton and Bobby Seale, called the Black Panther Party for Self-Defense.

The Black Panthers organised within African-American communities, and as well as providing armed self-defence, they also provided services such as free medical centres, free legal centres and free breakfasts for school children. At its peak the party had 45 chapters and branch organisations throughout the country and its newspaper had a circulation of a quarter of a million. There were already many diverse African-American organisations ranging across the political spectrum, of course, but it was only the Panthers and other radical groups, such as the League of Revolutionary Black Workers in the auto plants in Detroit, that were prepared to meet violence with violence.

The prospect of an armed, organised, revolutionary African-American working class was altogether too threatening. It was also a bad example. Puerto Ricans, Mexican-Americans, Native Americans and the Untouchable caste in India were among those who followed the Panthers' lead. Bobby Seale, Huey Newton and Angela Davis were all eventually jailed — on trumped-up charges. The Panthers were harassed, infiltrated, destabilised, intimidated, arrested, incarcerated and assassinated. In 1969 alone 27 Panthers were killed and 749 jailed. By the 1970s they were in decline and by the early 1980s they had ceased to function; this was when crack cocaine became the drug destabilising the ghettoes.[140]

By the early 1960s the pharmaceutical companies had added Valium to the amphetamines, analgesics and barbiturates that were available as chemical companions to modern living. 'Better living through chemistry' could well have been the description of what they had to offer. But it wasn't. It was the slogan that both justified and celebrated LSD. The contested terrain between the acid pioneers and the pharmaceutical industry was freedom of drug choice. The view expressed by Clare Booth Luce (who, with her husband Henry Luce, president of *Time-Life*, had turned on to LSD in the late 1950s and early 1960s) — that acid should be restricted to the middle classes because you couldn't have 'everyone doing too much of a good thing' — clearly had significant support.[141] As early as 1962, long before LSD was made illegal in the United States, underground chemists were manufacturing acid in direct competition with the drug companies. Initially, at least, they were motivated as much by turning people on as by turning a profit.

The improbably named Augustus Owsley Stanley III and his assistants first produced their underground acid in early 1965. They went on to produce enough for four million trips in California in the mid-1960s. Principally distributed in Haight-Ashbury, when it wasn't given away it sold at US$2 for a 250 microgram tablet; this was stiff competition in the marketplace ... until Owsley was arrested in late 1967. The Brotherhood of Eternal Love, a psychedelic church set up on the advice of Timothy Leary, distributed 10 million trips of the famous 'orange sunshine' acid, which was manufactured by two underground chemists in less than six months in California in 1969 and found its way all around the world. The Brotherhood also helped distribute the 50 million trips made by Ronald Hadley Stark, who recognised the international dimension of the LSD market when he set up acid labs in Paris and Brussels in the early 1970s.[142]

Stark was not an acid guru into love and peace and pretty flowers; he was a businessman plain and simple. He sold LSD because it was profitable. He sold cocaine for the same reason, and his arrival on the drug-making scene was indicative of how it was changing. He was a conman who managed to convince the Brotherhood that he'd invented a new way of making acid. He also managed to convince them to entrust their considerable investments to his care. When the Brotherhood's network was broken up by the authorities in the early 1970s, they found that most of the money and property the Brotherhood had accumulated was in Stark's name.

A cheap and easy way of making good-quality acid had, in fact, been discovered in 1970 by Stark's one-time assistant, a British chemist named Richard Kemp. Setting up shop on his own account in the United Kingdom, Kemp's exported acid accounted for half the world's total supply by the mid-1970s. By 1977 the Vietnam War had been over for two years and the era of radical politics was well and truly over in the United States and elsewhere. Kemp was arrested that year, and the era of those who produced and distributed LSD for radical political purposes also came to an end.[143]

Australia had its own anti-war movement and Nimbin, the site of Australia's somewhat belated Woodstock, the festival of

Aquarius in 1973, became a centre of counterculture lifestyle. LSD was a part of the scene just as it was in the United States, and even though the student newspaper *Honi Soit* published a recipe for making acid, Australia's supply in the 1960s and 1970s came mostly from California, just as it does today.[144] More than one million Australians have used hallucinogens during their lives, mostly LSD, and more than 175,000 use them each year. They rank not far below cannabis and amphetamines as Australia's most frequently used illicit drugs and are particularly popular with young people and high school students.[145] What has changed these days is the dosage. Oswald's acid, typical of the times, came in 250 microgram lots. Today it's more likely to be 100 micrograms (which suggests a sensible market adjustment) and to cost around $20 a tab, which is well within the occasional budget of most ... but, like today's politics, it's a different experience from the 1960s.[146]

Ecstasy: 3, 4 methlylenedioxymethylamphetamine (MDMA)

If LSD was associated with social upheaval, ecstasy, its popular successor, was firmly associated with apolitical hedonism. From the late 1970s it became popular with 'clubbers' in the United States out for their version of a good time, which centred on hours of frenetic dancing to music of such rhythmic intensity that it almost demanded chemical assistance. During the following decade and beyond, the combination caught on in lots of other places around the world.

Ecstasy is structurally similar to both amphetamine and mescaline, and combines some of the properties of both drugs, which is why it is often referred to as a hallucinogenic stimulant or a psychedelic amphetamine.[147] Yet another product of the German pharmaceutical industry, it was first synthesised in the

Darmstadt laboratories of Merck in 1912, but thereafter seems to have remained in the laboratory for want of commercial application.[148]

Nearly 40 years after it was first synthesised, the US Army began experimenting with it at the Edgewood Chemical Warfare facility in Maryland and at the University of Michigan in the early 1950s. Carried out at the request of the CIA as part of the search for greater truth through chemistry, the experiments appear to have been limited to animals. Showing little promise, they were discontinued in favour of LSD by 1953.[149]

The drug once again returned to the laboratory shelves until the 1960s, when Dr Alexander Shulgin, a US biochemist with an uncommon interest in psychoactive drugs, began his experiments with it. Born in Russia, Shulgin served in the US Navy during World War II, gained his doctorate in biochemistry at the University of California in 1945, and thereafter worked as a research chemist for the Dow Chemical Company. Although he worked on successful commercial projects for Dow, most notably inventing the first biodegradable insecticide, Zectran, Shulgin's preference for research into psychedelics (he began with mescaline) led to a mutual parting of ways in 1965, at which point he set up his own laboratory at his home in Berkeley. Shulgin invented a number of psychedelics and undertook groundbreaking research into two classes of mind-altering drugs: phenethylamines (MDMA belongs in this group) and tryptamines (the psilocybin mushroom belongs in this one). Together with his wife Ann, he wrote two books that detailed their work: *PiKHAL: A Chemical Love Story*, published in 1991, and *TiKHAL: The Continuation*, published in 1997. Both titles are acronyms for phenethylamines and tryptamines 'I have known and loved' and reflect the fact that, in the heroic tradition, the Shulgins' experiments were carried out on themselves.[150]

Shulgin's early work on MDMA led to its use by hundreds of US psychotherapists, starting in the mid-1970s, on patients who were suffering from conditions such as anxiety, trauma and depression. Its most obvious therapeutical benefit was to facilitate open and honest communication between doctor and patient, enabling specific problems and their causes to be better identified and treated. It was then thought that the cathartic nature of this experience meant that it could be practised without the drug and extended to other significant relationships that the patient had in order to resolve existing and future conflicts. It was in this medical setting that some 500,000 doses were administered in the United States between 1977 and 1985.[151]

While it was being administered by psychotherapists to thousands of patients in the United States, it was being self-administered by many more thousands of people for its pleasurable effects. In fact recreational use, first identified by US authorities in 1972, predated its use in medical practice by several years. And as it became more common in medical practice, MDMA also became much more prominent as a recreational drug — known as E, X or XTC before 'ecstasy' was settled on. Produced by some of the same chemists who had manufactured LSD in the 1960s, consumption rose from 10,000 doses a year in 1976 to as many as two million doses a month in 1984.[152] By the late 1970s ecstasy was a part of the club scene in New York, where the dance music that accompanied it was known as house (from a venue in Chicago called the Warehouse).[153] At this point ecstasy was a perfectly legal drug, but as its use within the club culture spread from New York and hit Texas it ran into trouble.

A letter to the editors of the *American Druggist* in 1894 is the earliest reporting of recreational cocaine use in the United States. The city at which this dangerous habit was spreading was Dallas, Texas and the drug was held to have a special appeal to African-Americans and others among the 'lower orders'.[154] In 1984 the drug that was spreading through Dallas and capturing the headlines was ecstasy, and its special appeal was not to the lower classes or African-Americans but to those patrons of establishments like the Starck Club, where it could be bought over the bar for US$15 plus tax to complement a fun night out. When the pampered sons and daughters of oil-rich Texan society began copying the clubbers and consuming ecstasy, they did so in the same way that they consumed alcohol. They added binge ecstasy-taking to their binge drinking, and according to one contemporary observer, it was their behaviour that hastened the drug's prohibition. These were 'politicians' kids. Their parents were all friends with George Bush (then vice president of the United States), for God's sake. They were the death knell for legal ecstasy, those kids.'[155]

And so it proved. In July 1984 the US Drug Enforcement Administration (DEA) initiated proceedings to prohibit ecstasy, to take effect the following year. In the 12-month period before its complete prohibition, the sale of the drug was illegal but its possession was not. During that year there were stores in Dallas where you could buy a plastic disposable pen for US$25 that came with a 'free' ecstasy pill.[156]

Making ecstasy illegal only increased its consumption in the United States, and its notoriety and subsequent popularity elsewhere. By this time it was being exported to Britain, where it had been illegal since 1977. In early 1987 it was becoming popular in London nightclubs and in the summer of that year young British holidaymakers in Ibiza were dancing the night away on ecstasy. In London in the following year there weren't enough nightclubs to accommodate all those who wanted the ecstasy and Acid House experience, so the 'rave' filled the market gap. Inventive entrepreneurs hired or simply took over disused warehouses and even aircraft hangars where patrons could party from Saturday night to Sunday afternoon with a steady supply of ecstasy to hand. Demand was such that the rave had to head outdoors, to huge open spaces in the countryside where 10,000 might gather at locations kept secret until near opening time — the organising capacity of mobile phone technology was essential to this. A new squad of police, the Pay Party Unit, was formed to respond, and in 1990 it became a criminal offence in Britain, punishable by a 6-month jail term, to organise an illegal party.[157]

After swallowing a typical ecstasy pill (75–125 milligrams), the desired ecstasy experience will normally come on within 20 minutes, with a 'rush' that might be accompanied by nausea. This peak 'coming-up' is followed by a plateau period which lasts from two to five hours, and a come-down which can last a day or longer.[158] Euphoria is complemented by a loss of inhibitions and a heightened sense of touch and empathy with others, which has led to it being labelled a 'love-drug'. Reports of it being an aphrodisiac, though, seem unfounded. Male users often complain that while it makes you want to cuddle up it's often difficult to get it up. It also increases blood pressure and heart rate, causes jaw clenching, teeth grinding and dryness in the mouth, and can lead to tiredness and depression. More importantly, it can lead to hyperthermia (overheating), which can be exacerbated by frenzied dancing activity over many hours, and hyponatraemia (low blood sodium concentration), which can lead to brain-swelling and coma.[159] These latter conditions have led to a number of deaths which, in turn, have led to lurid headlines about 'killer ecstasy'. These have had little effect on those who use the drug, but they tend to provoke a reaction akin to panic in those who don't. As the *New Scientist* pointed out several years ago, panic is hardly a substitute for an honest assessment of the risks associated with the drug's use.[160]

There are about eight million ecstasy consumers around the globe according to the 2005 World Drug Report, and between them they are currently managing to get through something like 92 tonnes of the drug each year. Almost two-thirds of consumers are in the United States and western and central

Europe, but Australia, where the drug became illegal in 1987, has more consumers on a per capita basis than anywhere else.[161] More than 1.25 million Australians have used the drug, with 500,000 doing so on a regular basis. The cost of an 'eckie' pill has come down in recent years to $35 in most places, and the number of consumers increased by more than 100,000 between 2001 and 2004.[162]

Despite the fact that the drug is often adulterated, consumers keep coming back for more. For many young people, at least, it seems to be connected with the idea of having a rollicking good time on the weekend. This impulse is hardly new. As Engels observed of the English working class in the early 1840s, 'On Saturday evenings, especially when wages are paid and work stops somewhat earlier than usual, when the whole working class pours from its own poor quarters into the main thoroughfares, intemperance may be seen in all its brutality.'[163] So if a little pill named ecstasy provides the promise of a short but happy release from the brutality of everyday life, it's not surprising that it has plenty of takers.

6
Opium and the masses

Opium and its derivatives, morphine and heroin, have undisputed claim to predominance in the history of drugs. It is a history that stretches back to the shores of the Mediterranean 10,000 years ago.[1] Opium was the ancient world's miracle drug, indispensable because of its capacity to relieve pain at a time when life expectancy was short and suffering was a daily hazard difficult to avoid. As the medicinal use of opium increased and it spread around the globe, it came to be used recreationally; this led to increased production and marketing. For those who controlled supply, this had the beneficial effect of increasing profit. The use of opium made a few people rich and many more ultimately miserable. Opium revenues were to sustain colonial states. Wars were fought over it, and according to one account, the British Empire would probably not have existed without it.[2] Certainly the licit/illicit division of drugs originates with opium.

There are more than 250 different species of the poppy plant, but *Papaver somniferum*, a species classified by Linnaeus in 1753, is one of only two species that produces opium, and is the only one commercially exploited for this purpose.[3]

The Sumerian civilisation in Mesopotamia cultivated opium — and has claims to the invention of writing. In what is probably the first written evidence of opium use, Sumerian ideograms of around 4000 BCE refer to opium as the 'plant of joy'.[4] Knowledge of opium spread from the Sumerians to the Egyptians, and from Egypt, opium found its way to Greece and Rome. Arab traders took opium to North Africa, Persia, India and China, establishing an international trade that was later carried on by the Venetians and the Portuguese.[5] Homer's *Odyssey* contains references to opium, as do the works of the Roman poet Virgil, and later Chaucer and Shakespeare.[6] By the end of the 15th century there was a body of writing on the use of opium dating back more than 3000 years. Among others, Arab, Greek, Roman and Chinese physicians and scholars had all made significant contributions to it.[7]

By the early 16th century, the German physician Paracelsus (a much more succinct title than his full name, Philippus Aureolis Theophrastus Bombast von Hohenheim) became renowned for the curative powers of his 'stones of immortality', an opium concoction otherwise known as laudanum.[8] In the 1660s the English physician Thomas Sydenham developed a tincture of opium; it was this preparation, also known as laudanum, which was increasingly used from the 18th century. It was also in the 18th century that several important works on the medical use of opium were published in England. Some of these were translated and subsequently published in a number of other European countries.[9]

All of this further popularised opium, and it came to be used in a variety of ways for a variety of complaints. Cholera and dysentery were two of the more common diseases of the time that were treated with opium. Self-medication extended its use for the amelioration of symptoms associated with coughs, colds, rheumatism, diarrhoea, and aches and pains of any description (such as earache and toothache). Its general use as a remedy for fatigue, depression and sleeplessness was complemented by its use for 'hysteria' and 'women's ailments'.[10] Opium was tried and trusted because it had a capacity for relieving pain that no other drug could match. Its popularity was assisted by the fact that it was readily available and relatively affordable. There was hardly any alternative at the time; it was, as might be said today, the only game in town.

The dangers of opium use were well known to those earlier physicians and scholars who had written about the drug from their experience of administering it and observing its effects. The propensity of users to demand progressively larger amounts was well recognised as was its poisonous nature if taken in too large a dose. Addiction was a problem that demanded attention, but it was only in the latter half of the 19th century that the use of opium came to be regarded as morally reprehensible and subject to reproach. Even then it was as much to do with who the users were as with what they were using.

The opium poppy doesn't seem to be too difficult to grow, as sightings in suburban gardens around the country attest, but optimum conditions are to be found in temperate climates with low humidity, light rainfall in the early growing period and long hours of sunlight.[11] The areas known as the Golden Triangle (encompassing Burma, Thailand and Laos) and the Golden Crescent (the mountain areas of Iran, Afghanistan and Pakistan) produce most of the world's opium today, but it is also grown in Turkey, Lebanon, Mexico, China, Colombia and India. Tasmania has produced commercial quantities of licit opium from poppy straw since 1970. It is, in fact, the world's largest producer of opium alkaloids for the pharmaceutical industry, supplying around 40 per cent of the world market.[12]

The use of opium for non-medical reasons — for recreational use — is probably as old as its medicinal use. Given its availability and the prevalence of self-medication, recreational use could easily have been confused with medicinal use in the early days; however, the danger of poisoning is likely to have somewhat militated against its becoming a pervasive practice.

Certainly recreational use of opium in producing countries such as Turkey and Iran was known of and written about by European travellers in the 16th century.[13] In India its non-medicinal use varied by region and class. The Hindu soldier caste used it as a paregoric before hostilities, whereas in central India the labouring classes used it as an aid to toil. In the Mogul Empire it was the preserve of the aristocracy, who used it purely for pleasure.[14]

When used recreationally at this time, opium was simply eaten (or taken as a drink). The Chinese were to perfect a much more efficient method of ingestion — smoking — which, with the considerate assistance of the British merchant class and the East India Company in particular, eventually led to mass addiction on a scale not seen before or since.

Portuguese and Dutch traders introduced tobacco to China, and the Spanish were also involved with its importation early in the 17th century,[15] in yet another example of the Columbian exchange. The practice of smoking tobacco with opium appears to have begun with Dutch sailors during the middle of the century as a supposed antidote to malaria, and seems likely to have reached Chinese coastal ports from Formosa (now Taiwan),[16] although some accounts record Chinese in Indonesia smoking opium with tobacco as early as 1617.[17]

Chinese smokers adapted the tobacco smoking pipe, altered the way in which opium was prepared and eliminated the tobacco.[18] By 1729 the extent of opium smoking was of such concern that an Imperial edict was issued banning the practice and prohibiting the sale of opium except under special licence for medical purposes.[19]

The opium used in China came from India, supplied first by the Portuguese and then by the Dutch. At the end of the 18th century control of the trade was in the hands of the British, and their version of free trade took precedence over mere edicts of the Celestial Empire.[20] For the better part of the next 200 years

China's fortunes were largely determined by British policy in India which, in turn, was dominated by the interests of the East India Company.

On 31 December 1600 a group of merchants who had incorporated themselves into a trading organisation known as Governor and Company of Merchants of London trading into the East Indies were given monopoly rights to the East Indies trade by courtesy of royal charter issued by the reigning monarch, Queen Elizabeth 1. The company came to be known more simply as the East India Company. Its immediate objective was the profit to be made from the spice trade, which had hitherto been the preserve of first the Spanish, then the Portuguese and Dutch traders. The latter, in the face of this new competition, formed the Dutch East India Company two years later.

The Portuguese had been granted a trading port in China in 1557 — Macau — and began exporting opium from their Indian territory (Goa) to Macau in the early 1600s. The East India Company began trading into China in 1678 using the facilities they had been allowed to establish in Macau 12 years earlier.[21]

The establishment of a dominion in India, first envisaged by the East India Company in 1689,[22] proceeded apace in the 18th century, thanks in no small part to Robert Clive and his victory at Plassey in 1757 following the deaths in custody of scores of British subjects in a Calcutta dungeon that came to be known as the Black Hole.[23]

From the outset, the occupation of India by the East India Company was concerned with ensuring a favourable balance of payments, from England's perspective — more money coming in than going out. To this end the company, at the start of its operations, was limited to exporting gold, silver and foreign coin to an annual value of £30,000.[24] The company's mercantilist approach, together with its anomalous administrative system, 'a blended character of merchant and sovereign',[25] meant that it had to both fund a governmental structure and make a profit in its own right — allowing exports of Indian goods into Britain that would tilt the balance of payments in India's favour did not fulfil this requirement. (During the Seven Years' War [1756–63] the East India Company went from a commercial to a military and territorial power in India. Robert Clive commanded the troops of the East India Company and they waged a number of wars which gave them control over Indian territory. To avoid funding government administration in this expanding territory, which would be at the expense of profits, they operated a 'subsidiary system' of 'agreements' with Indian princes whereby the princes were obliged to pay for the company's troops to be stationed in their territory. The question of how a British company could hold territorial sovereignties independent of the Crown was never addressed.)

The China trade in tea and silk presented a similar balance of payments problem. The British demand for tea in particular escalated during the 18th century: they brought in under one million pounds of tea in the 1730s, but around 20 million pounds in 1789.[26] In return, the self-sufficient Chinese wanted only silver, preferably in the form of Spanish dollars.

The solution to this dilemma was as brutal as it was simple. The Indian cotton industry was emasculated so that India went from being a country that exported cotton manufactures to a country that eventually had to import them from Britain.[27] Taxes and duties on salt, tobacco and betel, plus a land tax so precisely calculated as to keep the cultivators in penury, were introduced by Clive to provide the revenue base for India's administration.[28] The export of opium to China provided the basis of company profits as well as reversing the outflow of silver bullion and coin.

The East India Company also ensured that it had a monopoly on the supply of Bengal opium, and the export trade to China went ahead in leaps and bounds. In the 1720s some 15 tons of opium had been exported to China. Fifty years later this had increased to 75 tons and by 1850 it had grown to 3200 tons[29] — so much opium that naval architects had to be pressed into service designing ships that could beat into the monsoon and carry three opium cargoes a year rather than one. They rose to the challenge by producing the famous opium clippers.[30]

It was an altogether efficacious trade insofar as balance of payments in Britain's favour was concerned. In the 1820s Britain's purchase of Chinese tea (£20 million) was more than offset by the goods she sold to India (£24 million), which in turn were offset by the goods, mainly opium, India sold to China (£22 million).[31]

The opium trade was also a corrupt and corrupting trade. In order to addict the Chinese in the pursuit of profit, the populace of India first had to be subdued, and officials of the East India Company were just the people to do it. As Karl Marx observed:

> The monopolies of salt, opium, betel and other commodities were inexhaustible mines of wealth. The officials themselves fixed the price and plundered the unfortunate Hindus at will. The Governor-General took part in this private traffic. His favourites received contracts whereby they, cleverer than the alchemists, made gold out of nothing. Great fortunes sprung up like mushrooms in a day; primitive accumulation proceeded without the advance of even a shilling. The trial of Warren Hastings swarms with such cases. Here is an instance. A contract for opium was given to a certain Sullivan at the moment of his departure on an official mission to a part of India far removed from the opium district. Sullivan sold his contract to one Binn for 40,000 pounds; Binn sold it the same day for 60,000 pounds, and the ultimate purchaser who carried out the contract declared that he still extracted a tremendous profit from it. According to one of the lists laid before Parliament, the Company and its officials obtained 6 million pounds between 1757

and 1766 from the Indians in the form of gifts. Between 1769 and 1770 the English created a famine by buying up all the rice and refusing to sell it again, except at fabulous prices.[32]

There was also the not inconsiderable matter of the legality of the trade to be contended with. The Chinese 1729 Imperial edict banning opium had been renewed with increased penalties in 1796, and in 1799 Emperor Kia King issued a further proclamation prohibiting domestic production and consumption as well as imports.[33] The response of the East India Company was to contract out the transport and sale of its opium in China to 'country ships' — ships owned and operated by individuals or independent shipping companies, not by the East India Company — and the response of the British government was to look the other way. (This turning a blind eye was necessary because any company caught transporting opium ran the risk of being barred from all trading in China. The tea trade in particular was enormously important to the East India Company, and being barred from it would have been catastrophic.) It mattered not that the opium was specifically produced for Chinese consumption; that it was sold by the East India Company on the condition that it be traded in China; that no British ships could trade to China without a company licence; or that the chests of opium bore the East India Company's name (demanded by Chinese importers as a sign of its quality).[34] The company insisted that they weren't in the drug trade. Once they sold the opium at Calcutta they neither owned it nor had a legitimate concern with what any new owners might want to do with their rightfully acquired property. The British government professed 'no knowledge of the existence of any but the legal trade'.[35]

British Prime Minister William Gladstone, who was fond of a drop of laudanum and knew firsthand about addiction from his sister's opium habit, was being altogether too gentle in describing this absurd fiction as 'a miserable equivocation'.[36] Britain was well and truly in the international illicit drug trade, and doing very nicely from it. By 1840 trade with China amounted to one-sixth of the combined revenue of Great Britain and India.[37]

By this time the doctrine of mercantilism had given way to one of 'free trade', and this economic theory was used to provide the intellectual justification for continuation of the opium trade. Adam Smith's *Inquiry into the Nature and Causes of the Wealth of Nations* had been published in 1776 and David Ricardo's *Principles of Political Economy and Taxation* in 1817. Free men were free to contract. In trade there is an entitlement to offer goods for sale but no obligation to buy. Indeed the obligation on those buying is to beware of those selling. On this basis there was a free and fair exchange of goods with certain of the Chinese population. The fact that the exchange involved opium was testimony to the freedom in free trade. If there was a sustainable moral objection to the opium trade it could only be remedied by China: first, China could open up its market of 400 million potential consumers to other, preferably British, exports, and second, it could discourage the opium trade by the imposition of taxes. Unfortunately for the British, the Chinese were unimpressed by this line of argument. Taxing the opium trade meant legalising it, which they resolutely refused to do, and they saw no need to import goods they were able to produce themselves. But in any event, the argument of the British free traders was contradictory, as it used the same set of principles to support both free trade and its direct opposite, a monopoly.

Monopolies are, in the ordinary course of events, so inconsistent with the principles of free trade as to represent their antithesis. When called upon to explain this apparent contradiction by a parliamentary committee of inquiry in 1832, the company were fortunate to have in their employ one James Mill and his son John Stuart Mill. James Mill, who had some years earlier published *The History of British India*, was a committed free-trader who counted the influential philosopher Jeremy Bentham as well as David Ricardo among his friends. His ingenious defence of the opium monopoly was that it wasn't actually carried out for profit but was in fact a revenue-raising tax that had the splendid virtue of being levied on foreigners rather than British subjects! It's difficult to determine what was more extraordinary, the defence itself or the fact that the parliamentary committee adopted it.[38] As Marx pointed out, Indian monopolists were the first preachers of free trade in England but it was a curious form of free trade, with monopoly lying at the bottom of its 'freedom'.[39]

Adam Smith's invisible hand contributed about as much to the general welfare of the desperate and dispossessed in India as it did to those in similar parlous circumstances in Britain. Free trade was nevertheless elevated to a status on a par with nature itself, so that even governments were not at liberty to reject it. This, at least, was the position advanced by the first drug barons, William Jardine and James Matheson, as justification for the first Opium War.

The Opium Wars

The increasing cost of importing the amount of tea needed to help maintain the productivity of Britain's Industrial Revolution, together with the increasing administrative costs of an expanding Indian Empire, were responsible for increasing the amount of opium being illegally trafficked into China. The greed of British merchants also played its part, particularly after the East India Company lost its monopoly rights to the China trade (but not opium production) as a result of the *India Act 1833*.

Between 1820 and 1840 the opium flowing into China increased from 270 tons to more than 2500 tons. Included among the three million addicts in China were large numbers of her armed forces, and the three sons of Emperor Tao Kwong, who were all to die as a result of their addiction.[40]

In these bleak circumstances, the emperor and his advisers were entitled to the view that the spreading addiction had precipitated a crisis, and that it would only get worse if left unattended. They also had to face up to the uncomfortable fact that the opium trade could not have been carried on without the corrupt assistance of local officials in the trading ports.

The decisive step in attempting to bring the trade to an end came with the appointment of Lin Tse-hsu as special commissioner for Canton in 1839. A provincial viceroy above corruption, Lin had devised a comprehensive plan to eradicate both opium smoking and the smuggling operations. Opium stocks would be seized and destroyed and foreign ships would be prohibited from trading in the drug. Chinese officials collaborating in the illegal trade would be severely punished, but in an enlightened move, addicts would receive sympathetic assistance in giving up the habit. The experienced opium merchants had heard most of this before and assumed that it was just another display for show purposes and that it would soon pass, enabling the trade to resume.

This was an incorrect assumption. To be fair to the British, although the trade was overwhelmingly carried out by them (they accounted for more than 80 per cent of it) it wasn't exclusively so: a number of mainly European maritime nations had a small percentage and the Americans had around 10 per cent.[41] Even before the Calcutta auction of 1834, the Americans had established close to a monopoly on the supply of Turkish opium. (Before the 1833 *India Act*, the East India Company had sold its opium by auction at Calcutta to private British merchants, who were the only ones allowed to bid. In 1834 the Americans, and others, were allowed to bid.[42]) The American merchant fleet was the second largest in the world (after Britain's) and even at this point of unprecedented British hegemony, it was clear that the United States was emerging as a rival force.

In March 1839, Lin demanded that the merchants hand over all their opium stocks and undertake to renounce the trade. Refusal to do so would mean expulsion from the legal trade in tea, silk and other commodities. The response of the merchants was to hand over a token amount; they thought this would placate the new commissioner. It did not. He knew full well how much opium they had in their possession and he wanted every grain of it. In May, following a series of incidents, the merchants eventually handed over their stock: more than 20,000 chests of opium.[43]

British representation in China was in the hands of Captain Charles Elliot, who held the office of Chief Superintendent of Trade. When he advised the merchants to surrender their opium he assured them, without authority, that they would be compensated. He also thought that China had to be taught a lesson, given that 'its government has taken the unprovoked initiative in aggressive measures against British life, liberty, and property, and against the dignity of the Crown'.[44]

The foreign secretary, Lord Palmerston, and the prime minister, Lord Melbourne agreed. Palmerston had a decidedly odd view on the rights of sovereign states to enact their own laws. He argued that the Chinese law banning opium was effectively invalid because it had been broken by Chinese nationals and not impartially enforced. To enforce it without warning against the British was therefore unjust.[45]

An expeditionary force was duly put together. It was commanded by Admiral George Elliot, Charles Elliot's cousin, under the supervision of Lord Auckland, governor-general of India. Palmerston's instruction to the admiralty on the size and composition of the force was that it should comprise two men of war, two frigates, two river steamers and troopships sufficient to transport 7000 troops. By happy coincidence William Jardine, who at the time was back in England, had advised Palmerston of the need for an expeditionary force of precisely this composition.[46]

The expeditionary force demonstrated, as historian Eric Hobsbawm has said, that 'the Chinese Empire was helpless in the face of western military and economic aggression'.[47] In a military sense it was no contest. As to the behaviour of the British troops, suffice it to say that the Bengal word for plunder, 'loot', entered the English lexicon as a result of this first Opium War.[48] The war ended with the signing of the Treaty of Nanking in August 1842. Under its terms the British had five 'treaty ports' opened up for foreign trade, the merchants were compensated for the destroyed opium and Hong Kong became a British colony. What the Chinese got was more opium, despite the fact that they still refused to legalise it. Over the next 16 years illegal opium imports almost doubled, reaching 4810 tons in 1858.[49]

The second Opium War, fought between 1856 and 1860, is sometimes called the Arrow War after the Chinese-owned but British-flagged ship that was used as the excuse to start it. The Chinese had impounded the vessel after making accusations of piracy, and the war started when the Chinese refused British demands for its return. In truth there had been escalating tension between the two countries over what the Chinese saw as the unfair imposition of the Nanking Treaty. This time the French joined in on the British side and the result was even bloodier than the first time around.

The war was settled by the Convention of Peking, signed after that city's Summer Palace and hundreds of other buildings had been burned to the ground. The British negotiator was Lord Elgin, the man whose father had managed to extract certain sculptures from the Parthenon in Athens, much to the displeasure of many Greeks. What his son extracted from the Chinese was the effective opening up of the whole country to foreign trade and the legalisation of opium. What the Chinese got was, again, more opium. By 1879 the amount of opium being imported from India reached 6700 tons.[50]

For the British free-traders the tantalising prospect of supplying the manufactured wonders of the Industrial Revolution to 400 million Chinese consumers was at last opened up. Whether the Chinese wanted them or not was hardly a consideration, but the free-traders' prospects did rest on one important consideration: the capacity of the Chinese to pay for these goods. Between 1814 and 1850 the Chinese Treasury had already been drained of 13 per cent of its total stock of silver by paying for increasing supplies of opium.[51] This was a matter considered by Karl Marx in a leading article for the *New York Daily Tribune* during the war. His caustic characterisation of the relative moral considerations of the opium trade was: 'While the semi-barbarian stood on the principle of morality, the civilised opposed the principle of pelf.' With his habitual insight, Marx observed:

> *by raising dreams of an inexhaustible market and by fostering false speculations, the present treaty may help prepar[e] a new crisis at the very moment when the market of the world is but slowly recovering from the recent universal shock. Beside its negative result, the first opium war succeeded in stimulating the opium trade at the expense of legitimate commerce, and so will this second opium war do, if England be not forced by the general pressure of the civilised world to abandon the compulsory opium cultivation in India and the armed opium propaganda to China ... The Chinese cannot take both goods and drug; under actual circumstances, the extension of the Chinese trade resolves into extension of the opium trade; the growth of the latter is incompatible with the development of legitimate commerce.*[52]

Cotton and other textiles represented more than 70 per cent of British exports to the rest of the world in 1830, and although these items were in decline from the middle of the 19th century as a percentage of exports, they still, in 1870, accounted for more than 50 per cent.[53] However, China was self-sufficient in cottons and woollens, and the second Opium War didn't appreciably change this state of affairs. There was a market for British cottons and woollens in China, but it was primarily because they were sold down and traded for tea. The British products that China did import more of after 1860 were arms, ammunition and war material, principally to suppress the Taiping Rebellion, which in itself owed much to the consequences of the opium trade.[54]

The Chinese would in due course work out that they could grow their own opium rather than rely on Indian imports, and the British would in due course work out that they could source their tea supplies from India. It was, of course, also open to the Chinese authorities to legalise the trade and profit from it by way of taxes and charges earlier. This course was in fact seriously considered, but it was retreated from for fear of encouraging the evils of mass addiction. And they did have a point. At the beginning of the 20th century China's estimated 13.5 million addicts were managing to smoke their way through 39,000 tons of mostly Chinese opium each year.[55] By this time opium smoking was no longer confined to China or other parts of Asia. Chinese seamen and emigrant labour had taken it around the world with them and opium had met modernity, enabling a different but altogether more potent use of opiates.

The Chinese Empire collapsed in 1911 and the country was thereafter dominated by a succession of regional warlords who continued to rely on opium revenues. By the late 1930s, 40 million Chinese were addicted to opiates of one form or another. In 1949 Chairman MaoTse-Tung's Communist Peoples Republic of China set about tackling the opiate problem with some determination — and a vigour that at times seriously abused human rights. The result, at least, was an impressive one: by 1960 the addict population was negligible and a decade later China was producing just 100 tonnes of medicinal opium a year.[56] By the end of the 20th century, however, an illicit drug problem had re-emerged, coinciding with China's move to 'controlled capitalism'.

Opium among the civilised

The British were also using large amounts of opium during the 19th century, but very little of it was being smoked. At a time when professional healthcare ranged from limited to non-existent, particularly among the working class, self-medication was the only alternative. The sick had to heal themselves and their medicine of choice was opium, which was consumed in considerable amounts in England. Between 1827 and 1860 the five-year average home consumption of opium was between 2–3.3 pounds for each thousand of the population. Estimated consumption fluctuated, but reached much higher levels over the next 45 years. Opium was readily available in its pure form and in the form of laudanum. It was stocked by pharmacists and grocers and sold in corner shops, markets and even pubs. Widely advertised and enormously popular proprietary medicines contained opium, laudanum and morphine. Opium was available in the form of pills, powders, lozenges and confection. Opium wine was on sale, as were opium liniments and enemas. Opium preparations were 'everywhere to be bought'.[57] Opium suitable for smoking was about the only type not on general sale.

The pattern of opium consumption in Australia was similar to that in Britain. Access to healthcare in Australian cities would have been, at best, no better than in England during the 19th century and, in the more remote areas of the bush, much worse. The fact that there was a system for the registration of doctors from the mid-19th century didn't prevent the practice of medicine by those who weren't registered. Chemists, druggists and midwives were in the medical labour force in far greater numbers than doctors, and any professional consultations concerning medical problems that did occur were likely to be with chemists.[58] Self-medication was the order of the day. As the historian Geoffrey Blainey put it, 'Opium in the 19th century was not simply a dangerous drug of addiction but a general painkiller welcomed from time to time in millions of Christian households.'[59]

Australia even had its own opium-growing industry to supplement imports. Opium was grown in Tasmania in the 1820s and 1830s; in New South Wales in the 1830s; and in Victoria from the late 1860s. As late as 1893 there were 23 growers at Bacchus Marsh in Victoria with 66 acres (26.7 hectares) of opium poppies under cultivation supplying local manufacturers that had begun producing opium-based proprietary medicines in the 1880s.[60]

Some indication of the amount of opium used at the time can be had from examining import figures. Victoria, for example, imported more than 18 tonnes of opium, principally from India, in 1880. 'Refining houses', processing imported raw opium, had been established in Melbourne under the supervision of the Customs Service five years earlier.[61] In 1890 the value of opium imported by all of the states was more than £126,000, with Queensland taking a much larger share than either New South Wales or Victoria.[62] In the year of Federation, New South Wales imported slightly more than 13 tonnes of opium and Victoria 3.5 tonnes.[63] In 1820, when the first retail pharmacy in the country was opened in Sydney, it was stocked with opium-based medicines such as the ever-popular Godfrey's Cordial.[64] In March 1844, you needed to do no more than open *The Sydney Morning Herald* to know that Ambrose Foss, Chemist, Druggist etc of 313 Pitt Street had to hand a good supply of opium and poppy heads that were 'absolutely of the best quality and free from every kind of adulteration'.[65]

Opium smoking

Tens of thousands of Chinese came to Australia from the 1850s, attracted by the prospect of making their fortunes from gold. Most of those who hadn't already acquired the habit of smoking opium either picked it up on the way or developed it while here; among those who spent any appreciable time in Australia, an estimated 90 per cent smoked opium.[66] They smoked in opium houses which came to be pejoratively called 'dens'. As historian Eric Rolls described them:

> *The better houses had tiers of bunks for the smokers, and attendants to prepare the pipes. Most of them were sparsely furnished. In the centre on a low table stood a small lamp full of peanut oil with its flame burning through the top of a short, bell-shaped glass chimney. That functional lamp was the only source of light. Beside it was a small round horn pot of opium, long wire needles sometimes flattened into narrow spatulas at the end, thin wooden torches and several bamboo pipes, 60 centimetres long and 3.5 centimetres in diameter. An acorn sized clay or iron bowl with a central pinhole was fixed in at a point about one third the length of the pipe from the base. Cool air from the bottom of the pipe was thus drawn in with the smoke. Mats lay about for the smokers to recline on, with pillows against the wall for those who had smoked their ration, against the table for those preparing their pipes. Even in Australia the pillows were usually squat, heavy, concave wooden blocks.*[67]

The use of opium in Australia attracted little comment, and even less criticism when it involved white Australians. Its use by Chinese immigrants and Indigenous Australians was a different matter entirely, and ubiquitous as opium use was, it seems beyond doubt that the majority of opium was consumed by Chinese. By the end of the 1870s, according to one estimate, more than 100 tonnes of opium was coming into Australia (some of it smuggled in illegally to avoid duty), with most of it used by the Chinese. As late as 1902, the three eastern states, New South Wales, Victoria and Queensland, imported 19 tonnes of opium: probably only 5 per cent was used for medical reasons, with the rest smoked by the Chinese, whose numbers by this time had declined to less than 30,000.[68]

The NSW and Victorian governments had introduced an import duty on opium as early as 1857 — a hefty 10 shillings per pound weight. It was a duty aimed squarely at Chinese smokers, as laudanum users had their imported drugs treated as duty-free medicines. By 1905, the year when collecting the duty ceased, smoking opium attracted a duty of 30 shillings per pound weight, but all items of European consumption were taxed at least two-thirds lower.[69]

Chinese in Australia experienced hatred, harassment and violence from the time they landed. The outcome of the inquiry resulting from the murderous events at the Eureka Stockade in December 1854 is for some a cause of celebration: a vindication of the miners' just cause, a condemnation of unjust laws and their oppressive enforcement, a victory for militant action. Perhaps. But Chinese miners trying to earn a living would be entitled to a different view. Besides the abolition of licence fees, the inquiry led to the introduction of legislation with the disingenuous title of 'An Act to make Provision for Certain Immigrants'. Its purpose was to restrict the number of Chinese brought to Victoria by ship to one person for each 10 tons of a ship's registered tonnage. For good measure, each Chinese landed had to pay a poll tax of £10, an enormous sum at the time. There was little that the Chinese could do about this blatant act of discrimination except land in South Australia and walk to the Victorian goldfields, which is what they did. And when the SA government introduced similar restrictive measures, Chinese immigrants came in via Sydney.[70]

The racist and xenophobic reaction to Chinese immigration is demonstrated by the events surrounding a ship called the

Afghan in 1888. The *Afghan*, together with several other vessels, was refused the right to disembark Chinese passengers in Melbourne in early 1888. It sailed to Sydney, where landing rights were similarly refused. This action by the two colonial governments was plainly illegal. Among the nearly 600 Chinese passengers, many had undisputed right of entry. Indeed some of them were simply returning to Australia; they had been here for many years and operated businesses and lived here just like other citizens.[71] But the law proved a mere bagatelle when confronted by the reality of racism. While the Afghan and its Chinese passengers were quarantined at anchor in Sydney Harbour, the NSW government passed the *Chinese Restriction and Regulation Act 1888*. As Premier Sir Henry Parkes said, 'I care nothing about your cobweb of technical law; I am obeying a law far superior to any which issued these permits, namely the law of the preservation of society in New South Wales.' White society, that is, of a civilised 'pure British type'.[72]

Alleged unfair competition for labour, fear of miscegenation and the habit of opium smoking were all used to demonise the Chinese. Australia's first drug laws were aimed at the immigrant Chinese and that even more demonised and despised race, Aboriginal Australians. Chinese in Queensland and the Northern Territory were alleged to be unfairly procuring Indigenous labour by the inducement of opium, thus denying those pioneering descendants of the stout yeomen of England access to a convenient and cheap workforce. That Aboriginal people might prefer to work for half-decent Chinese employers than to be ill-treated and worse by racist whites never seemed to be considered. A white farmer in Queensland in the late 1890s complained that he had done his bit to settle the land by 'shooting thirteen or fourteen niggers', yet couldn't get one to work for him when he was in need: 'they all go to the Chinaman'.[73]

The *Sale and Use of Poisons Act* introduced in Queensland in 1891 and the *Opium Act* introduced in South Australia four years later were aimed at those 'persons' (that is to say, Chinese) who supplied opium to 'any aboriginal native of Australia or half-caste of that race'.[74] As many as 20 Chinese were imprisoned or fined each month in the Northern Territory following the promulgation of the South Australian legislation.[75] White Christian settlers shook their heads disapprovingly at these vulgar transgressions … while reaching for the laudanum bottle.

7
Drug laws and changes in supply

The origins of suppression

In the latter half of the 19th century opium use in the United States increased more than fourfold, from an average of 12 grains annually per person in the 1840s to 52 grains in the 1890s.[1] But, as in Australia, it was the Chinese opium smokers and the non-Chinese who smoked with them who attracted the attention of the lawmakers.

Chinese labourers began arriving in California during the gold rush that began in 1848 and their numbers increased rapidly, from less than 100 in 1849 to considerably more than 100,000 in 1876, by which time they made up a quarter of the state's immigrant population.[2] But if racist maltreatment in Australia was trying for the Chinese, the Californian experience was literally large-scale murder. In 1853 and 1854 a total of 82 Chinese were murdered on the goldfields, and in the downturn of 1862, 88 were murdered.[3] Securing a conviction against any alleged perpetrator faced the difficult hurdle of Chinese witnesses' evidence being disallowed by the Californian Supreme Court on the grounds that testimony from an inferior race of people was inadmissible.[4]

San Francisco was the port through which most Chinese entered California and the place where many of them stayed for varying lengths of time. And it was the San Francisco authorities who passed the first anti-opium laws, in 1875. The San Francisco prohibition, which was followed in 11 states over the next 15 years,[5] was aimed at the keeping and frequenting of opium shops, and at the consumption of opium. It was, of course, the Chinese who kept such establishments and who, in the main, frequented them. The opium shops were not segregated, though, and non-Chinese were as free to come and go as Chinese were.

The fear that Chinese opium shops would attract growing numbers of marginalised whites — and, even worse, corrupt the white middle class — is said to be the rationale for the San Francisco ordinance.[6] The prohibition nevertheless occurred in an environment of blatant racial discrimination against Chinese. Left to their own devices, white Americans were quite capable of finding all manner of intoxicating substances to consume. It's difficult to escape the conclusion that what the US authorities really wanted was to get rid of the Chinese. Once Chinese labour had helped build the rail system they were able to do this, by passing a series of Exclusion Acts, beginning in 1882. The violence continued, though, with 28 Chinese miners murdered in Wyoming in 1885. Not surprisingly, news of US restrictions on Chinese immigration was favourably received in Australia and led to calls for the introduction of similar laws.[7]

Prohibition from the Philippines

The Arab and Portuguese traders who brought opium to China in the 16th century had established a limited trade in the drug with those Southeast Asian ports en route, and over the next two centuries the Dutch established a somewhat more substantial trade with their Javanese colony.

In the 19th century the hundreds of thousands of Chinese who migrated to the area brought with them the opium habit they had acquired back home courtesy of the British. By the time San Francisco was passing its anti-opium ordinance, there were large opium-smoking populations throughout the region: in Rangoon, Saigon, Bangkok, Singapore, the Malaysian states and Manila. The local inhabitants were imbibing as well, and opium smoking spread out from the ports and capitals.

The British, Dutch, French and Spanish colonial administrators were not, as might be imagined today, disposed to discourage the practice; they were rather more concerned with making a profit from it. To this end, they established monopoly control over the importation of opium, followed by a monopoly on its retail sale in the thousands of opium shops throughout the region. Opium revenues weren't merely a boon to these colonial economies; they represented in some cases almost 60 per cent of state revenue, and it's true to say that much of the early infrastructure of Southeast Asian countries was built on opium.[8]

It was the Spanish American War of 1898 that changed this state of affairs, and the events that followed led to international drug controls. This 'splendid little war',[9] which gave the United States a naval base at Guantanamo Bay in Cuba, also provided an excuse for the invasion of the Spanish colony of the Philippines. More than 200,000 Filipinos died in the conflict and when the fighting had eased somewhat and the US Navy was ensconced in Subic Bay, the occupying forces found that what came with the territory was a profitable opium monopoly that the Spanish had had the foresight to establish in 1843.[10] The Spanish imported opium and then auctioned contracts to sell the drug to the highest bidders — this system raised about US$600,000 annually. They allowed the drug to be smoked in dens and other authorised establishments.

The Americans abolished these arrangements. Opium

imports were prohibited, as were opium shops and opium smoking. This resulted in an increase in opium smoking that caused the US colonial administrator (and future president) William Taft to rethink the ban and press for the monopoly to be reintroduced. US missionaries had different ideas. The prospect of gaining a foothold in Roman Catholic Cuba and the Philippines had generated a good deal of enthusiasm for the Spanish-American War among Protestant religious bodies in the United States. One of the country's Methodist publications claimed that, in support of such a just cause, 'Every Methodist preacher will be a recruiting officer.' Spreading the gospel of both God and mammon, they had come to expect, to paraphrase one contemporary commentator, that the US military would 'stand by with fixed bayonets while they preached peace on earth and goodwill to men'.[11]

The Episcopalian bishop of the missionary district of the Philippines, Charles Henry Brent, had arrived in the country in 1901. An outspoken critic of Taft's proposed policy reversal, he was determined to ensure that matters of such high moral concern not be left solely to administrators. He was able to organise enough support in Washington to prevent Taft from proceeding, and the matter was referred for further investigation to a three-man committee that he was a member of. The Philippines Opium Committee went on a tour of the region that could only have confirmed Brent's view of the character deficiencies of Orientals: 'The constitutional fault of the Filipinos, a fault common to all Orientals, is sensuality, which in this case finds vent in laziness, concubinage and gaming.' He thought opium smoking 'the most horrible vice of the Orient'. Following the committee's report in 1904, an official policy of opiate prohibition (except for medicinal use) became effective from 1908.[12]

The result, again, not surprisingly, was an illicit market supplied by opium smuggled in from China and Borneo.[13]

Undeterred by this, Brent was next influential in persuading US President Theodore Roosevelt to convene an International Opium Commission in Shanghai in 1909, which Brent chaired.[14] Before this commission convened, the United States established the bona fides of its prohibitionist position by passing the *Smoking Opium Exclusion Act*, which mirrored the Philippines legislation.[15] However, delegates from the 13 countries that attended went no further than to advise a policy of gradual suppression implemented by the government-controlled opium monopolies.[16]

Two years later, the International Conference on Opium at The Hague, which Brent again chaired, led to a more tangible result: the International Opium Convention of 1912. This convention, sometimes known simply as The Hague Convention, determined that the recreational use of opium, morphine and cocaine be prohibited (albeit gradually), and mandated countries to introduce anti-drug legislation. Serbia and Turkey baulked because of their interest in the opium trade; Germany did too, because of its cocaine-processing industry. It was therefore agreed that the convention, with its promise to restrict opium imports and exports to medical use, would only come into force when signed by 35 nations.[17] Momentum was certainly with the prohibitionists in the United States, and led to the *Harrison Narcotic Act 1914*, but for most European countries World War I (1914–18) meant that there were more pressing matters to attend to.

However, the Versailles Peace Treaty of 1919, which settled the terms on which the war ended, also bound its signatories to The Hague Convention. By 1921, 38 countries were signatories[18] and Australia had managed to become a party to it twice: first, when the United Kingdom signed up on its behalf in 1912, and second, on signing the Versailles Treaty in 1919.[19]

The opium conferences held in Shanghai and The Hague paved the way for the Geneva Conference of 1925 and the subsequent regime of international drug prohibition authorised by the League of Nations. As these controls were further expanded under the auspices of the United Nations, member states introduced complementary drug laws into their domestic jurisdictions. Australia, consistent with its international obligations, introduced drug prohibition laws in both state and Commonwealth jurisdictions.[20]

Together with Brent, the other prominent architects of prohibition in the Philippines were those US missionaries who had earlier promised to be recruiting agents for the war of occupation. They were typical of that puritan US tradition that has a profound distaste for a long list of sinful behaviour, including indolence and the liberty to allow intoxication. Its political expression was assured early in the 20th century because it happily coincided with US business interests. Being 'tough on drugs' was judged to be good for trade, particularly the China trade.[21] Equally, protection of commercial interests in the drug trade was behind the opposition to controls voiced by Britain and Germany (among others).

But the United States had more to gain than most in the early decades of the 20th century. An international prohibitionist regime would buttress US domestic prohibition laws and, importantly, reflect its growing international hegemony.

At the time of the Geneva Convention of 1925, a policy of alcohol prohibition had been in force in the United States for five years, and would somehow survive another eight.

What is clear now, and was equally clear then, is that alcohol prohibition didn't succeed in stopping consumption, it simply criminalised its sale. It was a social disaster in drug control that even the United States failed to export. Within nine years the number of alcohol-related convictions had doubled and six new jails were under construction to house the offenders.[22] It gave control of a significant sector of the economy to gangsters in circumstances where the states' regulatory apparatus was reduced to policing; it had no ability to use the tools available in a licit market — taxes, import restrictions and licensing, plus education and rehabilitation programs — to discourage consumption. The illicit market developed a crude mechanism of internal self-regulation based on thuggery and murder, and this usurped the state's monopoly on violence. Where the newly created illicit economy intersected with the licit economy it was able to corrupt it at almost every level. Its corrupting influence, developed during the 13 years of Prohibition, proved enduring beyond the repeal of the Volstead Act. Once the prohibition on alcohol was lifted in 1933, there was no return to the old normality. The fortunes made under the cloak of criminality were wisely invested in the mainstream economy. The profits made from Prohibition sustained a large criminal class, and their fortunes were put to good use opening up yet more illicit markets.

The international drug controls that came from Geneva in 1925 did have some initial success in limiting production and dampening demand.[23] But sufficient demand persisted to fuel a profitable international market, and US gangsters were prominent in exploiting it.

The suppliers

In countries where smoking opium was banned, it continued to be smoked, just as alcohol continued to be consumed in the United States during the prohibition years. In Melbourne in the early 1960s an elderly Chinese market gardener was fined £10 for doing what he had been doing since he arrived in the country in 1894: smoking opium. In Sydney's Chinatown opium smoking was still going on in the 1970s.[24] The opium that was prepared for smoking had a morphine content of less than 9 per cent, but much less than that was actually ingested. Most of it went up in smoke and what wasn't vaporised was left as residue in the pipe bowl, to be used again later. And, of course, not all of the morphine in the smoke entered the bloodstream.[25] But modern science would change the nature of the opium experience forever, and the medical profession would be the first to demonstrate how.

By 1840, after opium had been subject to scientific scrutiny and analysis earlier in the 19th century and its active ingredient, morphine, isolated, the new drug had been accepted into medical practice. Several times more powerful than opium, morphine's effects were much more rapidly felt when injecting became possible following the development of the syringe in the 1850s.[26] Then in 1874, at St Mary's Hospital in London, the pharmacist C R Alder Wright created a substance that he named tetra-ethyl morphine. It was renamed diacetylmorphine in the next decade, as several papers were produced on its effects. In the Bayer laboratories in Elberfeld, Germany in 1898 it was renamed again; this new drug, which was somewhere between five and eight times more powerful than morphine, became known as heroin.[27]

The medical use of opium gave way to its more powerful derivatives; first they were popped in pill form, later they were injected. One-quarter of a grain of morphine has the same effect as 1–1.5 grains of opium,[28] so morphine was particularly suited to the relief of pain that came from war injuries and illnesses. More than 600,000 died in the American Civil War of 1861–65, and if they were lucky they were treated with opium before they breathed their last. Close to 400,000 were wounded but survived, and the more serious of them were treated with morphine. In Germany, the injecting use of morphine was popularised shortly after the war with Austria, in 1866. These war veterans continued to use morphine after the peace, either for pain relief or because they were addicted.[29] This addiction became known as the 'army disease' but, if anything, addiction to morphine — morphinism, as it was then known — might better have been called a 'doctors' disease'. Not only were doctors over-represented among male addicts, but their less than judicious practice of injecting their mainly female patients was the main cause of addiction as a whole.[30] Among the long-suffering Chinese, morphine pills were referred to as 'Jesus opium' after the missionaries who promoted it as a cure for opium addiction.[31]

If morphine worked well, so the thinking went, heroin should work even better on the killer respiratory diseases that dogged the times. It proved particularly useful as a suppressant of the cough associated with two of the predominant illnesses of the period, pneumonia and tuberculosis.[32] By the end of the 19th century, heroin was available over the counter in several easy-to-take forms, including pills, lozenges and cough mixtures. Doctors could administer it by syringe, as they'd done with morphine, and could even instruct you on how to do it yourself. The good news for morphine addicts was that heroin was now on hand to cure their troublesome little problem.[33]

It took the medical profession almost four decades to realise and write about the dangers of morphine addiction, and several more decades were to pass before they started to do something about it. With heroin it took a mere decade, but by then its recreational use was established in the United States, and by 1919 heroin use was known as the 'American disease'.[34]

Iatrogenic addiction aside, many of the heroin users in the United States in the early 20th century had previously smoked opium or taken cocaine. They turned to heroin because it was more readily available and, as with cocaine, the method of taking it was by sniffing. New York was the heroin capital of the world, and the new recruits to the drug were typically young males of an immigrant background, from the more squalid districts of the city. They were mostly white and working class, with a tendency to belong to gangs and be associated with criminal activity.[35]

New York Jewish criminals controlled much of the illicit activity in the city, in competition with others that included the Irish and the Italians. They profited from gambling, prostitution, cocaine and heroin. Between 1920 and 1933 alcohol was added to the list. Irving 'Waxey Gordon' Wexler, Benjamin 'Bugsy' Siegel, and Arthur 'Dutch' Schultz were prominent among them. Arnold Rothstein was even more prominent, powerful enough to fix the 1919 World Baseball Series by bribing players from the Chicago White Sox.[36] But the most important of them all was Meyer Lansky.

Lansky's background was strikingly similar to that of New York's emerging heroin users, except, of course, that he was on the other side of the fence — in the supply department. Born Maier Suchowljansky in Grodno, Poland, in 1902, he arrived in New York in 1912 when his family fled persecution. By the tender age of 16, together with the even younger Bugsy Siegel, he had taken part in all forms of violence, up to and including murder.[37] Lansky became associated with the Lepke and Gurrah mob, who dominated much of the New York heroin trade,[38] and later teamed up with Rothstein, who was dealing in both illicit alcohol and heroin.[39] Lansky demonstrated his ruthlessness in the Prohibition period when a crew working for him relieved fellow bootlegger Joseph P Kennedy, father of future president John F Kennedy, of his booty of Irish whiskey, murdering 11 of Kennedy's men in the process.[40]

Lansky was a genius with figures, but his great insight, learned in Manhattan's Lower East Side, was that corruption was not incidental to, but rather an integral part of, the American way of life. Although not beyond the expediency of bribery, he preferred partnerships to payoffs,[41] and his most lucrative partnership was with Charles 'Lucky' Luciano.

It was a partnership forged in 1918 in unusual circumstances; in the back of a paddy wagon following their arrest, when Lansky objected to Luciano's too vigorous beating of one of his 'working girls'. Lansky convinced Luciano of the considerable benefits to be had from the heroin trade; senior Mafia leaders had had till then a considerable aversion to such activity. Their partnership came to dominate the trade and Luciano certainly got lucky in 1929, when the more conservative dons decided to put him out of business on a permanent basis. Luciano was kidnapped, hung from a beam in a New Jersey warehouse, flogged with a baseball bat and had his throat slit. For good measure he was stabbed with an icepick.[42]

Unfortunately for the dons, Luciano lived up to his nickname. He survived, and went on with Lansky and others to murder more than 70 of them in the course of the following four years. His position thus consolidated, he was able to add the resources of the Mafia to an international crime organisation that Lansky structured on the same basis as the pre-eminent enterprise of the time, the Standard Oil Trust established by John D Rockefeller.[43]

The heroin that was being peddled on the streets of New York and elsewhere was sourced, in various illegal ways, from local pharmaceutical companies that were licensed to produce the drug, until manufacturing was prohibited in the United States in 1924.[44] Thereafter it was supplied from different parts of the world — this syndicate, an alliance of Jewish and Italian gangsters, had a global reach. Pharmaceutical companies such as Merck in Germany, Hoffman-La Roche in Switzerland and Roesler & Fils in France were all sources of illicit heroin. It was also imported from Japan, China, Hong Kong and the Middle East. Manufacturing plants that were established in the opium-growing countries of Serbia, Turkey and Bulgaria were another source. Persian, Turkish and Chinese opium was smuggled into the United States to be manufactured in situ, though this could be a dangerous process if not properly handled. In 1935 a New York apartment being used to manufacture heroin by a Jewish criminal syndicate exploded, bringing unwanted attention to the enterprise and leading to the conviction of the chemist involved.[45]

The 1920 decision by US authorities to cease maintenance programs for addicts meant that addicts had the choice of either going cold turkey or going to the illicit market.[46] Many chose the easier option of getting their drugs on the street, thus adding to the syndicate's consumer base. Profits were also increased by the simple process of adulteration. The Mafia operatives who had taken over the street supply were much greedier than their Jewish counterparts. As purity levels dropped below 30 per cent, users had to compensate by switching from the sniffing method to the needle.[47] The net result was that by the outbreak of World War II in 1939, the heroin business was one of the biggest in the United States. It generated in excess of $1 billion a year — Lansky's claim that the syndicate was 'bigger than United States Steel' was no idle boast.[48]

In the middle of the 'roaring twenties' there were some 200,000 heroin addicts in the United States. In the next decade they came to include many of the prostitutes working in the 200 New York brothels that Luciano controlled; this was a profitable precedent that would be widely emulated.[49] But old habits died hard with Luciano, and it was his mistreatment of the women in his employ that eventually brought him undone. Their evidence led to his conviction on 62 charges of forced prostitution in a case brought to trial in 1936 by district attorney and future New York governor Thomas Dewey. Luciano was sentenced to 30–50 years' imprisonment.[50]

The heroin business also fell on hard times in the war years. Supplies from Europe and Asia proved all but impossible to procure and Lansky and Bugsy Siegel were reduced to smuggling opium across the border from Mexico into California.[51] By 1945, the number of heroin addicts in the United States had dwindled to 20,000.[52]

8
The Cold War and the CIA

After war comes peace, and with it the difficult task for the victors of shaping peace terms that guarantee their security and, at the same time, ensure that the vanquished have no good cause to resume hostilities. In 1945 the lessons of recent history had to be heeded. After all, the onerous reparations that Germany had had to pay to England and France following the 1914–18 World War had contributed in no small way to Adolf Hitler's rise to power and World War II, which followed in 1939.

Leaders of the Big Three nations that fought the 1939–45 war against Germany and her Axis partners turned their minds to these vexing questions when they met in Teheran in November of 1943, in Yalta in February of 1945 and again in Potsdam in July of that year, following the German surrender in May. When Winston Churchill, Franklin D Roosevelt and Josef Stalin first met in Teheran it was Stalin who had the upper hand. In the summer offensive of that year his mighty Red Army had already recovered two-thirds of the Soviet territory previously lost to the Germans. The military production facilities that had been moved thousands of miles to the east to shield them from Hitler's invading army would provide increasing and continuous war supplies from the following year.[1]

The war in Europe was being fought on the eastern front with somewhere between 80 and 90 per cent of German land forces deployed against the USSR. Moreover, the 260 German divisions in the east represented the cream of Hitler's troops, and they could not be reinforced from the 59 inferior divisions to whom the protection of the Atlantic coast was entrusted.[2] In early 1944 the Russians were still engaged in a desperate fight to break the German blockade of Leningrad. Before the year ended they had blockaded the German garrison of Budapest.[3] The Red Army was on an unstoppable march to Berlin and the thought must surely have occurred to Stalin that he could defeat Hitler without the help of Britain or the United States. The same thought must have also exercised the minds of Churchill and Roosevelt.

This is perhaps why Churchill presented Stalin with a piece of paper at their meeting in the Kremlin in October of 1944 on which was written his proposal for the postwar division of Europe. The USSR was to have 'ninety per cent predominance' in Romania; Britain the same in Greece. Hungary and Yugoslavia were to be an even split, with Bulgaria going 75 to 25 in the USSR's favour and Britain controlling the Mediterranean. Stalin concurred, and privately Churchill conceded Poland and all of the Balkans.[4] The declarations of the Yalta conference may well have spoken of 'free elections' in the soon to be liberated countries, but as Stalin saw it, he had an agreement whose practical effect meant that he was as free to define the term 'free election' in his zones of influence as Churchill and Roosevelt were in theirs.

At the end of hostilities 55 million were dead. Europe, much of it in ruins, was partitioned, its eastern countries claimed in the name of communism, its western countries in the name of capitalism. Then the recriminations began.

At Potsdam, Churchill complained to Stalin about the 'iron fence' that was placed around His Majesty's representatives in

Bucharest.[5] Eight months later, in Fulton, Missouri, the home state of then US President Truman, the fence became an Iron Curtain that had descended across Europe from the Baltic to the Adriatic. Throughout the entire world, communist parties and their fifth columns posed a 'growing challenge and peril to Christian civilisation'. The only exceptions, it seemed, were the United States and the British Commonwealth, where communism was in its infancy.[6]

Harry S Truman assumed the presidency from the position of vice president when Franklin D Roosevelt died in April 1945, and was elected resident in his own right in 1948, when he defeated Thomas E Dewey. A year after Churchill's Iron Curtain speech, on 12 March 1947, he launched the Truman Doctrine: its aim was to contain and resist the spread of communism. This was the formal declaration of the Cold War. Accompanying it would be an arms race. In September 1949 the USSR detonated its first atomic bomb, wiping out the nuclear advantage that the United States had demonstrated with the bombing of Hiroshima and Nagasaki in August 1945.[7] This was a war that would shape the political landscape of the entire planet for the rest of the 20th century.

Was it all worth it? Was it even necessary? About the only certainty is that opinions on these questions will forever differ. Opinions certainly differ as to the nature and extent of any agreements made among the Big Three (the United States, the USSR and Britain). Isaac Deutscher, journalist, economist, literary critic and author, probably summed up the situation as well as anyone when he said, 'The pledges of the allies, had, anyhow, been so vague and contained so many loopholes that by reference to the text each side could justify its conduct.'[8] To be strenuously fair to Stalin, there were indications at the time that he would stick to what he, at least, thought was the bargain. At the end of World War II there were some very powerful communist movements in Europe that Stalin had effective control over, despite their nominal independence. It is not implausible that the communists in France, Italy and Greece could have successfully gained power — with his encouragement and support. The major political force in both Italy and France was the Communist Party. The French Communist Party had a membership of almost one million, the Italian Communist Party closer to two million.[9] And they knew something of the sharp end of struggle through their role in the Resistance. But under Stalin's influence the leadership of the French and Italian parties had a curiously accommodating accord with the Big Two whose zone of influence they were now in. It was an accord at odds with the views of their membership, and that strained the links of internal democracy. Stalin was able to convince a leadership that knew about seizing power that they should participate in coalition governments, conceding the military and police organs of the state to their minority partner. That was the agreement.

If there was a policy of appeasement in France and Italy, there was nothing short of a sell-out in Greece. When British forces arrived there in 1944 they found the communist-led ELAS in control.[10] Stalin had already agreed to look the other way when the British found it necessary, in conjunction with the royalists, to oust ELAS by force, and during the next two and a half years, while they tried to do so, he kept his word. Indeed it was when an exhausted Britain was forced to withdraw, leaving a certain communist victory in Greece, that the Truman Doctrine was enunciated and the United States intervened.[11] Outside Europe, Stalin was on the side of Chiang Kai-shek in 1945 and he was still there on the eve of communist victory four years later, advising Mao Tse-tung to reach an accommodation with the Kuomintang.[12]

Despite his own accommodation with the west, or perhaps in some cases because of it, there was an enormous level of support for Stalin in the immediate aftermath of World War

II. 'Joe for King' was a sentiment that British troops in Europe didn't shy from proclaiming.[13] It was a sentiment not long in evaporating.

Disputes as to its origins notwithstanding, the Cold War was off and running from 1947. By its very nature, such a war demanded a level of international intelligence activity hitherto unprecedented. This would become the province of the Central Intelligence Agency (CIA). Created with the passing of the *National Security Act 1947*, the CIA was inevitably influenced by the military intelligence organisations that preceded it and the domestic institutions that had an intelligence-gathering capacity (the Federal Bureau of Investigation and the Federal Bureau of Narcotics). The Office of Strategic Services (OSS) and the Office of Naval Intelligence (ONI) had already adopted Harry Anslinger's methods — using criminals as paid informants and sanctioning undercover agents to engage in criminal activity — and applied them internationally.[14] These useful, practical precedents would become standard operating procedure for the CIA.

Liberating Lucky Luciano

At the end of February 1942, more than 70 allied merchant ships carrying supplies vital to the war effort in Europe had been sunk off the Atlantic coast in just two and a half months by German U-boats. Earlier in the month the liner *Normandie* caught fire and sank while moored in New York's Hudson River. Spies and sabotage were suspected. Tighter security on the New York waterfront was called for. The anti-fascist union leader from the west coast, Melbourne-born Harry Bridges, had a different solution. New York's waterfront workers should leave the corrupt, Mafia-controlled International Longshoremen's Association and join the International Longshoremen and Warehousemen's Union that he led. A cleaned-up waterfront could be relied on to support the war effort through democratic politics in a democratic union. But Bridges was suspected of being a communist, so the authorities spent their efforts trying to deport him and stood by while his supporters were bashed and murdered by Mafia thugs.[15] The gangsters remained in control and the ONI turned instead to Meyer Lansky. Lansky became the intermediary to the imprisoned Lucky Luciano as the ONI tried to enlist the aid of Luciano's lieutenants in enforcing control on New York's docks. The OSS had previously made contact with a Sicilian Mafia decimated by Mussolini, trying to get their support for the planned 1943 invasion of Italy. Luciano became involved in this project too. His reward was freedom from incarceration. Luciano was freed on the authority of the Governor of New York, his old nemesis, Thomas E Dewey, who would shortly be the Democrat nominee for the US presidency.[16]

The decision to involve the Mafia in domestic dock security and the liberation of Europe would very quickly contribute to a resurgence of America's heroin problem. Deported to Italy in early 1946, Luciano wasted no time in establishing heroin laboratories in Sicily and exporting the drug to New York via Cuba. The US heroin market, comprising fewer than 20,000 addicts at the end of World War II, was rejuvenated, with the complicity of the OSS and the ONI. CIA complicity in the trade would ensure that heroin became an enduring problem, both in the United States and beyond.

The heroin for Luciano's European operation was initially sourced from the Italian pharmaceutical company Schiaparelli. When this supply was eventually cut off, the operation relied on raw opium from Turkey that was refined into morphine in Beirut and finally processed into heroin in Sicily, ready for export.[17] The Sicilian operation proved the weak link in the chain: a number of couriers were arrested,[18] largely due to incompetence and an arrogance that came from being in a position of power courtesy of the OSS. The heroin laboratories were shifted to Marseilles, establishing a supply link that became infamously known as the French Connection. By 1952 the number of addicts in the United States had tripled.[19]

The financial details of the shift were organised by Meyer Lansky when he travelled to Italy and Switzerland in 1950.[20] Lansky had learned the importance of money-laundering when America's most notorious gangster, Al Capone, was jailed for tax evasion in 1931.[21] By 1950, in a brilliantly inspired move, he had already begun to establish the casino business in a small town in the Nevada desert called Las Vegas, which would go on to become the Mecca of the gambling world. Casinos were perfect for Lansky's purposes. They were legitimate enterprises that could be built in the first instance from drug profits. Drug money in the form of cash could then conveniently be passed through them, coming out suitably laundered. The casinos would themselves contribute to profits in the proper course of business and improperly (and illegally) through the cash skimmed off the top.

The banking arrangements were the tricky part, but as long ago as 1932 Lansky had had this in hand: he had set up a Swiss bank account for Huey Long, the Governor of Louisiana, in exchange for allowing the mob access to gambling facilities in New Orleans.[22] The offshore arrangements would later include banks in the Bahamas, and Lansky and his criminal colleagues would, by the mid-1950s, control their own banks in Miami. Enormous sums of money were involved, which meant that within the banking system generally there were many establishments keen to do discreet business. As one authority put it, 'Lansky had enough banks in his pocket to qualify for the presidency of the American Bankers' Association.'[23] In a neat symmetry, profits from wartime opium production in Mexico helped build the Las Vegas casino business and the skim from the casino business financed the French Connection. The profits from the French Connection were then laundered in the casinos and passed through US banks to Switzerland and the Bahamas. The accumulated and drycleaned capital was then reinvested in legitimate businesses such as casinos.[24]

Marseilles was chosen as the location for Lansky and Luciano's heroin production and distribution network for reasons beyond its geographical location. Although well suited from this perspective, what Marseilles also had to offer was a well-developed criminal class. As well as giving France Napoleon Bonaparte, Corsica had also provided a criminal group centred in Marseilles, where Corsican immigrants made up 10 per cent of the population. They specialised in prostitution and nightclub ownership from the 1920s, and dabbled in opium smuggling and heroin production in the 1930s. They also acted as paid thugs for the French fascists in their battles against the French communists in the lead-up to World War II. During the war, though, they joined the Resistance movement in Marseilles, in patriotic protest against the planned annexation of Corsica by Italy. The Resistance in Marseilles was split into two groups, communist and non-communist. Given their previous involvement with fascists, the Corsicans were, not surprisingly, on the non-communist side. They stayed there after the war, again providing the muscle for the right-wing forces that were battling the communists for political control of Marseilles.[25]

In 1947 both sides in Marseilles were affected by events happening elsewhere. In June of that year the Marshall Plan for United States aid to Europe was announced. This was something the United States was obliged to consider, irrespective of the Cold War, in order to protect its own economic interests. The Cold War just made its introduction more urgent. The intention of the plan was to rejuvenate the economies of western Europe so that these countries could compete in a postwar global trade system that the United States would nevertheless dominate. Without the kick-start provided by US dollars, European countries, economically weakened by war, would be unable to pay for US imports. This in turn would mean high levels of unemployment — and probably also social unrest — in the United States. There was also the danger of social unrest in Europe because there, too, there would be high unemployment and lower spending on social services as finance was diverted to industry restructuring.[26] Again, the Marshall Plan would alleviate this, funding Europe's transitional phase to international competitiveness.

The poverty that would continue in Europe in the absence of a Marshall Plan would also increase the possibility that countries such as Germany, as well as France and Italy, would look to the Soviet Union and become more attracted to the idea of a communist-led government. To combat that threat, the CIA channelled funds through the US labour movement, the AFL-CIO, to right-wing French unions, who in return would support a cooperative approach with capital and oppose the communist unions.[27] In Moscow, Stalin was aware of the danger that the Marshall Plan posed, so the French and Italian Communist Parties were directed to obstruct it.

On one account this resulted in the French general strike which lasted from 18 November to 9 December in 1947;[28] however, there were also spontaneous strikes born out of austerity. Indeed the response of the French and Italian Communist Parties has been described as 'feeble and incoherent'.[29] This description couldn't be applied to the communist-led workers in Marseilles, who were already on strike when the general strike was called. They too returned to work on 9 December, but only after a series of bloody battles in which a number of strikers were murdered by Corsican gangsters and their colleagues.

Corsican gangsters consolidated their position in 1948–49, but it wasn't until after the 1950 strike that they were able to control the Marseilles waterfront. In 1950 the militant waterfront unions in Marseilles were again on strike, banning the loading of ships that were supplying the French military in their war with Vietnam. It was a tactic that Australian waterfront unions were to repeat 20 years later as the war dragged on, with US forces having replaced French ones. The Vietnamese communist leader Ho Chi Minh had popular support among the Vietnamese community in Marseilles and elsewhere in France. He was a founding member of the French Communist Party, and had attended the Versailles Conference in 1919, arguing for Vietnamese independence.[30] Other workers in Marseilles stopped work to stop the war, and once more the strike was broken by Corsican gangsters and CIA money, this time with the addition of imported Italian scabs.[31]

The choice between communist militants and gangsters was as easy for the CIA in Marseilles as it had been for its predecessor organisation in New York. Control of the Marseilles waterfront, together with political influence in municipal affairs, left Corsican gangsters free to export heroin to the United States for the next 20 years.

The rise of the Golden Triangle

The decline of opium production in Turkey from the late 1960s and early 1970s deprived Marseilles' heroin laboratories of their supply of raw material. Together with a breakdown of discipline among the Corsican gangsters that resulted in heroin being sold in France rather than reserved for export, this eventually led to the demise of the French Connection.

European heroin laboratories didn't disappear completely, and nor did Corsican criminals or members of the Sicilian Mafia suddenly become unemployed. But there was a shift in the centre of illicit opium production to the Golden Triangle, the name given to the area that encompasses the hills of eastern Burma, the mountain crests of northern Thailand and the high plateaus of northern Laos. By the early 1970s it was producing around 70 per cent of the world's illicit opium.[32] The area also developed refineries that produced morphine base, and laboratories that went on to manufacture high-grade heroin.

Opium was being cultivated in the Golden Triangle area from at least the late 19th century, but until World War II annual production was relatively modest, as the state monopolies that supplied Indochina's opium shops relied on opium imported from India, China and Iran. During the war years, these sources of supply were cut off; this led to local production increasing from less than eight tons in 1940 to more than 60 tons in 1944. By then the region's addict population was more than 100,000.[33]

After the war, as opium smoking was made illegal and the state monopolies were being dismantled, the illicit market and opium production in the Golden Triangle steadily increased. In little more than a decade after the war ended, the area was producing 700 tons of raw opium annually, about half the world's illicit supply. By the late 1980s it was producing more than 3000 tons a year, and had also become the world's main supplier of heroin.[34] Towards the end of the century it was the world's number one producer of both opium and heroin.[35] In an ironic twist, it was the Golden Triangle that helped supply China's growing population of heroin addicts — officially one million in early 2004, but by some estimates as many as 12 million.[36]

The rise of the Golden Triangle to pre-eminence in world opium and heroin production was largely due to the way the Cold War unfolded in Asia and, in particular, how it went on to become a 'hot' war in Indochina.

In 1911, as the political fragmentation of China descended into chaos, the Manchu dynasty was overthrown. In the following year a new republic was declared, led by Sun Yat-sen and his nationalist party, the Kuomintang. The Kuomintang formed an alliance with the Chinese Communist Party and in 1925 began a military offensive from South China aimed at ousting the warlords in the north and uniting the country. Chiang Kai-shek had succeeded Sun Yat-sen as leader of the Kuomintang, and as his army approached Shanghai in 1927 the communist unions began a series of supportive strikes and demonstrations that resulted in a bloody confrontation with the opposition warlords. Chiang Kai-shek deliberately delayed his entry into Shanghai as the communists suffered heavy losses. After taking the city with the help of still-loyal communists, Chiang Kai-shek teamed up with the 'opium king' Tu Yueh-sheng, leader of the notorious Green Gang, in a massacre of his communist allies that became known as the 'white terror'.[37]

The Green Gang, together with the Chiu Chau triad syndicate, owed their prominence to the management of opium concessions for the British and French monopolies when Shanghai was opened up to them after the first Opium War. When the trade went underground, the two groups fought for control until Tu Yueh-sheng was able to broker a peace … and in the process become Shanghai's most influential gangster.[38] Tu's reward from a grateful Chiang Kai-shek for his part in the slaughter of Shanghai's communists was to be made a general in the Kuomintang Army. The Green Gang leader was thus able to ensure that the opium trade financed both the Kuomintang and his own ostentatious lifestyle.[39] When the Japanese invaded Manchuria in 1931, Tu showed his commitment to a perverse internationalism by supplying them with opium, which they then refined into heroin to help quell the northern populace.[40]

As World War II ended and the Cold War began, the United States provided large-scale aid and military assistance to Chiang Kai-shek; this went as far as co-opting the defeated Japanese forces still in China. In 1946 there were around 100,000 US military personnel in China, and between 1945 and 1949, US economic assistance to the Kuomintang of almost US$2 billion was complemented by the provision of a further US$1 billion's worth of military equipment.[41]

Despite this effort, Mao Tse-tung's communists prevailed and, in 1949, took control of the country. Chiang Kai-shek beat a hasty retreat to Taiwan, taking remnant Kuomintang forces with him — as well as the country's entire gold reserves, looted from the vaults of the Bank of China.[42] Tu Yueh-sheng, the Chiu Chau triads and the Green Gang departed to Hong Kong.[43]

But not all of the defeated Kuomintang forces fled to Taiwan. Several thousand crossed the border from China's Yunnan province to Burma's Shan states. From 1950 these forces were fed, organised and armed by the CIA in an attempt, more naïve and desperate than ambitious, to invade China and re-take the southern provinces from Mao's People's Liberation Army. Their incursions across the border were more an irritating insult to sovereignty than an imminent threat to the collapse of the new People's Republic, but for the Kuomintang, they were a decidedly more serious threat to life, limb and liberty. As casualties mounted they took up the less dangerous and considerably more profitable alternative of reorganising the Shan State's opium production.[44]

The evacuation of the remaining Kuomintang from Burma to Taiwan in 1953 following UN intervention proved something of a sham: between 5000 and 6000 stayed to further their interests in the opium business. They stayed until 1961, when a joint Burmese and Chinese military offensive drove them out, but they were only pushed as far as Laos and Thailand. From these new locations in the Golden Triangle it was business as usual, but better, when their activities expanded to embrace heroin as well as opium production.[45]

CIA support for and collaboration with the Kuomintang didn't mean that they entered into a joint venture in the opium business from which they directly profited. What it meant was a degree of financial autonomy for an ally that would, as a consequence, require correspondingly less CIA support, thus freeing up funds for more expansive operations. What it also undeniably meant was complicity in an illegal venture that was at its best hypocritical and morally bankrupt, and which would eventually contribute to rising levels of addiction among US troops abroad and citizens at home, all of whose interests the CIA was supposed to be protecting.

In comparison, the operation of the French intelligence agencies in the opium trade in Vietnam was much less subtle. Strapped for cash, they simply expropriated the trade. When the Japanese occupied French Indochina in 1941, it was not entirely without French opposition. But for the most part it was close to business as usual for the French in Vietnam. The Japanese left the French colonial administration intact, but beholden now to Tokyo rather than Paris. It was very much oppression as usual for the long-suffering Vietnamese, two million of whom the Japanese starved to death in 1944.[46]

Resistance to the Japanese was led by a coalition of communists, Catholics, Buddhists, small-businessmen and farmers, collectively known as the Vietminh.[47] At their head was the dissident communist Ho Chi Minh.[48] Ho Chi Minh's admiration for the United States as an anti-colonial power was evident in his adoption of the US Declaration of Independence principles of equality and inalienable rights when he proclaimed the Democratic Republic of Vietnam in Hanoi in September 1945, after the Japanese surrender to the Allies.[49] The OSS had also worked in Vietnam against the Japanese, and many of them thought that the US should back Ho after the Japanese surrender.

In Saigon the Vietminh had already formed an administration and begun to celebrate their new role in government the previous month.[50] The French, however, had a different view of the future shape of Vietnam following the Japanese defeat, to which they had contributed so little. The legacy of Napoleon III would not be as easily given to Vietnamese nationalism as it had been to Japanese imperialism. Less than a month after the Saigon celebrations, a company of French infantry, together with 1400 Ghurkhas from the 20th Indian Division, under the command of Major-General Douglas Gracey, were airlifted into the city from Burma. After re-arming the surrendered Japanese troops they forced the Vietminh withdrawal from Saigon.[51] The British Ghurkhas withdrew and the Japanese were repatriated as reinforcements arrived from France to continue a war that, for them, would last until 1954.

The French attempt to re-establish control of Vietnam was long on colonial ambition but short on financial and military support. To combat these deficiencies, the French intelligence organisation, Service de Documentation Exterieure et du Contre-Espionage (SDECE) devised a strategy of recruiting mercenaries from among the hill tribes in the north and the criminal gangs in the south, and financing both the recruiting and the subsequent fighting with the profits of the opium trade.

The fact that the French colonial administration abolished the state opium monopoly in 1946 and was thereafter seriously attempting to wean the region's addicts off opium presented no moral or legal dilemmas. Rather, it was a market opportunity for the SDECE, as they matched supply with demand.

The northern mercenary force of predominantly Hmong tribes that were recruited was 40,000 strong by 1954, and it was their opium that the SDECE bought and then transported in French military DC-3 planes to the airbase at Cap Saint Jacques near Saigon. From here it was processed and retailed by the Saigon mercenaries, who were recruited from a criminal gang known as the Binh Xuyen.[52]

The Hmong, at the wholesale end, were paid handsomely for their raw opium, and the Binh Xuyen, at the retail end, were pleased with the profits they shared with French intelligence. The latter, in turn, were more than pleased that they were now able to finance an operation which saw the Vietminh harassed by mercenaries in the north and suppressed by the French in Saigon and its surrounds in the south. There was even a surplus available for sale to the Chinese syndicates, who exported it to Hong Kong, and the Corsicans, who exported it to Marseilles.

But not all the Hmong tribes were happy with their share of the opium trade. Those in the northwest of Vietnam considered themselves exploited by the French-appointed regional leader, who was from a minority tribe and who enriched himself and his supporters by securing their opium at below market prices. As a result, these disaffected Hmong sided with the Vietminh and gave them significant logistical support, which helped them defeat the French in the decisive battle at Dien Bien Phu in May 1954.[53]

A peace was negotiated in Geneva soon after Dien Bien Phu, by the 'great powers' — Britain, France, the United States and the USSR. Under its terms the French were to cease hostilities and withdraw to the south of the country for two years, at which time national elections would take place, uniting the country under one government. With something like 80 per cent support, Ho Chi Minh was destined to become the leader of Vietnam in the July 1956 elections. He never did, though, because the elections were never held. The United States simply couldn't accept a communist-led Vietnam bordering a communist China that they had just fought to a bloody draw as the Cold War erupted into a hot war in Korea. So they created a new country called South Vietnam and stepped into the breach vacated by France.[54] After the French withdrew, the United States set up what was in effect a puppet regime headed by Ngo Dinh Diem, who had spent the previous four years in the safety of catholic seminaries in New Jersey and New York.[55]

The South Vietnamese armed forces battled the Vietminh (who in 1960 re-formed as the Front for the Liberation of South Vietnam, or NLF) for the next 20 years, until Saigon fell on 30 April 1975. Assisted first by US military 'advisers', they were ultimately buttressed by 500,000 US troops. With the help of the CIA — under the direction of Edward Lansdale, whose activities in Vietnam were later portrayed in *The Quiet American*, by Graham Greene, and *The Ugly American*, by William J Lederer and Eugene Burdick, they undertook a campaign of military and psychological warfare that, among other things, encouraged migration of Vietnamese from the north to the south, infiltrated paramilitary forces in the north, contaminated the oil supply of the bus company in Hanoi and sabotaged railways — Diem turned South Vietnam into a police state,[56] while his brother and chief adviser, Ngo Dinh Nhu, resuscitated the opium business, with the help of Corsican gangsters, in order to finance it.[57]

Opium from Laos was transported to Saigon courtesy of a unit of the South Vietnamese Air Force led by the then Colonel Nguyen Cao Ky. After Diem and his brother were murdered in a US-backed coup — the United States was frustrated with their corrupt rule, which included opium dealing, and their inability to rally the people in the fight against the communists, and so gave their full support to a group of Vietnamese generals to launch a coup in November 1963 — Ky became an air vice-marshall and both premier and vice president of South Vietnam. The South Vietnamese Air Force continued ferrying opium and competed with the country's army, navy, customs officials, politicians and the national police for control of the trade.[58]

There are two enduring images of the Vietnam War that remind us of its brutality. One is of a little girl fleeing a US napalm attack, her face framed in terror; the other is of a suspected NLF member being shot through the head on a Saigon street by the chief of national police, General Nguyen Ngoc Loan. When not carrying out summary executions, Loan's main job was to organise the opium business in Saigon on Ky's behalf. Following Ky's fall from favour — he was involved in a power struggle with Thieu which he lost, largely because his organisation, which was built on opium profits, was decimated during the Tet offensive — this task was taken over by General Dang Van Quang on behalf of the country's president, Nguyen Van Thieu.

From late 1969, Hong Kong chemists associated with the Chiu Chau syndicate began refining opium into no. 4 heroin, which was up to 99 per cent pure, in the Golden Triangle. Like opium, it soon found its way to US troops, and within 18 months it was estimated that between 10 and 15 per cent of them were using it. Later estimates went as high as 34 per cent.[59]

These troops took the habit back home with them, and some of them became involved in the trade itself. By this time, the US addict population had climbed to 500,000 and Australia was seeing the start of its own heroin problem. By the time the war was over, Vietnam lay in ruins, and Golden Triangle heroin was being exported all around the world.

Large amounts came through Thailand, where a long tradition of corruption among the military and police nurtured the narcotics trade. Bangkok was a major export centre. In Laos, the CIA created a clandestine army of 40,000 Hmong fighters, and generously allowed the Hmong commander, General Vang Pao, to use the CIA airline Air America to transport opium to the region's heroin refineries. One of the biggest opium entrepreneurs in Laos was the ex-head of the army, General Ouane Rattikone; the level of corruption in the country was illustrated by the attempt by the Laotian ambassador, Prince Sopsaianna, to smuggle 60 kilograms of heroin into France in 1971 (Sopsaianna returned to Laos after the matter was covered up, and France refused to recognise his diplomatic credentials).[60]

By the mid-1970s, the United States' Cold War policy of 'containing communism', spearheaded by the CIA, had contributed to an unprecedented worldwide heroin problem. Time to take stock and even for some collective hand-wringing at Langley, one might have thought. Well, not quite. When the pre-eminent historian of the period, Alfred W McCoy, was about to publish his exposé of heroin politics in Southeast Asia, the CIA said that it posed a national security threat and demanded that the publisher cancel the contract. The publisher refused to do so. McCoy himself was subjected to a period of harassment that included the tapping of his phone. The CIA placated the US Congress by promising an internal review of the charges McCoy had detailed. The report has never been released in its entirety, but what was released proclaimed the CIA's innocence of any charge of complicity in the opium business.[61] It was a denial reminiscent of that issued a century earlier by the British government concerning their complicity in the opium trade with China.

The rise of the Golden Crescent

Barely two years after the fall of Saigon, a military dictatorship headed by General Zia-ul-Haq seized power in Pakistan with US approval. The country's elected leader, Zulfikar Ali Bhutto, was imprisoned and later executed, and Islamic fundamentalism was recruited into brutal government service.[62] The Cold War was by now 30 years old, and the last major conflict between the United States and the USSR was under way in the Golden Crescent. Pakistan became the base for the US-backed opposition to the pro-Soviet government of Afghanistan that ruled the country before the Soviet invasion of December 1979.

Pakistan went from a country that was barred from receiving US aid because of its nuclear development program — this ban was imposed unilaterally by President Carter in April 1979, and removed in December the same year — to the largest US aid recipient country in the world after Israel and Egypt.[63] It also went from a country with fewer than 5000 heroin addicts in the early 1980s to one with more than 1.6 million in 1996.[64]

The war in Afghanistan was financed by US dollars in the form of direct US aid, much of it channelled by the CIA through the Pakistan intelligence organisation Inter Services Intelligence (ISI), and in dollars that were the profits of heroin sales. By 1981, just three years after General Zia seized power, heroin from Afghanistan and Pakistan had captured 60 per cent of both the western European and US markets.[65]

The US and Pakistan-backed forces fighting the Soviets and their supporters on the ground in Afghanistan were headed by a group of tribal warlords who had varying degrees of influence in various parts of the country. When not engaged in hostilities against a common enemy, they were often engaged in hostilities among themselves. Included among them were those who controlled Afghanistan's poppy production and operated heroin refineries on the border between Afghanistan and Pakistan. The hundreds of refineries in Pakistan itself were controlled by a corrupt elite within the Pakistani political, military and intelligence apparatus. ISI's man in Afghanistan was Gulbuddin Hekmatyar, a heroin merchant who led a small organisation called Hezbi-i Islam and whose contribution to the struggle included the urging of his followers to throw acid in the faces of women refusing to wear the veil.[66] Thanks to CIA funding, Hezbi-i Islam became the largest of the warring groups in Afghanistan and Hekmatyar the most prominent heroin merchant.[67]

From the start of General Zia's dictatorship in 1977 until the Soviet withdrawal from Afghanistan — its equivalent of Vietnam — in 1989, the armies of the warlords in Afghanistan were supplemented by religious Muslim students trained in Pakistan. Some 2500 religious boarding schools (*madrasas*) were established in Pakistan; they attracted the children of Afghani refugees and Pakistani peasants. The curriculum was intended to produce fundamentalist fanatics, and included training provided by the ISI in weapons and bomb-making techniques.

The better performing students, known as *taliban*, went on to receive further specialist instruction before being sent back into Afghanistan as holy war warriors.[68]

They were assisted by other fundamentalist fighters recruited from around the world, including Osama bin Laden, who was part of the contingent contributed by Saudi Arabia. Following the Soviet withdrawal in 1989, the Afghan warlords fought among themselves for control of the country and its opium crop and heroin-producing facilities. Unable to secure victory for Hekmatyar, the Pakistan military switched its support to the Taliban movement that had emerged from the madrasas. They eventually gained the upper hand and imposed a misogynist brand of religious terror under the leadership of Mullah Omar. Poppy production continued apace, unaffected by the agreement that the Taliban came to with the United States in 2000 to eradicate production in the areas under their control in return for US$43 million. This merely handed control of the industry to the rival Northern Alliance, for whom the Russian Mafia provided an export facilitation scheme.[69] Taliban extremism was condemned throughout the region, from Cairo to Qom, by Sunni and Shia clerics alike.[70] US condemnation began the day after 11 September 2001.

After the US-led invasion that followed the atrocities in New York and Washington, the Taliban were deposed and Osama bin Laden and his al-Qaeda forces were dispersed. Hamid Karzai became the interim leader of Afghanistan and was confirmed as president in the October 2004 elections. But outside Kabul, the real power is in the hands of warlords, who still control the heroin trade and now hold influential positions in the central government. More than 60 per cent of the Afghan economy is accounted for by drug exports. The industry employs 2.3 million people and now produces 87 per cent of the world's heroin. Meanwhile, Osama bin Laden is still at large, with recent attempts to capture him centred on advertisements that air on

Pakistani television. This strategy doesn't seem to take into account the fact that the mountain regions that are his likely place of refuge (and the likely source of information as to his precise whereabouts) are unable to receive television broadcasts because they lack electricity.[71]

As these events were unfolding in Afghanistan, Pakistan's nuclear development program, which had once caused the United States to withdraw its aid to the country, had progressed to the point where in 1998 it was able to test explosive devices. Dr Abdul Qadeer Khan, the head of the nuclear program, was said to be personally responsible for assisting Libya, Iran and North Korea to develop their nuclear programs. For his sins of commission he was pardoned by the Pakistani government.

Cocaine and the Contras

Not content with pursuing Cold War policies that led to an increase in heroin consumption at home and elsewhere, the US intelligence apparatus managed to turn its hand to cocaine as well.

In what came to be known as the Iran-Contra affair, first revealed in the Lebanese media in November 1986, a scheme was hatched in the White House to secretly sell US weapons to Iran in the hope that the government of that country would then assist in freeing US hostages held in Lebanon. The profits from the enterprise would then be directed to the Contras, a right-wing group of Nicaraguans attempting to overthrow the left-wing government headed by Sandinista commander Daniel Ortega, who was elected president in 1984. The one problem in aiding the Contras' activity was that it was illegal. From 1982 the US Congress had first limited and then expressly prohibited the appropriation of funds to undermine the Nicaraguan government.[72]

Lieutenant-Colonel Oliver North, a deputy of the White House National Security Council, was convicted for his part in organising the Iran-Contra affair in 1989 but the conviction didn't survive appeal. Caspar Weinberger, the US Secretary of Defense who was indicted for perjury and obstruction of justice over the affair, had the good fortune to be pardoned by President George Bush before his case came to trial. President at the time of the scandal, Ronald Reagan (Bush was vice president), subsequently denied any knowledge of the fact that profits from the arms sales to Iran were going to the Contras. This was despite admitting to secretly authorising the sales[73] and telling his national security advisor, Robert McFarlane, that the Contras had to be supported at all costs.[74] To be strenuously fair to Reagan, he may have simply forgotten, given that he was later diagnosed with Alzheimer's disease, named after the German psychiatrist and neuropathologist Alois Alzheimer, who first described it in 1906.

Whatever else might be said about the CIA and the various other arms of the US defence and intelligence networks, it is rarely claimed that they lack state funding. More often than not they are accused of having more money than intelligence. Funding for the Contras' activities from 1983 to late 1986 seems to be the exception. The amendments to the Defense Appropriations Bill restricting and then prohibiting US government funds being used to assist the Contras were introduced into the House of Representatives by Edward Boland from Massachusetts and were effective from fiscal year 1983. The so-called Boland amendment expired on 17 October 1986. On that date the CIA was free to use its budget allocation, which was US$100 million, to assist the Contras, which it duly did; in contrast, the total funding for the three years 1982, 1983 and 1984 amounted to just US$64 million. In 1985, as a consequence of the CIA's illegal mining of Nicaraguan ports, the funding allocation was zero.[75] The years from 1983 to 1986 were unusually lean years for the US security and intelligence services. They were in a position not dissimilar to that of the

French intelligence service in Vietnam in the late 1940s. Their solution also bore some striking similarities.

When the Nicaraguan dictator Anastasio Somoza was deposed by the Sandinistas in 1979, the Carter administration provided support to an opposition organisation initially known as the Fuerza Democratico Nicaraguense (FDN). It consisted of members of the former National Guard and other cronies of Somoza and was formally established in 1981 across the border from Nicaragua in Honduras, with CIA seed-funding.[76] The Contras, as they came to be known, would go on, with US assistance, to establish supply bases in neighbouring El Salvador and Costa Rica as well. Honduras, though, was particularly well suited as a base for illegal operations. In 1978 a military coup financed by drug profits had installed a Somoza supporter, General Policarpo Paz Garcia, as head of a ruling junta, and the Honduran military and intelligence services had become involved in the Colombian drug traffic. From the time it became a base for the Contras, it also had a US ambassador, John Negroponte, who declined to report to Congress human rights violations of the Honduran military that would ordinarily have resulted in a cessation of US military aid.[77]

Before Oliver North became involved with the Contras, they were financing their operations (and themselves) through cocaine that emanated from the Medellin cartel in Colombia and was smuggled into the United States. Colombian cocaine was peddled in California by US-resident Nicaraguan Contra supporters from 1981 on, and some of the profits were sent to the Contras in Honduras. In 1982, cheap cocaine from the same source began finding its way into South Central Los Angeles and being turned into crack, which resulted in the 'epidemic' of the 1980s.[78] These illicit cocaine profits supplemented official US aid during 1982 and 1983. Benefits of the Iran venture notwithstanding, cocaine profits were a significant source of income for the Contras during the drought years of US aid, which lasted until 1986. It was during this period that North recruited retired air force general Richard Secord, who teamed up with his ex-CIA comrade from Laos, Thomas Clines, to organise funds for the Contras.[79]

The logistics of the arms-for-cocaine operation were relatively simple. Air transport would be hired to take weapons and ammunition from various locations in the United States to Contra bases in Honduras, El Salvador and Costa Rica. For the return flight to the United States the freight would be Colombian cocaine. Sold throughout the United States, the cocaine then provided the finance for the purchase of further arms, allowing the cycle to begin again. All that was needed was for the authorities to look the other way while this was going on. The CIA made sure that this occurred: the outgoing arms shipments and the incoming freight were both protected.[80] Oliver North's own records reveal knowledge of flights to and from New Orleans being used to ship both arms and drugs, and on one occasion he was told by Richard Secord of a single arms procurement worth US$14 million being financed entirely by drugs.[81]

Senator John Kerry of Massachusetts began a congressional investigation into the links between the Contra operations and cocaine trafficking in 1986. The report was published in late 1988 and concluded that:

Individuals who provided support for the Contras were involved in drug trafficking. The supply network of the Contras was used by drug trafficking organisations, and elements of the Contras themselves received financial and material assistance from drug traffickers.

And what were the various authorities doing while this was going on? According to Senator Kerry, 'US officials in Central America failed to address the drug issue for fear of jeopardising the war effort against Nicaragua.'[82]

From 1986 on, cocaine profits ceased to be crucial in providing financial support for the Contras. In February 1990 the Sandinistas were voted out of office. Was it simply coincidental that Oscar Danilo Blandon, who looked after the wholesale side of the Contras' cocaine business, wasn't the subject of serious police attention until after official US aid to the Contras was resumed?[83] In 1991 he was arrested, and he was later convicted of cocaine trafficking. Despite a life sentence and a US$4 million fine being called for by the prosecution, he received a four-year term. He was freed after just over two years, in return for becoming an informant.[84] The year that Blandon was arrested was also the year that the bank the US National Security Council used to launder money in the Iran-Contra affair — the CIA also used it to launder money for its Afghanistan operation — went belly up. When the Bank of Credit and Commerce International (BCCI) was shut down by the governors of the Bank of England for fraudulent activity in July 1991, some US$9.5 billion went missing.[85]

The effect of the Contras' cocaine trafficking in the United States was dramatic. Between 1982 and 1985, cocaine imports increased by 50 per cent and the number of users increased by 38 per cent, reaching almost 6 million.[86] Cocaine was generating sales of US$30 billion a year. The Medellin cartel alone was selling some US$10 billion worth of cocaine; in 1988, two of its principals, Pablo Escobar and Jorge Ochoa, made it to the *Forbes* magazine list of the world's richest men.[87]

The CIA was never called to account for its part in flooding US cities with cocaine, but it did come in for unprecedented criticism for its failure to prevent the September 11 attacks in 2001. It came in for even more criticism for supplying the false intelligence that Iraq had weapons of mass destruction, which was used to justify the second Iraq War. A US Senate investigation described the claims as a 'global intelligence failure', and one of its authors, Senator Jay Rockefeller, said that had the claims been known to be false at the time, Congress would not have authorised the war.[88] As part of the White House response to this criticism, President George W Bush established the office of Director of National Intelligence. The director is vested with the authority to control the budgets of all of the US intelligence agencies, provide daily briefings to the Oval Office and ensure that there is a single, coherent intelligence strategy. President George W Bush nominated the man who had been US Ambassador to Honduras from 1981 to 1985, John Negroponte, as the inaugral director.

9
Australia's heroin market

In 1966 a young and enterprising NSW Special Branch police officer, John Wesley Egan, decided to go into the heroin business. The heroin would come from the Chiu Chau triads in Hong Kong and be sold to Mafia operatives in New York with whom Egan had contact through a former CIA employee he had become acquainted with through his work. Egan was able to persuade several other NSW police officers to join in the venture, and in a mere six months they managed to land US$22.5 million worth of heroin in New York. The operation was essentially a freelance courier business. Egan organised duplicate passports for couriers, who would fly from Sydney to Hong Kong to pick up the heroin and then enter New York from London or other European cities, disguising their Hong Kong stopover. The heroin was concealed in specially designed corsets or vests which earned Egan's crew the nickname the Corset Gang. Egan made a lot of money in a very short period ... before being sentenced to eight years in a US prison.[1]

One of the significant things that the Corset Gang's operation reveals is the state of the world heroin market in 1966. It would have been much simpler and less risky to have sold the heroin in Europe, but in the mid-1960s there was insufficient demand there. It would have been easier still to import the heroin directly into Australia, but there was no demand there either. Of the advanced economies, it was only in the United States that demand was strong enough to make heroin trafficking profitable. Within a decade this would change dramatically: by the late 1970s Sydney alone, according to some estimates, would have as many as 10,000 heroin addicts.

Heroin use wasn't unknown in Australia in 1966. In the previous year there had been the first 'sensational' case of heroin use, involving a 19-year-old prostitute in Sydney's Kings Cross. The fact that the person convicted of selling her the drug was of Chinese origin is consistent with the fact that until then the only source of heroin in Australia was criminal elements within the Chinese community.[2] From the time of Prohibition, opium had trickled into Australia to service the small market of Chinese smokers. The supply invariably came from Chinese seamen working on ships that traded with both Australia and the west coast of the United States. As heroin replaced opium in ports of origin such as Hong Kong during the 1950s and early 1960s, small amounts of the drug found their way into the Chinese communities of Sydney and Melbourne. From the early 1960s some of this heroin was sold in the red light districts of Sydney's Kings Cross and Melbourne's St Kilda.[3] Despite the odd front-page sensation, though, heroin use was an occasional experience confined to a limited few.

This changed in 1970, assisted in part at least by a patriotic promotion that the US airline Pan American World Airways had begun in early 1966. Pan Am thought it would be a good idea to give US servicemen in Vietnam a week-long holiday at one of several regional destinations — Bangkok, Hong Kong, Manila, Taiwan or Sydney. Hundreds of thousands of US troops chose Sydney for their R & R trips, and they brought their money and their drugs with them. The Kings Cross area was where most spent their time and the local economy boomed as strip clubs, brothels, restaurants and bars such as the Bourbon and Beefsteak and the Texas Tavern tended to their travel needs. When they first arrived they brought high-grade cannabis, which the locals acquired a taste for. From around 1970, they brought the heroin that they had acquired a taste for in Vietnam. By 1972, when R & R ceased, there were several hundred addicts in Sydney. The market for heroin had been established and would continue to expand.[4]

Pan Am and US servicemen played their part, but insofar as these things are possible to predict, it is likely that Australia would have developed a heroin market, at the very least on a limited scale, without their assistance. Compared with Europe or the United States, Australia is a small market for consumer goods, but a nicely profitable one. Australians have demonstrated a very healthy appetite for everything from motor vehicles to mobile phones. And, of course, when it comes to drug consumption of almost any description, Australians are generally hard to beat.

Another important element that is needed to sustain an illicit market like heroin is a culture of organised criminal activity, and here too Australia has a good pedigree. Sly-grog shops and SP bookmaking, with the corruption of politicians and police that go with them, have a long history. The illicit abortion racket also provided opportunities for the criminal entrepreneur, as did poker machine fraud and illegal casino operations, though the latter two were mainly confined to New South Wales. The criminals involved in these activities were Australians of Anglo-Irish extraction, plus some of a criminal bent from southern Italy, who had arrived in the large waves of postwar immigration. Later on a distinct criminal element would emerge from the South Vietnamese and Lebanese communities.

By the late 1960s Australia had all the basic elements necessary for the growth of a heroin market. As in many other advanced economies, a drug subculture had emerged, with people dabbling in speed, LSD and cannabis. Some in Sydney, and fewer in Melbourne, had developed a taste for heroin by the early 1970s, but the factors that led to rapid market growth were the development of a mass market for cannabis, which was taken over by criminals, and the crackdown on heroin entering the United States from the Golden Triangle.[5]

The local supply of cannabis — from backyard gardens, small crops in the bush and rather larger crops produced in alternative communities — that became available from the early 1970s failed to keep pace with growing demand. Operators of the homegrown cannabis industry were part-time gardeners who tended to be customer focused and operate on small profit margins. For $100 each, three customers could jointly purchase a weighed half-kilo of good-quality cannabis heads, enough to last the average consumer several months. It was an amount so bulky that it had to be delivered in an industrial-size garbage bag.

Word-of-mouth advertising proved particularly powerful, which meant that one of the effects of the way the cannabis cottage industry worked was increased demand. However, no amount of new age incantation could alter nature's gentle ways. Ploughing prodigious amounts of chemicals into the backyard plot didn't make the plants grow any faster. Productivity increases would have to await the development of hydroponics. In the interim, demand had to be supplied by imports and industrially organised domestic production. This obviously required significant amounts of investment capital and the other resources that are necessary to sustain complex illegal operations. The homegrown and hippie produce was muscled aside as organised criminal groups began to take control of the industry.

Although hashish was imported from Lebanon and, much less frequently, from Durban in South Africa, the main source of imported cannabis was Thailand. The Thais produced a particularly potent variety of the plant. Compressed and fastened around small pieces of bamboo, it was ideally suited for export. Millions of these buddha sticks appeared on the Australian market throughout the 1970s, with Sydney being the principal importing port. Increasing amounts of heroin were being imported at the same time, sometimes by the same people. Another former NSW policeman, ex-Detective Sergeant Murray Stewart Riley, was one of those engaged in diversified drug importing. He received a 10-year sentence in 1978 for his part in the importation of 4.5 tonnes of buddha sticks from Bangkok, and according to two official inquiries he was involved in importing heroin from the same region on six different occasions during 1976 and 1977.[6] Riley was also prominent in the Sydney criminal scene, which had strengthened its international connections by forging links with organised crime figures in the United States that led back to the legendary Meyer Lansky.[7]

Large-scale domestic cannabis production began in the early 1970s on plantations scattered throughout the eastern states, ranging in size from 10–50 hectares (around 25–125 acres).[8] It was most conspicuous in the Riverina district of New South Wales, centred on the town of Griffith. Thanks to irrigation from the Murrumbidgee River, the area around Griffith produces most of Australia's rice crop and a significant amount of its citrus and stone fruit. It produces something like a quarter of Australia's wine grapes, so there are also a number of wineries, including those of McWilliams, Orlando and De Bortoli. From 1971 it became the centre of Australia's cannabis production, thanks to the organising capacity of Robert Trimbole and Antonio Sergi, both of whom were later identified by a royal commission as leaders of a group known as L'Onorata, the Honourable Society.[9] Almost equidistant from Melbourne and Sydney, Griffith was ideally placed to service both markets, and over the next six years production and profits soared. Trimbole did particularly well. Though he was declared bankrupt in 1968, by the early 1970s he had managed to purchase a supermarket in Sydney and a clothing store in Griffith.[10] But the activities and the newfound wealth of the cannabis farmers of Italian descent (Calabrians had first settled in the area in the early 1920s) were difficult to disguise in a small town like Griffith.

Donald Bruce Mackay, manager of a furniture business in Griffith and prominent Liberal Party member, was the most notable public critic of the local cannabis trade and those he thought were caught up in its web of corruption. In late 1975 he informed the Sydney Drug Squad, rather than local police, of a 21.5 hectare (53 acre) cannabis plantation. This resulted in a number of arrests. In July 1977 Mackay disappeared, presumed murdered on the instructions of Trimbole, who later fled the country. The resultant furore led immediately to two royal commissions on drug trafficking and a major police drive aimed at eradicating large-scale cannabis production throughout the country.[11] What followed was a cannabis drought, the effects of which were felt widely, due to the recent growth of the market. In the normal course of market operations the local supply problem would have been eased by imports, but the importers now faced an increasing risk due to the crackdown, so they deleted cannabis from their manifests and increased the supply and promotion of what was now a less risky and more profitable product: heroin.

During this period the Southeast Asian syndicates were having problems accessing the US market (the number of users had declined from 500,000 in the late 1960s to 200,000 in the mid-1970s),[12] so they had begun to target the Australian and European markets that had been unavailable to them in the mid-1960s.[13] One of the more conspicuous of the heroin importers was the ruthless Mr Asia syndicate, led by Christopher Martin Johnstone and Terrence John Clark. Between 1976 and 1979, apparently untroubled by much police attention, they managed to import 85 kilograms of the product. Clark, who was also responsible for several murders, was an associate of Robert Trimbole and demonstrated that there is little honour among heroin wholesalers — he was convicted of Johnstone's murder in the United Kingdom in 1981.[14]

The cannabis drought led to a massive increase in price and a sharp decrease in quality. Heroin, in contrast, stayed at a steady price and was of superior quality — far better than the heroin that consumers in the United States, for example, were used to. The heroin sold in Australia had a purity level of some 22 per cent; that in United States ranged between 3 and 6 per cent.[15] It became the drug of availability rather than choice because of the ease with which supply could be manipulated in an illicit market. As an informed commentator said of similar circumstances in the United States some years earlier, 'The government line is that the use of marijuana leads to more dangerous drugs. The fact is that the lack of marijuana leads to more dangerous drugs.'[16]

Two other factors contributed to the rise in heroin use. On the supply side, decisions by organised criminal groups in New South Wales to enter into or expand their activities in the highly profitable heroin trade were made easier because profits from existing ventures were being squeezed. United States R & R revenue dried up in 1972, then revenue from poker machine and other licensed club fraud also dried up after exposure by the Moffitt Royal Commission. The abortion racket collapsed after the procedure was effectively legalised in 1974, and illegal casinos were being closed down from 1977.[17] The elimination of SP bookmaking would eventually follow. In the early 1970s the market for heroin was dominated by risk-taking middle-class youth. From the mid-1970s, overall rates of unemployment began to rise sharply and the youth labour market collapsed. By 1979, a third of all unemployed were aged between 15 and 19.[18] A growing number of unemployed youth in the western suburbs of Sydney and Melbourne became heroin users[19] and as unemployment spread to other capitals and regional areas, so too did heroin use.

Nugan Hand

The extraordinary affair of the Nugan Hand Bank demonstrates the extent of corruption in the 1970s that allowed the heroin trade to flourish.

In early February 1978, on the strength of a claimed turnover of $1 billion, the *Australian Financial Review* reported that 'at this sort of growth rate Nugan Hand will soon be bigger than BHP'.[20] Two years later, on 27 January 1980, one of the group's two founders, Frank Nugan, was found dead near Lithgow in New South Wales from a gunshot wound to the head, apparently administered by his own hand; at the same time, the other founder of the group, Michael Hand, was busy shredding documents in the bank's Sydney office, documents that included 'files identifying clients regarded as sensitive'.[21] By June 1980 Nugan Hand Ltd was in liquidation, with around $15 million identified as being owed to creditors, and Michael Hand had fled to the United States, never to be seen or heard of again.[22]

As some of the activities of the Nugan Hand group unfolded, following its collapse and the appointment of a royal commission of inquiry, numerous stories ran in Australian and US print media about the connection between Nugan Hand and the CIA.[23] Allegations regarding drugs and arms trafficking were also made.

Frank Nugan and Michael Hand were not bankers, and they employed a number of prominent former US military personnel, who also lacked banking experience. The bank's president was Admiral Earl Preston Yates, who was deputy chief of staff, US Pacific Command during the final US withdrawal from Vietnam.[24] General Edwin Fahey Black, the group's representative in Hawaii, commanded the US troops in Thailand during the Vietnam War, having previously served with the National Security Council and the OSS, the predecessor organisation to the CIA. Lieutenant-General Leroy Joseph Manor, who worked for the Nugan Hand Bank in the Philippines, was also a Vietnam veteran, and was at one time chief of staff of the Pacific Command. General Erle Cocke, a World War II veteran and former brigadier general of the Georgia National Guard, was engaged as a consultant for the group in Washington.[25]

Two other people employed by the group had clear CIA connections. Walter Joseph McDonald worked for the CIA from 1952 to 1979, including a period as deputy director, and thereafter was a 'special adviser' to Nugan Hand, opening an office for the group in Annapolis, Maryland.[26] William Egan Colby was the US Ambassador to Vietnam from 1968 to 1971, and was executive director, then director of the CIA from 1973 to 1976. Introduced to Frank Nugan and Michael Hand by Walter McDonald, Colby was retained by the group to provide legal advice on taxation matters and on a refugee resettlement program in the Turks and Cacios Islands in the Caribbean.[27] Conveniently located to take advantage of the Colombian cocaine trade (the 'sinister option' that occurred to the Commonwealth–NSW Joint Task Force on Drug Trafficking), these islands were the intended new home for 3000 Hmong tribesmen living in Thai refugee camps.[28] Colby described Michael Hand as 'a very energetic, good American fighting man now making a life in business'. His card, on which were written the dates when he would be available to meet Frank Nugan in Hong Kong or Singapore in March of 1980, was found in Frank Nugan's possession after his death.[29]

To complete the CIA connection, Richard Secord had a business relationship with the Nugan Hand Bank,[30] and the bank's representative in Saudi Arabia, Bernie Houghton, had a business relationship with two former high-ranking CIA officers,

Ted Shackley and Thomas Clines, former chief and deputy chief respectively of the CIA station in Vientiane in the mid-1960s.[31] Houghton also held a series of business meetings in Geneva with Edwin P Wilson, another ex-CIA operative, in an effort to convert Libyan letters of credit to the tune of US$22 million into a Nugan Hand Bank loan. The money was supposedly to enable Wilson to finance a supply of Korean-made uniforms to Libya. Wilson managed to raise the finance elsewhere and in 1982 was sentenced to life imprisonment in the United States for illegal arms sales to Libya. In the same year Clines was indicted for defrauding the US government of US$8 million. He was luckier than Wilson, escaping with a US$10,000 fine and a US$3 million restitution payment.[32]

It is probable that the intimate details of Nugan Hand's relationship with US intelligence services will never see the light of day. The CIA is unlikely to reveal what it knows of the matter and the Nugan Hand principals who knew are either dead or have disappeared. The royal commission that was set up to inquire into the activities of Nugan Hand seemed a little bemused that such a 'powerful agency of the United States Government' would have dealings with the 'inept individuals' who ran the Nugan Hand group.

Those who ran Nugan Hand Ltd were not so much inept as crooked, and the operation that they ran was a sham from the start. Shortly after the company was incorporated in July 1973, its accounts showed a paid-up share capital of $1,000,005. The shares were held by Frank Nugan and Michael Hand, 'paid' for with cheques drawn by Frank Nugan totalling $1 million. The company then 'repaid' Frank Nugan $999,900. When these cheques were passed around the boardroom table there was no money to cover them in the relevant accounts. All this created the illusion that the company was worth $1 million, when in fact its paid-up share capital throughout its life amounted to just $105 and it was at all times insolvent.[33]

The apparent success of the company was attributed by the royal commission to 'sheer fortuity'.[34] They were certainly fortunate in acquiring the services of a money market manager who was skilful enough to trade without any money. Using his market contacts he managed to trade on short-term extended credit each day, racking up sales of $2.4 million that resulted in a trading loss of $18,373, but which nevertheless gave the impression of a company doing significant business in its early days.[35] Nugan Hand was also said to be 'purely fortuitous' in finding auditors who were willing to certify accounts without checking them, and later, in obtaining a banking licence.[36]

The company obtained a banking licence in the Cayman Islands — well known as a tax haven — in 1976, after it had been refused a licence in Panama. The newly established bank was then able to collect deposits, which were used to pay for the inflated expenses and ostentatious lifestyle of its principals. It also enabled the group to establish offices around the world and go into the heroin trade. One of the offices it established (a helpful suggestion from Murray Stewart Riley) was in the heart of the Golden Triangle in Chiang Mai. Its principal purpose, according to the employee who set it up, was to attract deposits from those involved in the drug-trafficking trade; these were said to have been Michael Hand's instructions. It was apparently not too inconvenienced by its location next door to the US Drug Enforcement Agency.[37]

The company was also fortunate in obtaining the services of Bernie Houghton, a Texan who had worked in Saigon and Bangkok between 1964 and 1967 — in the construction business, he said.[38] According to the Joint Task Force on Drug Trafficking, the intelligence community and others, he had traded in anything that came along, including, but not limited to, opium.[39] Houghton arrived in Sydney in 1967 and opened the Bourbon and Beefsteak bar and restaurant in Kings Cross. The following year he purchased shares in a company that owned a private hotel in the area; this later became the Texas Tavern. Later on still he was a member of a partnership that bought the Aquatic Club in Kings Cross. In yet another partnership — this one including Sir Paul Strasser, a lawyer from Hungary who migrated to Australia in 1948, became a property developer and was knighted by Sir Robert Askin, then the premier of New South Wales — in 1973, he opened the Sydney restaurant Harpoon Harry's.[40]

It was at Houghton's Bourbon and Beefsteak and Texas Tavern that a good number of those associated with Nugan Hand first met.[41] Michael Hand, like many other US servicemen on R & R in the late 1960s, was a frequent visitor to the Bourbon and Beefsteak.[42] Houghton was good enough to find Hand his first job in Australia, with Sir Paul Strasser's Parkes Development, and Hand later repaid the favour by lending Houghton significant amounts of money — interest free and without security.[43] Admiral Earl Preston Yates was a guest of Houghton's at the Bourbon and Beefsteak on a number of occasions from 1972. Other guests included such luminaries as the Australian head of the CIA, John D Walker, Sir Robert Askin and Abe Saffron, at the time a prominent Kings Cross nightclub owner.[44] Houghton introduced Admiral Yates to 'several political and financial figures in the Sydney area', including Frank Nugan and Michael Hand, who made him an 'attractive offer' to work for them. Admiral Yates testified to the royal commission that he inquired into the bona fides of Nugan Hand by checking with Sir Robert Askin and Sir Paul Strasser, among others.[45] Unfortunately, he did not have some information that award-winning journalist Evan Whitton would later publish: a report following Askin's death 'noted claims that Askin had sold knighthoods for up to $60,000 during a decade of corrupt rule' and had 'extorted hundreds of thousands of dollars from criminals running illegal casinos'.[46]

Frank Nugan was impressed enough by Houghton's connections to ask him to prevent one of his (Nugan's) company employees being searched for drugs in Hong Kong (this had already occurred once). But according to Houghton it was Admiral Yates who encouraged him to join the Nugan Hand group. The office that Houghton opened for them in Saudi Arabia did good business attracting deposits from US nationals working there in the construction industry.[47] When the bank went under in 1980, more than $5 million of their hard-earned money went with it.[48]

The other fortuitous circumstance in the apparent success of Nugan Hand was the prosperity of its Hong Kong operation, which owed much to the endeavours of Michael Hand.

Michael Jon Hand was born and brought up in the Bronx, New York, and served in the US Army in Vietnam from 1963 to 1966. He was a highly decorated member of the elite Green Berets, who worked for the CIA with the Hmong guerrillas in northern Laos.[49] The royal commission noted claims that Hand had worked for one of the two CIA contract airlines operating in Laos and Vietnam, Continental Air Services and Air America, 'dropping food to the natives'.[50] It was, of course, these food drops, principally rice, that allowed the Hmong to concentrate their limited resources on growing opium,[51] and it was Air America, sometimes known as Air Opium, that obligingly transported it to market for them.[52] The royal commission also noted allegations made in the *Wall Street Journal* and various Australian newspapers that Hand was involved in drug trafficking, and had knowledge of heroin being smuggled into the United States in the bodies of servicemen killed in Vietnam.[53]

Hand teamed up with Frank Nugan in Sydney in 1968. The two were initially involved in buying and selling real estate, share dealing and a mining venture in Western Australia.[54] When Nugan Hand was formed in 1973, Hand continued his involvement in real estate, buying back the land in Brunswick Heads that he had originally sold to US servicemen, at prices said to have been between one-quarter and one-third of their value, then reselling it at its true value.[55] Hand was often flown to Brunswick Heads by an ex-American Airlines comrade from Laos, Kermit Walker King. The Australian Bureau of Narcotics was informed that King was also flying heroin into Australia for Hand, and King shortly thereafter fell to his death from the tenth floor of a Sydney building.[56]

From late 1974 until early 1976, Hand was in apartheid South Africa attempting to procure arms for the UNITA rebels in Angola as the Cold War came to southern Africa.[57] Back in Sydney in early 1976, Hand immediately got busy setting up the financial arrangements on which much of the importation of heroin from Southeast Asia would depend. Taking its name from a company called Yorkville Nominees that Frank Nugan had established in 1970, Hand operated a scheme known as the Yorkville Contra, a fraudulent system of transferring funds between the Hong Kong and Sydney branches of Nugan Hand without the necessary approval of the Reserve Bank of Australia, and in breach of Banking (Foreign Exchange) Regulations. The scheme operated thus: first, money was lodged with Nugan Hand in Sydney or Hong Kong, and second, the equivalent amount was then available in Hong Kong or Sydney respectively — without any money actually being transmitted.[58] Hand arranged for Murray Stewart Riley to use the scheme on several occasions commencing in April 1976.[59] After Riley deposited money in Sydney, one of his Hong Kong employees would pick up the equivalent amount from the Hong Kong office and use it to pay for heroin which was then dispatched to Sydney. The Mr Asia syndicate also availed itself of this convenient money transfer system to fund some of its heroin imports.[60] Starting in 1975 and accelerating when Michael Hand returned to Australia and organised the Hong Kong and Singapore branches of Nugan Hand from 1976, the bank was responsible for arranging the financial transactions of at least 26 known drug dealers before its demise in 1980.[61]

Following the collapse of Nugan Hand, Bernie Houghton left Australia on 2 June 1980 in the company of an unnamed American — later identified by the Joint Task Force on Drug Trafficking as Thomas Clines.[62] Twelve days later Michael Hand also left Australia, in the company of an American known only as 'Charlie' at the time. Charlie turned out to be James Oswald Spencer, a former Green Beret colleague of Hand's from Laos.[63]

Hand left the country on a false Australian passport, entering the United States from Canada, at which point he disappeared from view. He had previously been granted Australian citizenship as the spouse of an Australian citizen, despite a number of 'irregular circumstances', including the fact that his US passport was not collected from him and returned to US authorities, a matter on which he sought legal advice from William Colby.[64] It was this irregular — not to say illegal — retention of his US passport that allowed Hand to enter and then go to ground in the United States. Admiral Earl Preston Yates dutifully tried to assist the royal commission by delivering to Hand's father a cassette tape requesting Michael Hand to submit to an interview, and asking him to pass it on to his son.[65] It is not known whether or not Hand received the tape, but to this day his whereabouts are unknown.

The collapse of Nugan Hand was triggered by events that followed the murder of Donald Mackay in July 1977. Frank Nugan's parents had established a fruit-packing business in the Griffith area in 1940. It was carried on by a group of companies known collectively as the Nugan Fruit Group.[66] Frank Nugan was at one time a director of the company, but the business was eventually run by his brother, Kenneth Nugan.[67] In the early days it was prosperous enough to enable Frank Nugan's parents to send him to study law at the University of Sydney. He graduated in 1963, then went on to postgraduate studies in the United States and Canada before settling in Sydney to practise as a solicitor.[68] He specialised in tax matters, a practice that he continued at Nugan Hand, where tax evasion schemes were promoted to clients, many of whom were from the medical profession.[69] Such schemes were greatly encouraged by a 1970 decision of the High Court of Australia — the chief justice at the time was a failed Liberal Party politician, Sir Garfield Barwick, who had been appointed by the then prime minister, Sir Robert Menzies, in 1964.[70] The decision concerned was fundamental in nullifying the tax evasion provisions of the Tax Act,[71] and the evasion schemes that proliferated were known as 'bottom of the harbour' scams, a reference to the final resting place of many company records. Frank Nugan's other important role at the bank was soliciting deposits, and to this end he specialised in long boozy lunches with potential clients in the Liverpool Street area of Sydney, where many a good Spanish restaurant is found. The Labor mayor of Leichhardt Council in inner-western Sydney was an attendee at some of these lunches, having been told that Nugan Hand was a Labor Party supporter. Over a number of years that council, along with others, would invest significant amounts of money with the bank.[72]

Frank Nugan had a weakness for getting into the booze even before lunchtime. A common consensus was 'that he was rarely sober after 11 am and as the day progressed he became slurred in speech and grandiose in ideas'.[73] The trying times that began for him in the latter half of 1977 did little to change this.

It was at this point that the Corporate Affairs Commission of New South Wales commenced a special investigation into the affairs of the Nugan Fruit Group, following allegations of voting and other irregularities surrounding an attempted takeover bid for the company. As the investigation proceeded, further allegations emerged, to the effect that the Nugan Fruit Group was involved in the Griffith cannabis trade. These allegations related to both Frank Nugan and Nugan Hand when they were referred to the Royal Commission into Drug Trafficking.[74] The adverse publicity was such that in November

1977 there was a 'run' on the Nugan Hand Group that, on one day, claimed almost one-third of the company's total deposits.[75] Things got worse in May 1978, when the Corporate Affairs Commission began a criminal prosecution of both Frank and Kenneth Nugan in relation to the Nugan Fruit Group. This dragged on for 18 months and resulted in a prima facie case being found against them in November 1979. The game was almost up, despite the fact that Frank Nugan had been transferring money out of Nugan Hand and into the Nugan Fruit Group, and paying for the legal costs of the various investigations and court proceedings in an attempt to avoid this outcome.[76]

Shortly before the November court finding, Frank Nugan made a belated attempt to 'clean up' the affairs of Nugan Hand, telling his staff that in 15 different business categories there were both legitimate and 'illegitimate' activities. His plan was to pass the illegitimate clients off to other banks.[77] But it was too late, and a few months later Frank Nugan drove his Mercedes towards Lithgow and left the rest to Michael Hand. In August 1982, having pleaded guilty to three charges of fraudulent appropriation of property by a director, Kenneth Nugan was sentenced to six months' imprisonment.[78]

Beyond the seventies

Despite some periodic difficulties with supply (often erroneously described as droughts), the pattern of heroin consumption that was well established in Australia by the late 1970s, thanks in no small part to Nugan Hand, has proved enduring. It is an experience that is by no means unique. In most advanced economies the consumption of heroin in the last quarter of the 20th century, and into the 21st century, caught up with the experience of the United States during the first three-quarters of the 20th century. In 2005 the UN Office on Drugs and Crime estimated the number of consumers in the world market for illicit opiates at 16 million, with around 11 million being heroin consumers.[79] As ever, and despite more than 90 years of prohibition, the US market remains the largest and most profitable, with at least one million consumers.

As heroin use increased in Australia in the 1980s and 1990s, so did research into market demographics, consumption patterns and related issues such as crime and the public health consequences of injecting drug use. Much of this research was prompted by the rising number of overdose deaths and rates of HIV/Aids infection. Nevertheless, estimates as to the number of consumers varied. In 2002, for example, a senior writer for the *Far Eastern Economic Review* put the number of addicts at 45,000 and the number of occasional users at 600,000.[80] The term 'addict', though, was by now largely confined to popular use; in the more serious literature the terms 'problematic' and 'dependent', intended to more accurately define compulsive drug use and determine patterns of consumption, were being used. One of the difficulties concerns capturing precise numbers of consumers through household surveys. Household surveys that endeavour to determine the number of illicit drug consumers face an obvious problem: respondents might well be a little reluctant to disclose the true nature of their illicit habits to researchers who say that they are from a government-funded body and have come to help. To complicate matters further, there are problems with definitions of what constitutes 'problematic' or 'dependent' use. These factors account for the variations that are seen in estimates of dependent heroin users in Australia — they range from as low as 27,000 to as high as 500,000 in the popular press.[81]

In the global illicit drug market it is clear that heroin consumers are a relatively small percentage of total consumers, somewhere around 5 per cent. Compared with the 11 million heroin consumers, there are more than 160 million cannabis consumers and close to 30 million amphetamine consumers.

Cocaine is the drug of choice for more than 15 million consumers and ecstasy for eight million. This pattern seems to be broadly reflected in Australia, where the figures suggest that the number of young adults who have used heroin at some point in their lives is no higher than 4 per cent. Contrary, perhaps, to popular belief, only about one in four people who try heroin become dependent on it, which means that the likely rate of heroin dependence is somewhere between 0.5 and 0.7 per cent of the adult population.[82] Research published in the *Medical Journal of Australia* in November 2000 — it involved the application of a number of statistical techniques to all the available data — concluded that the number of dependent heroin users (essentially defined as daily users) was at the higher end of the scale, 0.7 per cent of the adult population aged 15–54 years. In the period that was under review, the late 1990s, this translated to about 300,000 heroin users, 74,000 of whom were dependent on the drug. This in turn was more than double the number in the previous decade.[83] Before 2001, heroin use in Australia was significantly higher than the world average. Interruptions to supply from the Golden Triangle in 2001 and 2002 led to a reduction in use that saw Australian consumption moving closer to, but still above, the global average.

Although heroin consumption is not unknown in rural areas, it is concentrated in urban areas in Australia, as it is in the rest of the world. New South Wales has the highest number of dependent heroin users (48 per cent of the Australian total) and Victoria has the next highest concentration (around 27 per cent). The other states together account for the remaining 25 per cent.[84]

The Australian heroin trade has, from the start, been centred on Sydney, which is the major point of entry for the drug and has the largest concentration of consumers. The Golden Triangle has, from the start, been the major source of Australia's heroin. The other consistent aspect of the trade has been the involvement of Chinese criminal groups and triads as brokers and wholesale suppliers. The criminal groups who collaborated with the Chinese syndicates and organised distribution were, up until the early 1990s, mostly Australians of mainly Anglo-Irish extraction; they have a criminal lineage that reaches back beyond Ned Kelly's time. The post-World War II activities of Sydney's criminal world have been extensively documented by a long series of official inquiries, beginning with the Liquor Royal Commission of 1951–54. A lucrative business like heroin will also attract other organised criminal entrepreneurs. The Russian Mafia tried their hand — a shipment of heroin from Vladivostok was intercepted in 1993.[85] Organised criminal groups from Lebanon have met with a greater degree of success than the Russians, due in large part to their direct connections in Bangkok; a significant number of Lebanese entrepreneurs settled there in the 1970s following the bloody events in their homeland.[86] But the real successors to the heroin distribution business in Australia have been Vietnamese criminal gangs.

After the Vietnam War ended in 1975 and Saigon was renamed Ho Chi Minh City, hundreds of thousands of Vietnamese, including many of Chinese origin, fled the country. Vietnam, having defeated the military might of France, the United States and the countries allied with them (which included Australia), now became a political pawn in the Cold War being played out between China, the United States and the Soviet Union. In February 1979, with the tacit approval of the United States, more than 600,000 Chinese troops invaded Vietnam, causing even more people to flee the country, many in ill-equipped boats that headed into the South China Sea bound for Hong Kong.[87]Some of the boats even made it to Australia, where, at the time, it was politically prudent to accept 'boat people' seeking refuge — there were people who had worked for the United States and their allies and were afraid of the repercussions and economic refugees. By the mid-1980s, between the boat people who had arrived under their own steam and those accepted from regional refugee camps such as those in Hong Kong, Australia had become home to more than 100,000 people from Vietnam. Those who came to Sydney were initially housed in the old immigration hostels in the western suburbs around Villawood; these hostels had previously been used to accommodate the first intakes of postwar migrants. Many thousands subsequently settled in the nearby suburb of Cabramatta.[88] Many were subjected to racial abuse, but most simply got on with things as best as they could … and managed to enrich Australian culture in the process. Others, though, went back to old habits. They began operating prostitution and extortion rackets and, inevitably, became involved in the much more profitable heroin distribution business.

The alienated young Vietnamese men these experienced hands recruited were quick to organise themselves into gangs. They gained a reputation for ruthless efficiency and violence. The two members of the notorious 5T gang who were murdered in Cabramatta in 1995 were just 19 and 20 years old. These 'older' gang members recruited boys who were barely old enough to be in high school as street sellers.[89] The word was soon out on the street that Cabramatta was the place to score the best smack in town; if you took the train ride out west, there were sellers touting for business before you left the station.

The suburb's new status as the centre of Australia's retail heroin trade didn't escape the attention of the local state MP, the Labor Party's John Newman. Like Donald Mackay in Griffith before him, he became an outspoken critic of the ethnic-based criminal activity in his electorate, and went as far as to suggest that migrants convicted of serious crimes should be deported to their country of origin. Like Donald Mackay, he too was murdered, gunned down outside his Cabramatta home in September 1994 in what was said to be Australia's first political assassination.

It was impossible not to notice the heroin dealing in Cabramatta and the NSW police eventually controlled its more visible aspects. But in 1994 the NSW police service had problems of its own. A few months before Newman's murder a royal commission had been set up to inquire into the service's activities. Its final report was released three years later, indicating that it had much to inquire into. The commission found that there existed within the service 'a state of systemic or entrenched corruption' that was widespread and longstanding.[90] The 'corrupting influence of the trade in narcotics' was emphasised throughout its inquiries and it found that police were using as well as supplying drugs.[91]Of all the corrupt behaviour that the commission uncovered, it came to the view that, 'Perhaps most disturbing of all was the extent to which police admitted being directly involved in the supply of cocaine, heroin and cannabis.'[92] The commission sought to dispel for all time the long-discounted notion that the problems of corruption were due to one or two 'rotten apples' in an otherwise uncontaminated barrel. One of its recommendations led to the establishment of the Police Integrity Commission, a permanent body charged with investigating serious police misconduct. The views expressed more than 20 years earlier by one who ought to know, ex-NSW policeman and heroin trader John Wesley Egan, had proved prophetic: 'Organised crime and highly placed policemen are often the same people.'[93] When, during the commission's inquiry, it became necessary to appoint a new commissioner of police, the NSW government thought it wise to look beyond not only the state of New South Wales but also every other state in the country, and appointed the former chief constable of Norfolk in the United Kingdom, Peter Ryan, to the position.

Unlike the cannabis trade, which was emasculated following the death of Donald Mackay, the heroin trade continued to flourish following the death of John Newman. Early in 2001

Commissioner Ryan asserted that the more than 40 criminal gangs fighting for control of Sydney's prostitution, extortion and heroin markets were predominantly Chinese, Lebanese and Vietnamese; he was said by some to be insensitive.[94] The synergy captured by bringing these three markets together, a connection first exploited by Lucky Luciano, was obviously well understood. The other lesson from criminal history that was well grasped was that drug money was easily laundered through casinos — this one was thanks to Luciano's partner in crime, Meyer Lansky. The lesson wasn't limited to criminal entrepreneurs. The illegal casinos of previous decades had given way to legal monopolies, and representatives from several of these establishments around the country began arriving in Cabramatta in the early 1990s, trying to persuade the punters holding heroin-trade cash to invest it at their gaming tables. In 1997 a Cabramatta businessman, Duong Van Ia, who in a two-year period was said to have unloaded somewhere between $20 million and $90 million at the Sydney Harbour Casino, was, much to the displeasure of casino authorities, prohibited by police from entering the premises on the suspicion that he was laundering drug money. Duong was one of the Vietnamese who arrived early in Australia. He went into business as a restaurant supplier in the Cabramatta area. He was also a heroin supplier, an activity for which he received an eight-year prison term in 1998.[95]

Three years before Duong's incarceration, global money laundering, much of it from the illicit drug trade, was estimated by the United Nations to be the equivalent of 2 per cent of global GDP — US$500 billion a year. Despite Australia's financial reporting laws, which are among the most stringent in the world, the money laundering associated with the heroin trade was estimated by the Australian Transaction Reports and Analysis Centre (AUSTRAC) at somewhere between $1 billion and $4.5 billion.[96]

And despite the best efforts of the Australian Federal Police

(AFP) and other enforcement agencies, the profits generated by demand continue to be worth the risks. It is difficult to conceive of any licit commodity that realises as much profit as heroin in its journey from producer to consumer. At the start of the new millennium, Golden Triangle farmers were receiving US$330 for the raw opium necessary to produce an export-size 700-gram unit of heroin — which would sell for just over $1 million when retailed in capsule form in Australia. At the transaction points along the way profits are equally impressive.[97]

The logistics of transporting heroin from the Golden Triangle have become more challenging as a greater emphasis has been placed on interrupting supply rather than on attempting to understand the dynamics of demand. Seamen working on vessels trading between Southeast Asian ports and Australia are probably the oldest source of supply; couriers carrying comparatively small amounts on commercial air flights from the same region have long been another favoured form of transport. As demand increased, the sea-borne container trade was pressed into service; it was later complemented by bulk supplies arriving by freighter off the Australian coast and being met by powerful small craft to complete the delivery. Postal and freight delivery services have also been a well-used importing method. Flexibility and innovation are key operational strategies. As policing resources are concentrated in one area, imports move to another. As methods of detection become more sophisticated, so do methods of concealing the drug, led by couriers inserting heroin-filled suppositories into their body cavities and swallowing heroin-filled condoms.

As importing strategies have changed in response to policing pressure, so too have trafficking routes. The traditional ports of departure for Australian-bound heroin have been Rangoon, Bangkok, Singapore and Hong Kong. Southern Chinese and Vietnamese ports have now been added to the list, as have ports in India and Bangladesh. The proximity of these two countries to Afghanistan raises the very real possibility that some of its supply will find its way to the Australian market. Indonesia, which has now become part of the trafficking route, has a large drug-using population: some estimates put the number of problematic heroin users as high as 1.3 million.

The drug couriers or 'mules' who first followed the example of John Wesley Egan and imported heroin into Australia on international airline flights in the 1970s were, in the main, young Australians motivated by the promise of big money with little effort in a short time. A profitable industry such as heroin can offer these opportunities. They were followed by those whose normal day jobs ranged from hairdressers to professional footballers, and those with no jobs at all. As people caught and convicted at the point of departure were either incarcerated in Southeast Asian prisons or executed, the business became less attractive to Australians. They were then replaced by nationals of other countries. The apparent increase in popularity of the heroin courier trade that the arrest of a number of young Australians in Southeast Asia and Indonesia in early 2005 seems to imply suggests a flawed risk assessment on their part, but clearly market demand continued to offer the same promise of quick wealth in 2005 as it did in the 1970s. And despite the publicity that heroin seizures attract, they have little impact on the overall level of imports. Towards the end of 2004, a supposedly lean year for imports, 86 per cent of heroin consumers are said to have found the drug either 'very easy' or 'easy' to obtain. This is hardly surprising given that Australians managed to consume somewhere between three and eight tonnes of heroin in that year and less than 10 per cent of that amount was actually intercepted.[98]

10
The triumph of the market?

In 1848, just four years after Karl Marx was writing of the opium of the people and Friedrich Engels was observing the part that opium played in the lives of the working class in England, they collaborated in the publication of a pamphlet that became famously known as *The Communist Manifesto*. In it they declared that the history of all hitherto existing societies was a history of class struggles between an oppressed class and an oppressor class. This explanation of history in terms of class struggles that formed a series of evolutions would, in Engels' view, do for history what Darwin's theory had done for biology. Moreover, there was but one inevitable outcome of this historical process: the victory of the oppressed over their oppressors, the victory of the proletariat over the bourgeoisie, the victory of communism over capitalism.[1] Less than 150 years after the publication of *The Communist Manifesto*, historian Francis Fukuyama was writing of the movement of a great number of countries 'in the direction of market orientated economies and [their] integration into the global capitalist division of labor'. It was a movement that constituted 'an end of history in the Marxist-Hegelian sense of History as a broad evolution of human societies advancing towards a final goal'.[2]

The Cold War was over. Capitalism had defeated communism. Not only had Engels' analogy with Darwin failed to materialise, but Darwin's theory of evolution was itself under attack by fundamentalist Christians who preferred the idea that it was a God that created the world in all its complexity, by a process that they liked to call 'intelligent design'.

From 1990, the ideology of economic liberalism has increasingly dominated the world. The collapse of the Berlin Wall in 1989 was quickly followed by the collapse of the command economies of the USSR and the eastern European countries behind Churchill's Iron Curtain. In the years since, China has opened up its markets to the world even as it struggles to contain the concomitant social costs and reconcile them with some hitherto unthought of version of communist ideology. There is the very clear sense that even if there is no change to the present structure of state political organisation and control in China, market influence will continue to grow there. Vietnam, denied the war reparations promised by President Nixon in 1973, then forced to repel Chinese troops — who invaded in even greater numbers than the United States had done after Vietnam rescued Cambodia from the murderous Pol Pot — somewhat wearily adopted a program of 'market socialism' in 1986. It is now the low-wage refuge of other Asian market economies.[3] India, with its days of Soviet trade agreements, five-year plans and mutual cooperation hardly a memory any more, has developed a growing base of consumers who have become integrated into the world market economy. Cuba remains a romantic oddity. For all its stoic resistance, it nevertheless gives the impression that if it were opened up to, rather than excluded from, the United States and other world markets it would become much more integrated into them. Instead it remains an island under siege. North Korea remains simply an oddity, if not an obscenity.

There are, naturally enough, a number of reasons for the

collapse of communism in the USSR and eastern Europe. The USSR's decade-long occupation of Afghanistan is one of them. Widespread corruption is another. But neither ill-advised wars nor systemic corruption are necessarily fatal to the continued operation of states, no matter what their underpinning ideology. What was central to the collapse of communism was the failure of the USSR's planned economy; an economy where free markets had no place. What, more than anything else, demonstrated the weakness of the Soviet Union's command economy was its inability to keep pace with the United States in the Cold War arms race.[4]

Nikita Khrushchev (1894–1971), the Soviet leader who succeeded Stalin in 1953, was confident enough of the superiority of socialist production methods over those of capitalism to promise, in 1961, that the USSR's production of industrial goods would overtake that of the United States within two decades. But by the time they had achieved superiority in cement production, the currency of growth was computer microchips.[5] Khrushchev was ousted in a bloodless coup in 1964, and under his successor, Leonid Brezhnev (1906–82), defence spending began to take an increasing share of the Soviet budget — later estimated at up to 25 per cent of GDP.[6] By the 1970s the Soviet economy was slowing down, and by the middle of the next decade oil and gas, rather than machinery, equipment and manufactured products, were its main exports. Under the notoriously corrupt Brezhnev, the Soviet managerial class, once held to be the driving force of the Soviet economy, had degenerated into an incompetent and corrupt elite.[7] The cooperatively owned economy, according to the black humour of the time, operated on the basis that workers pretended to work and the state pretended to pay them.

The dramatic increase in world oil prices in the 1970s brought about by the Organisation of Petroleum Exporting Countries (OPEC) was a boon to the Soviet economy that should have helped revitalise it, but in the end it merely disguised its inefficiency and postponed its collapse.[8] If anything, it had a negative effect, as it contributed to a confidence among the Soviet elite that they could continue to compete with the United States. The thinking seemed to be that the Soviet Union could import its grain requirements, subsidise its satellites, support friendly non-communist countries and still have a surplus with which to match the arms expenditure of the United States.[9] This reckoning may have made some sense, but it reckoned without the presidency of Ronald Reagan (1981–89).

Reagan was a fervent anti-communist who considerably upped the ante in the arms race. Early in his presidency he reduced the Cold War to a simple struggle between right and wrong, a contest between good and evil. Lest there be any doubt as to who was right and good and who constituted the opposition, the USSR was described, in an address to the National Association of Evangelicals, as an 'evil empire'.[10] Curiously, Reagan hadn't always been thought to be on the side of the angels. In 1946, apparently on the basis that his name appeared in the *People's World* (a communist newspaper circulating on the west coast of the United States) sponsoring the call for a free Indochina and withdrawal of support for Chiang Kai-shek, the FBI had come to the conclusion that he was a communist.[11] The bureau was also interested in his membership of a number of progressive organisations they thought were suspect, including the Hollywood Independent Citizens Committee of the Arts, Sciences and Professions (HICCASP), which Reagan's brother spied on for the FBI and warned him against. There was also the disturbing matter of the radio broadcast he had made attacking the Ku Klux Klan.[12] But Reagan had seen the light early enough. He became an FBI informer, and from his position as President of the Screen Actors Guild from 1947 to 1951, helped purge the Hollywood film industry of communists and their sympathisers.[13]

Even before he was elected president, Reagan had come to the conclusion that the USSR couldn't compete in an escalation of the arms race. He thought they would eventually be forced to drop out — or bankrupt themselves, given the toll that military spending was exacting on meeting the consumption needs of its citizens.[14] His calculation proved correct, but the truth of the matter was that the United States couldn't afford it either. During the presidential terms of Reagan and his immediate successor, George Bush, the United States went from being the world's largest creditor to being the world's largest debtor. The increase in its national debt in that 12-year period, US$3 trillion, is largely accounted for by increased defence spending. But unlike the USSR, the United States was able to finance its budget deficits with foreign capital.[15] Proof indeed of the superiority of free market forces.

The end of the Cold War marked the return of a laissez-faire approach to economic policy. The victory of free market capitalism championed by Reagan in the United States and Margaret Thatcher in the United Kingdom also marked the retreat of the social democratic project. It was a victory for the economic ideas of Friedrich Hayek (1899–1992) and Milton Friedman (1912–2006) and defeat for the now discredited ideas of state intervention and economic management in the pursuit of full employment, first systematically put forward by John Maynard Keynes (1883–1946).

As the titles of their various books illustrate, Friedman and Hayek successfully linked the idea of economic freedom to that of political freedom. In *Capitalism and Freedom* Friedman wrote that 'economic freedom is an indispensable means towards the achievement of political freedom'.[16] In *Free to Choose*, written three years after he won the Nobel Prize for economics in 1976, he wrote of the way in which government intervention in the United States had limited human freedom in that country.[17] For Friedman, economic and political freedoms were inseparable.[18]

For Hayek the road to socialism was also the road to serfdom. Writing before World War II had ended, he was already warning that even limited government intervention could lead to totalitarianism and that state planning was the scourge of competition.[19]For him, there was no Third Way between communism and capitalism.[20]

It had been a long hard road for Hayek, Friedman and their closed group of international followers, one that had begun in earnest in 1947. The idea of creating an international campaign for the defence of a free society against collectivism was first raised some years earlier, at a meeting Hayek attended in Paris in 1938 about the crisis of liberalism in Europe. At the conclusion of proceedings Hayek was given the responsibility of establishing a British section of the proposed organisation, but World War II intervened and the project proceeded no further. Hayek canvassed the idea once again in a paper he presented at Cambridge University in February 1944, entitled 'Historians and the Future of Europe'. The initiative finally took shape in the form of a conference held in Switzerland in 1947. This led to the formation of the Mont Perelin Society, named after the hotel where that first conference had been held.[21]

The work of the society — 're-establishing liberalism as the public doctrine of Western civilisation' — was carried out, without much initial success, by a small group of intellectuals. The most notable of these were Milton Friedman and the Chicago school, who took their name from the university where Friedman was professor of economics from 1946 to 1983.[22] Their ideas gained ground; gradually at first, and then rapidly from the early 1970s, with Hayek being awarded the Nobel Prize for economics in 1974. With the collapse of communism their victory was complete. Public ownership, that pillar of the welfare state that was being constructed when Hayek convened the 1947 conference, could now be ended; those assets could be divested, sold to private interests, because they would operate more efficiently under market conditions.

To the extent that public transport, airlines, public utilities (providing electricity, gas and water), port authorities, postal services, coal, steel, defence, shipbuilding and vehicle industries, banking, insurance and telecommunications were in public ownership, either partly or wholly, they were all subject to privatisation and market discipline. Public health authorities and public education institutions were, at the very least, subject to market accountability. Market authority and jargon became pervasive. Train and airline passengers were transformed into customers. If market relationships didn't exist they were created. Workers were organised into separate teams in production-line factories, with recipients of partly produced commodities the customers of those up the line who, in turn, serviced their new customers further down the line. Evidence of failure — fatally so in the case of Chile — was ignored as the world became a global marketplace. [23] People could only remain free if enterprise remained free.[24]

Friedman's political economy was a move backwards from Keynes to the laissez-faire and limited government of Adam Smith who, as it turned out, also had the answer to how capital could be civilised, way back in 1776:

As every individual therefore, endeavours as much as he can both to employ his capital in the support of domestic industry, and so to direct that industry that its produce may be of the greatest value; every individual necessarily labours to render the annual revenue of the society as great as he can. He generally, indeed, neither intends to promote the public interest, nor knows how much he is promoting it. By preferring the support of domestic to that of foreign industry, he intends only his own security; and by directing that industry in such a manner as its produce may be of the greatest value, he intends only his own gain, and he is in this, as in many other cases, led by an invisible hand to promote an end which was no part of his intention. Nor is it always the worse for the society that it was no part of it. By pursuing his own interests he frequently promotes that of the society more effectually than when he really intends to promote it. I have never known much good done by those who affected to trade for the public good. It is an affectation, indeed, not very common among merchants, and very few words need to be employed in dissuading them from it.[25]

The free market equivalent of intelligent design, the spontaneous order of markets would ameliorate the tendency to excess, and would work for the common good.

There is, of course, no such thing as a completely free market operating anywhere in the world. The state continues to have a monopoly on violence through its policing function, correctional system and military apparatus. A legal framework, rather than the market, enforces rights and usually acts against the tendency to monopoly by providing some standards for competition. Taxes continue to be collected and expended on public goods and welfare schemes (including corporate welfare) — the link between political and economic freedom seems to have gone completely missing in the new Russia, for instance, whose system of government has been called a 'kleptocracy'. Nevertheless, the change that began to take place in the 1990s is profound. The role of the state has been considerably reduced and those of its activities that remain are increasingly questioned by being held up against the 'efficiency test' of the market. The case for state intervention made out by social democracy (often enough with conservative support) has been stood on its head, with social democrats often enough leading the way.

However, the state doesn't seem to be in any immediate danger of withering away. Although some free market theorists have gone as far as to advocate the abolition of the state and its replacement, should it be thought necessary, by a market in the provision of private security, the idea has so far received scant support.[26] Proposals for market intervention that have attracted significant support seemed to reach their apogee in 2003, with the promotion of a market in terrorist activity by a section of the US Department of Defence. Adam Smith appears to have been silent on that subject.

The Defence Advanced Research Projects Agency at the Pentagon, having researched the matter thoroughly, concluded in 2003 that markets operate as 'efficient, effective and timely aggregators of dispersed and even hidden information'. What's more, they said, the capacity of futures markets to predict events is often superior to other expert opinion. For these reasons they proposed the setting up of a Policy Analysis Market that would enable anonymous investors to speculate on such matters as the assassination of political leaders and the likelihood of various forms of terrorist attacks. The attraction for investors would be the capacity to make money. By following the money trail Pentagon officials would then be better able to plan for future events. It was thought that the market would be particularly effective in the Middle East. However, public opinion proved fatal to the project and it was cancelled on the eve of its launch. The proposed market in terrorist activity was criticised on three counts: first, terrorists participating in the market could profit from their terrorist activities; second, terrorists could manipulate the market; and third, the market might not be viable given that government intervention would, more than likely, prevent its free operation (by, for example, providing extra security to prevent a political assassination that the market saw as highly probable and that they could therefore capitalise on).[27]

In today's age of markets, the underlying assumption of market superiority hasn't been widely challenged. After all, it rests on the simple unchallengeable proposition articulated by Adam Smith in the 18th century that, in the absence of coercion, an exchange between two parties was of equal benefit to both parties;[28] such market exchanges would not otherwise take place. The free market is now universally held by governments around the world (Cuba and North Korea excepted) to be the most effective distributive mechanism for ensuring that human needs and preferences are satisfied.[29]

The illicit drug market

The market in illicit drugs operates in the same way that markets in other commodities operate, but there are some points of difference between it and other commodity markets. The main difference is that exchanges in the illicit market involve a high degree of risk and aren't covered by consumer protection laws or the laws of contract.[30] But the basic exchange mechanism, as it was described by Adam Smith ('give me that which I want and you shall have this which you want'), is precisely the same and the laws of supply and demand are also equally applicable.[31] Although advertising of illicit drugs is restricted to word of mouth, drugs are nevertheless subject to the same marketing techniques as other commodities. In a marketing strategy like that used for designer-label clothing, LSD products have carried 'brand names' from the 1960s. Ecstasy products have similarly long carried brand names and, more recently, so too have cannabis and heroin.[32] The economics of packaging, where unit prices decline as the quantity purchased rises, have been shown to be little different for groceries purchased in supermarkets and illicit drugs purchased in less public surroundings.[33] To the extent that consumption of recreational drugs is a criminal activity, it is a 'market-based offence' rather than a 'predatory offence'. (A market-based offence involves mutual agreeable exchanges where value is offered for money, and there are no victims to complain, so police must initiate action; a predatory offence involves wealth being transferred from one person to another by the use of force or fraud, and the victim usually complains and thus initiates police action.) And the market is a buoyant one.[34]

Surveying the period which embraced the Cold War, the collapse of communism, the rise and fall of social democracy, and the victory of free-market capitalism, the World Drug Report of 2004 noted: 'The second half of the 20th century has witnessed an epidemic of illicit drug use.' During the 12 months preceding its report, there were some 185 million people around the globe consuming illicit drugs: 150 million people were consuming cannabis, 13 million cocaine, 15 million opiates, 30 million amphetamine-type stimulants and eight million ecstasy. More than 30 million people were consuming more than one of these drugs in the period under review. The report also noted the connection between increased urbanisation and illicit drug consumption. In 1950, 28 per cent of the people on the planet lived in urban areas; in 2003 it was 48 per cent. Urbanisation continues to increase rapidly; other factors aside, this implies an increase in illicit drug consumption.

In 2005 the number of people using illicit drugs increased by 15 million to 200 million, with cannabis use accounting for by far the most significant increase. The size of the retail market in illicit drugs, notoriously difficult to measure, was estimated at US$322 billion, a sum which is greater than the individual GDP of some 90 per cent of the countries of the world.[35]

As this epidemic of illicit drug use took hold in the second half of the 20th century, a number of states and state agencies became involved in their supply. The French intelligence service was, for a while, part of the supply network of opium. The US intelligence service, at the least, declined to intervene in the supply of opiates and cocaine. The intelligence service of Pakistan as well as the country's military became intimately involved in the heroin business. Heads of state, military leaders, government ministers and other high-ranking officials, particularly in Southeast Asia, Afghanistan and Pakistan, became involved in, and profited from, the illicit drug trade.

But none of these activities was responsible for creating

demand, and it is this failure to understand the basic economic laws of supply and demand that has contributed most to the rise in illicit drug use. The prohibition of abortion never eliminated demand, nor did the prohibition of alcohol, gambling or selling sexual favours. Attempting to control supply simply increases prices and, therefore, profits.[36] Far from being a solution to illicit drug consumption, prohibition is a net contributor to it. In the US market the price of heroin has been estimated as 200 times higher than it would be under free market conditions of supply and demand; the price of cocaine is estimated to be 20 times greater.[37] When tobacco was prohibited in Californian prisons in early 2005 the typical unit price went from US$11 to US$200.[38]

Marx and Engels, in *The Communist Manifesto*, underestimated the rate of development of markets, but the prohibitionists commit an error much more fundamental: failing to understand how markets actually operate. Marx and Engels could plead, in their defence, that they had not yet witnessed the 'creation of large new markets out of nothing'.[39] This occurred first following the discovery of gold in California and Australia (a state, according to Engels in 1851, 'consisting of undisguised rascals ... deported murderers, burglars, rapists and pickpockets'),[40] which happened after their manifesto was first published. Today's prohibitionists have no such excuse, since criminalising the supply of alcohol in the United States following World War I not only demonstrated the futility of such measures but also, legend aside, showed them to be 'the true incubators of modern organised crime'.[41]

There was one influential economist who, to his credit, did understand the nature of the illicit drug market and the role that supply and demand played in it. Friedman, always more logically consistent than Hayek (which perhaps explains why he has been more influential), entered into the debate on illicit drugs in a public way in the *Wall Street Journal* in September 1989.

This was occasioned by President George Bush's appointment of William Bennett as commander-in-chief of yet another war on drugs.

Friedman's intervention took the form of an 'Open Letter to Bill Bennett', in which he readily acknowledged the problems with illicit drug use that Bennett had identified. But he went on to invoke the words of Oliver Cromwell — 'I beseech you, in the bowels of Christ, think it possible you may be mistaken' — while asking Bennett to reconsider using increased penalties, more police and more policing, more jails and more jailing to deal with the problems. These measures, Friedman said, would only make matters worse. The root cause of these problems was demand and, in particular, the way in which demand operates in illicit markets: it gives rise to 'obscene profits' that finance the corruption that keeps the trade flourishing. Decriminalisation was the answer, with the case for state intervention limited to those measures (such as prohibiting advertising and sales to minors) which operate in the markets for alcohol and tobacco. These can actually work to reduce demand and are enforceable, whereas outright prohibition is not.[42] Friedman's views received support from the editor of the conservative *National Review*, William F Buckley Jnr, who supported licensing of the sale of drugs together with a campaign to educate and warn against consumption. In his view there was no solution to the drug problem, but legalisation in the form of licensing would strip away most of the profit that comes with illicit transactions, reduce the concomitant crime associated with such transactions and enable society to cease engaging in a futile exercise.[43] Bennett was unimpressed. Proposals such as these were 'morally scandalous' and 'irresponsible nonsense'.[44]

Friedman, long used to swimming against the tide, wasn't so easily put off. During the first term of office of the next president, Bill Clinton, he was involved in drafting a resolution for the police chiefs of San Francisco, Oakland and San Jose which said that the anti-drug effort had led to a race war and called for a strategy that focused on prevention and rehabilitation rather than arrest and punishment. Both the president and Congress were urged to establish a convention whose purpose would be to recommend a revision of US drug laws. The president, however, at least according to his press secretary, was not only against legalising drugs but not even interested in studying the issue.[45] For Republicans and Democrats alike Friedman was, it seems, as correct about the operation of markets generally as he was wrong about the operation of one market in particular, even though, as indeed those critics would anywhere else argue, they all operate in the same way.

State intervention in the marketplace

The case for state intervention in the drug market — that is, making drugs illegal — insofar as it is actually articulated these days, seems to rest on the idea of protecting certain members of the public from the harm they might do to themselves and others. The line of logic appears to be that certain drugs are dangerous and therefore those who might want to use them should be prohibited from doing so, both for their own good and for the good of others. This reason for state intervention in the drug market is a comparatively recent one. In today's age of markets some refer to its result as the re-formation of a 'nanny state'.

The first protective barrier that is erected in this scheme involves contracting out the control of drug use to the medical profession. There are few drugs whose use is totally prohibited by the state, so it is left to the medical profession to determine, in the course of medical treatment, which drugs the public should have access to. Limiting self-medication is largely a 20th century phenomenon, so this concession to medical authority is also of relatively recent origin. It is also one that has increasingly been shown to be problematic. Physicians have a habit of healing themselves. Some of them in Australia have been confident (or foolish) enough to want to remove their own appendix and haemorrhoids, but mostly they're stressed out, unable to communicate and have rates of depression, drug abuse and suicide three times higher than those of the general population.[46] General practitioners are heavily influenced in their prescribing decisions by the sales force of pharmaceutical companies. Their patients, in turn, report back to their GPs 10 million adverse reactions to these prescribed medicines each year in Australia. These adverse drug reactions are serious enough to account for up to 20 per cent of all admissions to hospitals.[47] Although the 1995 study which showed that there were up to 12,000 preventable deaths each year in hospitals has not been repeated, the safety standards have not changed, and according to the chairperson of the review body that commissioned the report, 'If we did the study again we would find just as many preventable deaths ... we haven't changed the system fundamentally, so why would the results differ?'[48] In the US, where such studies have been repeated, a study in 2000 identified up to 98,000 deaths caused by medical practitioners' negligence; in 2005 it was 100,000.[49]

The drug of choice for medical practitioners is a morphine-like drug, pethidine, but it certainly isn't the only one. A study in Victoria found that almost 40 per cent of GPs self-prescribed sleeping pills, opiate painkillers and antidepressants.[50] Long-term studies in the United States (going back to 1938) show that doctors consume mood-altering drugs they prescribe for themselves at a far greater rate than the general population does, and that over time their consumption increases.[51] It also seems that when GPs and surgeons consume some of the more common illicit drugs, such as cannabis and cocaine, their work is judged by their peers to be little affected and their treatment by the judicial system errs on the lenient side. A Sydney neurosurgeon who pleaded guilty to possessing a gram of cocaine, for example, had no conviction recorded against him but was instead placed on a good behaviour bond and ordered to undertake drug counselling.[52] An Adelaide GP addicted to valium who also consumed 10 cones of cannabis a day wasn't thought unfit for work by his psychiatrist. His habits came to light as a consequence of his seriously inadequate care of a patient he couldn't even remember treating. The patient died.[53] On the available evidence, the confidence that the state shows in medical practitioners by extending their monopoly privileges to authorising the prescription of designated drugs is misplaced. Indeed their overall performance suggests that it is time to revisit their monopoly on medical practice and reconstruct a medical marketplace. Milton Friedman is a long-time supporter of such an idea. In 1937 Friedman worked with the economist and future Nobel laureate Simon Kuznets (1901–85) on a research project that examined the professional structures of lawyers, doctors, accountants and others. This work formed the basis of Friedman's PhD thesis, which was completed at Columbia University in 1941. However it took another four years before the work, *Income from Independent Professional Practice*, was published, and it wasn't until 1946 that his PhD dissertation was accepted. What his evaluators found objectionable about the work was the findings Friedman had arrived at concerning doctors. He was able to show that organised medicine's restrictions on entry into the profession made the numbers in the profession grow at a rate far below that of population growth as a whole. The result of this restriction on supply in the face of rising demand was to increase the price consumers were forced to pay for doctors' services. The professed ideal of helping the sick get well seemed to have been subsumed by the goal of personal gain.[54]

What Friedman's PhD evaluators saw as an attack on doctors was for him an attack on state restrictions on occupational freedom. It was a theme that he returned to in *Free to Choose*, where he argued that an essential part of economic freedom was the freedom to enter into an occupation of one's own choosing. He went as far as to offer a solution in terms of a constitutional amendment: 'No State shall make or impose any law which shall abridge the right of any citizen of the United States to follow any occupation or profession of his choice.'[55] This suggestion has yet to be taken up even though it does represent a logical progression of free market economics. Doctors are also an important source of illicitly used drugs. Prescription drugs dispensed under their authority, such as tranquillisers, sleeping pills, barbiturates and analgesics, rank among the more commonly used illicit drugs in Australia after cannabis.[56]

Criminalisation

If doctors ought not control the supply of drugs on behalf of the state, neither ought those to whom the policing function has been entrusted as a result of criminalising drug use. Just a few years after the royal commission of inquiry into the NSW Police Force found that police in that state were both using and supplying illicit drugs, there was a similar inquiry in Western Australia that heard some similar evidence. It took just three months from the tabling of the royal commission report for the first police officer in Western Australia to be charged with drug-related corruption, in June 2004.[57] In Victoria in December 2001 the police commissioner disbanded the state's drug squad; 13 of its former members were subsequently charged with drug-related corruption offences.[58] In mid-2005 it was discovered that even the state's dog squad had been corrupted — the cocaine being used for training by its sniffer dogs had been replaced by talcum powder. At the same time an Australian Federal Police (AFP) expert on organised crime was suspended during an investigation into links with a cocaine smuggling ring.[59] Later in the year, the Commonwealth ombudsman identified the Victorian police force as one of Australia's most corrupt institutions.[60]

Despite the overall failure to enforce prohibition, the state does have some limited success, just as it did with alcohol prohibition. People are prosecuted and imprisoned, drugs are seized and removed from the market (in some cases, though, only to be later returned by corrupt police) and the threat of punishment presumably deters some prospective consumers from entering or continuing to participate in the market. But how can such small returns be justified when policy failures on such a massive scale in other areas would ordinarily result in a radical rethink of the failed policy?

Criminalising drug use has its origins in racism and fear. Opium smoking was first prohibited in San Francisco in 1875 and Queensland in 1891 in order to punish and marginalise Chinese immigrants. The fear of working-class use was an important consideration when the more general use of opium was curtailed in Britain in the 19th century.[61] Cocaine and heroin use were criminalised in the United States largely because the drugs were associated with African-Americans and working-class 'deviants'. Criminalising cannabis use in the United States was made easy, in terms of public acceptance, because of its link to Mexicans and African-Americans. The criminalising of amphetamine, LSD and ecstasy use in the second half of the 20th century had more to do with who the consumers were (bikies, hippies, radicals and ravers) and why they were consuming (for pleasure) than anything else. How then can a case for criminalisation still be made?

Douglas Husak, a US philosopher and legal scholar, has ruthlessly and systematically scrutinised the rationale for the criminalisation of drug use and the consequent punishment of illicit drug users in the United States. His reference points are established principles of justice and the moral rights of consumers.[62] He first points out that the rationale for prohibition must be assumed, since criminal laws are rarely accompanied by an official rationale.[63] The rationale that he assumes is that the various drug prohibition laws are meant to prevent people from harming themselves and others, and prevent addiction and crime, both of which are equally assumed to be accepted as undesirable in themselves. His inquiry investigates whether punishing recreational drug users protects children, safeguards health, prevents 'immorality' and a general 'deterioration of society' or reduces crime.[64] On no count can he find an answer that would justify criminalising drug use.

He describes the main kind of crime associated with drugs as systemic. That is, it occurs because drugs are illegal and bought and sold in black markets. Disputes concerning these illegal transactions, unable to be settled using normal legal channels, are dealt with by violence. These sorts of crimes account for about 75 per cent of all drug-related crime. The second type of crime associated with drug use he calls economic crime. This is largely attributed to heroin addiction: desperate acts are committed by desperate people who are unable to afford their drugs because of hugely inflated black market prices. Evidence of the third type of crime associated with drug use, which he calls psychopharmacological crime — crime that results from the actual effect of a drug — is inordinately high with one drug in particular: alcohol. These crimes are almost impossible to find with cannabis, rare with heroin, and marginal at best with cocaine. (Although amphetamines seem to be absent from his inquiry, it would be safe to assume that, particularly in combination with alcohol, they contribute significantly to the incidence of psychopharmacological crime.) He goes on to make the often overlooked point that the number of criminals who use drugs tends to disguise the fact that the number of drug users who are criminals is extraordinarily low, and he concludes that, on balance, drug prohibition probably causes more crime than it prevents.[65]

Husak isn't looking for an excuse to legalise drugs and he doesn't minimise the harm that they are capable of causing. He rejects the libertarian argument of total freedom of personal consumption and concedes that illicit drugs can be detrimental to the health of those who consume them. However, he notes that the role of the state doesn't ordinarily extend to punishing those whose health it is supposed to be protecting. Moreover, the sanction for illicit drug use — imprisonment — is in most cases infinitely more deleterious to health than drug use is ever likely to be. The extent of the harmful effects of illicit drugs is also questioned. There is apparently no data in the United States which shows that the health of the scores of millions of illicit drug users is readily distinguishable from the somewhat greater number of abstainers.[66] Not one to shy from controversy, Husak asserts that moderate drug use among adolescents is no great cause for alarm, and points to longitudinal tests which show that adults who experimented with illicit drugs as adolescents tend to be better adjusted in terms of psychological health than either abstainers or heavy drug users. Importantly, heavy drug users had also showed symptoms of maladjustment before their drug use, leading him to observe: 'Heavy drug use does not cause subsequent problems as much as prior problems cause heavy drug use.'[67]

The 'harm principle' is tested by analogy. Some 25,000 Americans die each year from using illicit drugs, a majority of them from hepatitis and AIDS contracted from shared dirty needles.[68] This compares with 100,000 who die from adverse reactions to prescription drugs, 430,000 killed by tobacco and 100,000 by alcohol. Obesity is responsible for 300,000 deaths, and more people are killed by melanoma than illicit drugs. On the principle of safeguarding health, alcohol, tobacco, fatty foods, prescription drugs and sunbathing should all be prohibited and their illicit indulgence punished.[69]

The seemingly laudable aim of preventing addiction also tends to contradiction on close examination. Addiction can be difficult to accurately define,[70] but if it's understood as obsessive and compulsive behaviour, the effects of the condition are real enough, as anyone who has taken the responsibility to care for a heroin-dependent person can confirm. So can those who care for an alcoholic or workaholic, for that matter. The difference between these latter two addicts and the heroin addict is that it is only the heroin addict who is liable to punishment as a consequence of their addiction. Moreover, the state, by its silence, appears to recognise a right to addiction: caffeine and a considerable number of prescription drugs are addictive, and people are said to be addicted to a variety of substances (such as sugar, chocolate and junk food) and a variety of recreational activities (such as sex, shopping, gambling, exercise, reading, watching television and surfing the internet), but none of these substances or activities is illegal. Nor is the most addictive drug of all nicotine.[71]

Very few illicit drugs are in fact addictive, and only a minority of consumers of those drugs actually become addicted to them. Heroin is probably the best-known addictive drug and a significant number of heroin addicts manage to overcome addiction on their own, without specialist assistance.[72] It is also obvious that the prospective health gains of prohibition (including the prevention of addiction) can only be made if criminal sanctions actually do deter illicit drug use. Rising rates of consumption indicate that they do not. If, on the other hand, prohibition is designed to prevent the medical condition of addiction, it fails entirely. A medical condition that causes a person to 'lose control' is, according to established doctrines of criminal law, sufficient to create a defence to criminal liability and punishment.[73] Insofar as the case for criminalisation based on preventing people from harming others is concerned, Husak describes the harmful qualities that a recreational drug would need to have before adults could justifiably lack a moral right to consume it, and goes on to explain the principles on which the state could justify prohibition. He concludes, however, that no such drug yet exists.[74] As the distinguished historian of US drug use, David Musto, has said, 'The history of drug laws in the United States shows that the degree to which a drug has been outlawed or curbed has no direct relation to its inherent danger.'[75]

Those who argue for prohibition on the ground of the harm that might be done to consumers can never explain why drugs are banned in inverse proportion to their harmful properties. Their struggle to do so usually results in the retort that the harm caused by alcohol and tobacco shouldn't be added to by making other drugs easier to obtain.[76] This response evades rather than explains the original contradiction in the harm principle, but its underlying assumption is also almost certainly wrong.

Adding to the harm caused by alcohol and tobacco by ending prohibition assumes that the patterns of consumption of alcohol, tobacco and illicit drugs would then remain unchanged. But in a free market for recreational drugs where product innovation would be naturally encouraged and preference freely exercised, it may well be that the consumption of some of the more dangerous drugs decreases and the consumption of some of the less dangerous drugs increases. Less harmful drugs, such as coca wine, and coca and opium teas, might well make significant inroads into the more harmful cocaine snorting and heroin injecting markets, and cannabis consumed as a drink or a food would be less harmful than smoking. The variety of products likely to be available could well reduce alcohol and tobacco consumption.

Research conducted at the University of Western Australia shows that if cannabis were legalised, consumption would increase among already frequent users without drawing in a substantial number of new users, and that for all types of consumers consumption would increase by 4 per cent, while beer, wine and spirit consumption would decrease by 1 per cent, 2 per cent and almost 4 per cent respectively.[77] The experience of decriminalisation in Holland seems to also point in this direction: the levels of cannabis consumption are lower in Holland than in the United States after more than a quarter of a century of decriminalisation. There have also been some encouraging signs with heroin addiction. In 1981, 14 per cent of Dutch heroin addicts were under 22; 15 years later, the figure was less than 5 per cent.[78]

In the final analysis, the case for criminalisation of drug use is a moral one. Drug use, according to William Bennett, destroys human character and makes a mockery of virtue.[79] It follows then, according to former administrator of the US Drug Enforcement Administration John Lawn, that the solution to drug use is character reconstruction,[80] although it's not entirely clear how the sort of character reconstruction recommended can take place in prisons, where drugs seem to be at least as readily available as in most other places. Nor is it clear why all immoral acts should be subject to criminal penalty. Violating the moral right to life, property or personal security constitutes an immoral act that invokes the powers of the criminal law, but recreational drug use doesn't violate the rights of anyone. Breaching a contract is an immoral act that has its remedy in restitution, specific performance and damages, not in the imprisonment of those who behave immorally by breaking such promises.[81]

People have widely different views on what constitutes proper moral behaviour, but the link between an individual's view of immorality and criminal punishment by the state demands a further reference point, and that point is usually found in an individual's right to protection of life, limb and property. These rights were determined by the English philosopher John

Locke (1632–1704) as inalienable rights that governments were granted a warrant to protect but had no right to infringe. America's Declaration of Independence in 1776 added the pursuit of happiness to this list of inalienable rights and William Bennett was bold enough to declare that the Founding Fathers never meant this to confer a right on citizens to go about in a drug-induced haze.[82] This is despite the fact that the Founding Fathers had ready access to now-illicit recreational drugs and that some of them at least were happy enough to indulge in them.

Controversy over what the pursuit of happiness might mean to one side, the extension beyond Locke's formulation to include state-sanctioned punishment according to people's various moral preferences needs to be explained, defended and supported within a legal and constitutional framework. However, the advocates and defenders of criminalising drug use simply insist that their moral prejudices have the virtue of good work being done in God's name. In 1977 the Senate Standing Committee on Social Welfare in Australia found that 'The current debate [on drugs] is distinguished by extreme views, marked hysteria and lack of perspective.'[83] By the early 1990s things hadn't much changed. Husak found that the moral right to recreational drug use was one of the small handful of issues that seemed almost immune to rational debate.[84] Little improvement has been observed since, and a large part of the reason is the central role organised religion has been able to carve out for itself in determining drug policy.

Religious beliefs rely on faith rather than reason, and the Christian faithful in the United States entertain some odd beliefs, some of which are to a lesser but still significant extent shared by non-Christians. According to various polls, 86 per cent of Americans believe in miracles, 83 per cent in the virgin birth, 45 per cent believe that there is a devil, 75 per cent of them do not accept Darwin's theory of evolution, and among evangelical Protestants the vast majority are convinced that the world will end in a battle at Armageddon between Jesus and the Antichrist.[85] Opposition to drug use, like opposition to abortion, is an article of faith with the faithful, and on a good day the best response that can be expected to a reasoned argument is the promise of prayers offered up on your behalf. As Husak puts it, 'Religious opposition to illicit drugs, like non-religious moral opposition, is a conclusion in search of a reason to support it.'[86] Here is a religious and moral framework that constructs harmless pleasure as pathological.[87] It makes the conclusion of Husak's long inquiry all the more difficult to resist: 'From a moral point of view, the case for decriminalisation is compelling.'[88]

'Deviants' and the dynamics of demand

The idea that began to seriously take hold in the United States in the early years of the 20th century that recreational drug users are of a 'deviant type' has been as enduring as it is demonstrably false. Recreational drug users can certainly be found among those whose lifestyles deviate from what might be, for others, commonly accepted norms, but like opium in the 19th century, recreational drug users are everywhere. Their individual reasons for using illicit drugs range from experimenting with 'forbidden fruit' to deliberately pursuing oblivion, and they embrace all points in between. There are some who believe that intoxicants function as medicines and that drug use for the purpose of intoxication should be properly regarded as self-medication.[89] But the pursuit of pleasure seems the most common theme among recreational drug users, and that clearly has no demographic limitations.

In the United States, the number of people who have used illicit drugs is probably close to 100 million. Those people range from presidents past and present to lesser politicians at every level of government. They include actors, artists, sports stars, lawyers, police, doctors, those in the armed forces, media workers, scientists, stockbrokers and at least one Supreme Court judge. Wage labourers of every description, the unemployed and the unemployable all use illicit drugs. In the United Kingdom in 2005, 45 per cent of those aged between 16 and 24 admitted to having used illicit drugs.[90]

In Australia considerably more than six million people over the age of 14 have consumed illicit drugs, and as in other advanced economies, they straddle occupations and social class, although there does seem to be a particularly high incidence of use in the armed forces and with prison guards.[91] Among politicians who have publicly self-reported illicit drug use are two former premiers of Western Australia, the former premier of Victoria, both the former chief minister and attorney-general of the Northern Territory, and at the national level, a former health minister, foreign affairs minister and Labor leader.[92] Random testing of professional footballers reveals recreational use of cannabis, cocaine, ecstasy and amphetamines. In a submission to a Senate inquiry into the setting-up of the Australian Sports Anti-Doping Authority in February 2006, the National Rugby League, supported by the Australian Football League Players Association, called for a distinction between performance-enhancing drugs — which they agreed should be prohibited by the authority — and recreational drugs, which they argued should not be. The inclusion of cannabis in sports anti-doping laws was denounced by the National Rugby League as 'social engineering'.[93] Selective recreational drug use by millions of mature, intelligent and often enough tertiary-educated and relatively high-income earning Australians shows that such behaviour, far from being deviant, is perfectly normal.

So why is it that so many people find pleasure in consuming mind-altering substances? For the very good reason, it's argued, that it is a biological characteristic of the human species: the impulse to periodically alter consciousness has been described as 'an innate, normal drive analogous to hunger or the sexual drive'.[94] It is a characteristic observable from early childhood, when children experiment with oxygen deprivation by holding their breath for as long as they can to experience the feeling of light-headedness. Spinning games, where children whirl around rapidly on the spot for the pleasurable giddiness that follows, are said to be a close to universal experience.[95]

The use of inhalants by children who are only slightly older seems to add weight to the contention that intoxication is a primal impulse. Nitrous oxide, the laughing gas inhaled so pleasurably by Sir Humphrey Davy and his friends in the late 18th century, is readily available today as the propellant gas in cans of whipped cream.

Glues, solvents, aerosols and hundreds of other common household products (such as disinfectants and nail polish removers) have a similar euphoric effect; so too do spray paint and petrol.[96] These sorts of inhalants, easily found around most kitchens, are frequently the first psychoactive substances that children, often between the ages of 11 and 13, use, and in the United States they are the only class of drugs whose use is significantly higher among younger children than older children. In one survey, nearly two-thirds of 10 to 17-year-olds indicated that they were about 12 years old when they first knew of fellow classmates using inhalants. Statistics show that the average age at which Australians used inhalants for the first time was lower than the age at which they first used other illicit drugs.[97]

Though food and drink are necessary to maintain existence, mere existence is often not enough. Some degree of modification is frequently called for, and intoxicants in one form or another are the agents that have been used throughout human history for this purpose.[98] Small wonder, then, that significant numbers of people graduate from spinning games to psychoactive drugs.

It would make little difference to the consumption of these drugs if, as Edward Kremers (head of the pharmacy program at Wisconsin University, who campaigned so vigorously against the misuse of the term 'drug') said in 1924, all the opium plants in the world (together with the coca and cannabis plants) could be destroyed; if they weren't substituted by synthetics, some other drugs would simply take their place.

Minimising harm from the more dangerous drugs

All drugs have a potential for harm; some clearly have a greater potential than others. However, a curious paradox emerges with public policy on drug consumption. Not only are drugs prohibited in inverse proportion to their harm, but the policing effort expended on illicit drugs is concentrated on the drug that causes the least harm. In the United States in the late 1980s and early 1990s, 750,000 drug users were arrested each year, more than three-quarters of them for simple possession of cannabis. In 2001, more people were still being arrested for cannabis offences than for heroin or cocaine, and of the 724,000 cannabis arrests, more than 90 per cent were again for simple possession.[99] In the United Kingdom, more than 80 per cent of all drug seizures between 1988 and 1998 were for cannabis, and in 1998, in terms of offenders the figure was closer to 90 per cent: 113,232 out of a total of 127,919.[100] In Australia in 2003–04, arrests for cannabis offences continued to represent by far the largest category of drug arrests: 72 per cent of the total. In 2005–06 they represented 71 per cent of the national total.[101]

Just as curiously, the limitations applied to the more dangerous recreational drugs — alcohol and tobacco — that actually have some success in reducing consumption are rejected in favour of a policy approach that has led to increased consumption.

Tobacco

From early in the 20th century the production of cigarettes came to resemble the production of the opium and cocaine-based proprietary medicines of the late 19th century. There was similar massive and false advertising, so their consumption increased in much the same way as it had for those earlier products. It took much longer, though, for the harmful effects of cigarettes to be recognised, despite the declaration of King James I of England in 1604 that tobacco was dangerous to the lungs. It wasn't until the early 1960s that most advanced economies began to take measures aimed at reducing consumption. These centred on education and the gradual prohibition of most forms of advertising. This was followed by the right of people to smoke being set against the rights of people to be in a smoke-free environment; in Australia, as in many other countries, this led to smoking being prohibited on public transport. As the dangers of passive smoking came to be better recognised, smoking was also prohibited in workplaces, restaurants and stadiums. By July 2007 smoking was prohibited in all Australian hotels. All of these measures, taken alone, have dampened consumption. In addition, workplace prohibition has reduced the daily consumption of those who continue to smoke by some 20 per cent.[102] The overall result is impressive, with daily smoking rates declining by 30 per cent between 1991 and 2004. Only 17.4 per cent of Australians aged 14 and over are now daily smokers, a clear majority have never taken up the habit and more than a quarter of the population have managed to discontinue it.[103]

While these trends are encouraging, they also point to shortcomings in the present policy approach. Much more could be done, and given that tobacco is responsible for some 19,000 deaths a year in Australia, a useful start would be to realign the public funds that are spent on drug programs so that they bear a closer relationship to the harm that various drugs cause. When more than 95 per cent of drug deaths are attributable to alcohol and tobacco, it makes no sense to direct more than 95 per cent of funding to attempting to control illicit drug use.[104] Funding needs to be allocated to more extensive and better targeted anti-smoking education campaigns, to programs that help smokers quit and to tackle the evident problem of female smoking. While male smoking rates decreased by 2.5 per cent between 2001 and 2004, female smoking rates showed a less marked decline (1.7 per cent) and smoking among 16 to 17-year-old females was almost double that of males.[105]

A more serious anti-smoking policy that paid a bit more than lip service to the prohibition on those under 18 smoking would abolish cigarette vending machines and all point-of-sale advertising and would ban tobacco advertising at televised sporting events. The retail sale of tobacco products could be restricted to specially licensed outlets so that the prohibition could be policed, and penalties for selling to those under 18 could then be enforced. The use of cigarettes in films, which still glamorises smoking, could be prohibited. At a more general level, the funds available for anti-smoking campaigns could be increased by forcing the tobacco companies to make a contribution.

The results of the US$246 billion settlement with the tobacco companies in the United States in 1998 have proved disappointing, with children still being bombarded by marketing and still taking up smoking at the rate of more than 3000 a day three years after the settlement was concluded.[106] Although they are not without some obvious merit, one-off settlements will continue to disappoint. They imply an end to litigation together with an assumption that a chastened industry will see the errors of its ways and begin to behave more responsibly. Such optimism is clearly misplaced. Tobacco companies have responded to the US settlement by promoting smokeless and 'reduced harm' products such as 'Eclipse', which looks like a cigarette but uses a special process to heat tobacco instead of burning it; this, it is claimed, reduces the harmful chemicals in smoke. Other new products include tobacco lozenges and cigarettes that use a carbon filter and special tobacco-curing process to lower toxin levels.[107] More than 900 million cans of smokeless tobacco — snuff, as it was once called — are now sold in the United States each year and 63 per cent of new users are smokers or former smokers.[108] Today's so-called reduced-harm products replicate the industry's use of the terms 'light' and 'mild', which goes back to the 1970s. Even health authorities initially agreed that these cigarettes were less harmful, until studies showed that smokers compensated by puffing harder and inhaling more deeply, the result of which was more cases of a new kind of cancer further down the lungs.[109] In early 2005, when the Australian Competition and Consumer Commission accused tobacco companies of misleading and deceptive conduct with the use of 'mild' and 'light' labels, the companies agreed to remove them from packaging and contribute $9 million to a consumer education campaign that emphasised that all cigarettes were equally dangerous. Later in the year the companies were accused by anti-smoking groups of breaking the agreement by using replacement terms and pack colouring.[110]

A more considered and potentially productive approach would be for state authorities to assume that a strategy that includes continued litigation is a necessary part of exercising some control over the tobacco industry and thereby improving public health. Following the 1998 US settlement, the US government again had the tobacco companies before the courts, under the provisions of the *Racketeering-Influenced and Corrupt Organisations Act* (the RICO Act), alleging a 50-year conspiracy to defraud and mislead the US public about the deaths and illnesses that they knew smoking caused. The penalty they demanded, US$280 billion, was an estimate of the profits the industry made selling cigarettes to minors over three decades when it had promised not to market its products to young people. The case failed when an appeals court ruled in 2005 that the intention of Congress in passing the RICO legislation was to make forward-looking orders to prevent future violations, not to pursue violations committed in the past.[111] The obvious remedy is for Congress to pass legislation making it clear that the tobacco industry is indeed liable for its past conduct. This appears unlikely, however, given that the US House of Representatives, in 2004, overwhelmingly voted for a Bill that will prevent people from suing the food industry for making them obese — this followed the release of a study that said that obesity was likely to overtake smoking as the country's biggest preventable killer.[112]

Legislation which limits smoking also reduces government revenue and governments often find the tension between the two difficult to resolve, although few of them are willing to admit it. The Indonesian government is something of an exception. When it increased the price and excise on cigarettes — which it has done on five occasions from 2001 — consumption decreased. One of the larger cigarette companies reported an 8 per cent fall in sales in 2003. But the accompanying decrease in government revenue led to a reversal of the policy: prices and excise were kept stable in 2004 instead of increasing again, with the hope that production and consumption would increase enough to meet the government's revenue expectations. This when there are 40,000 deaths each year in Indonesia caused by smoking-related illnesses.[113]

If a policy of prohibition can be made out for any drug it would be made out for tobacco, but revenue considerations, for both industry and government, are one good reason why it won't be adopted. But prohibition would also be wrong on moral grounds. If there is a moral entitlement to the consumption of drugs, even though they might cause harm to the consumer, it applies as much to tobacco as to any other drug. Moreover, prohibition of tobacco, just like prohibition of other drugs, simply won't work while there is demand for it. This is demonstrated in the case of tobacco by the effects of high taxation regimes aimed at limiting consumption (these also, of course, have the considerable attraction of increasing state revenue). This has significantly increased the retail price of tobacco products, and has contributed to the growth of an illicit market in Europe, the United States, Canada, China and Australia. According to some estimates, about one-third of all exported cigarettes find their way to the illicit market.[114]

In the United Kingdom, counterfeit cigarettes smuggled into the country from Asia and eastern Europe — made from tobacco treated with carcinogenic pesticides — have been found to contain between two and six times as much of some toxic substances as conventional cigarettes, which means they are a much greater health hazard.[115] In Australia, together with illegal cigarette imports, there is a growing market in an illicit tobacco product known as 'chop chop' or 'chop'. Initially sourced from the tobacco-producing regions of Victoria and North Queensland but now imported, illegal tobacco avoids the taxes imposed at the production level. Processed chop is then packaged and sold clandestinely through a network of retailers, avoiding retail taxes. The result is a product reliably reported to be little different from the commercial variety but costing less than half the price; some enterprising retailers will even deliver to your door. An indication of the size of the market can be seen by the Australian Tax Office seizures of illegal tobacco leaf and cut tobacco: 30 tonnes in 2001–02 to 68 tonnes in 2003–04.[116] Clearly, strategies to limit consumption have a limit beyond which illicit markets will emerge.

Alcohol

Unlike tobacco, sensible alcohol use has some beneficial effects on health. In small doses it protects against cardiovascular disease, and a study published in 2003 showed that even at levels above those recommended by health authorities, alcohol consumption was estimated to have prevented 3576 deaths in Australia between 1992 and 2001.[117]Although less easily quantified, the beneficial effects of consuming a relaxing few drinks shouldn't be underestimated either. And the mere fact that large numbers of Australians do not limit themselves to only one or two drinks a day shouldn't lead to the automatic condemnation of intoxication — as long as one is not harming others, intoxication is a matter for each individual. However, balancing a right to intoxication with the rights of others not to be surrounded by the intoxicated means that intoxication should be a private rather than a public activity.

The negative consequences of consuming immoderate amounts of alcohol, though, are hardly trifling. Between 1992 and 2001, sensible alcohol consumption prevented 3,576 deaths, but alcohol consumption also caused 31,133 deaths. And between 1993/94 and 2000/01, 577,269 hospitalisations were directly attributable to the drug.[118] The role of the state quite properly extends to disseminating this information widely and to educating consumers. It also extends further, to ameliorating, if not eliminating, the harm that alcohol consumers cause to others.

Unfortunately, such harm is not inconsiderable. The deaths in the 2003 study include 1,363 homicides; the hospitalisations include 76,115 due to injuries caused by violence and a further 47,167 from road crash injuries. Alcohol is linked to 34 per cent of all homicides, 50 per cent of domestic violence cases and almost half of all assaults.[119] Each year in Australia more than two million people are threatened by others who have drunk too much alcohol. This pattern of alcohol-related violence is similar in other countries. A study in Canada, however, found much higher rates of violence committed by people under the influence of alcohol than in Australia, and government research in the United Kingdom has found that 44 per cent of violent crime is alcohol related and that 70 per cent of hospital admissions on weekends are linked to the consumption of alcohol.[120] Yet, much like tobacco in earlier times, the view of alcohol that comes from its advertising is a celebration of the drug that refuses to recognise any dark side.

Although there is a visible and effective public education campaign against drink-driving, the educational resources devoted to warning against harmful alcohol consumption and the greater public menace of alcohol-induced violence are thinly spread. This allows those in the business of selling alcohol to assert that it is only a small percentage of the population that get so drunk that they become a danger to themselves and others.[121] The truth is, in fact, exactly the opposite. An estimate based on the 2001 National Drug Strategy Household Survey is that 80 per cent of alcohol consumed in that year in Australia was consumed in a way that put the drinker's health and safety at risk. Among females aged 14 to 24, 85 per cent of total consumption of alcohol was drunk at a risky or high risk level for acute harm, and in the younger female group, those aged 14 to 17, there was a striking increase in drinking at these dangerous levels, from 1 per cent in 1998 to 9 per cent in 2001.[122]

The ambivalence about public drunkenness which has been a constant theme in Australia since 26 January 1788 is perhaps best seen today in the annual event that has come to be known as Schoolies Week. Towards the end of November each year more than 100,000 school-leavers and high school students gather at popular locations from Queensland's Gold Coast to Western Australia's Rottnest Island in a serious attempt at week-long inebriation, where having a good time means having almost no memory of it. Public drunkenness and under-age drinking on a mass scale was until recently celebrated not for what it is, but as an innocent rite of passage, with only passing references, at best, to those damaged by the violent behaviour of others along the way.

Harm minimisation with alcohol is clearly a difficult

challenge. It is the original problem drug, and drunkenness was the first drug-induced condition to be medicalised, by the disease category of 'alcoholism' that the Swedish physician Magnus Huss (1807–90) created in 1849. Fittingly, perhaps, what was once a sin then came to be widely treated by a 12-step movement of group therapy (developed by William G Wilson and Robert Holbrook Smith in the United States in the 1930s and known as Alcoholics Anonymous) that is based on the Protestant religious tradition of bearing testimony. Applied since to other drug addictions, AA includes among its 12 steps a readiness to have God remove one's character defects.[123]

Fortunately there are measures the state can reasonably take to prevent alcohol-related harm to others that do not rely on this kind of intervention. Lowering to zero the blood alcohol concentration permissible for driving a vehicle would be a useful addition to the measures already in place. Providing much cheaper low-alcohol products to consumers by significantly lowering state-imposed taxes on them is also likely to have a positive effect on consumption patterns, as would the replacement of advertising that celebrates the drug by advertising that emphasises the link between alcohol consumption and violent and anti-social behaviour. However, the balance between short-term revenue collection and long-term public health benefits is often, as noted above, a difficult challenge for governments. In New South Wales, after a quarter of a century of judicial licensing laws the police commissioner complained that 75 per cent of all police engagements were as a result of alcohol. From July 2008 the state moved to an administrative system which allows for the imposition of restrictions on licensed premises on the basis of anticipated risk rather than proof of breaches.[124]

It is clear that measures taken to limit drug consumption can work, but when consumption is driven by an enduring strength of demand, prohibition has very little, if any, prospect of success.

Epilogue:
The defeat of communism and
the revenge of religion

Together with Ludwig Feuerbach (1804–72) and Sigmund Freud (1856–1939), Karl Marx is credited with being one of the three great pillars of the golden age of atheism, which spans the period from the fall of the Bastille in Paris in 1789 to the fall of the wall dividing Berlin 200 years later.[1] In 1841 Feuerbach, who was a former pupil of Hegel, published *Das Wesen des Christentums* (translated by George Eliot [Mary Ann Evans] as *The Essence of Christianity*). For Feuerbach the idea of a God was a 'consolation and a distraction', a human invention that was a misguided attempt at providing comfort during dark and difficult times. The mother of religion was darkness.[2] Voltaire had earlier said, in 1768, that if God did not exist it would be necessary to invent him, and Feuerbach advanced the idea that the human mind unconsciously 'projects its longing for immortality and meaning onto an imaginary screen, and gives the name God to its own creation'. Religion was a dream.[3] Feuerbach wrote: 'If man did not exist, God would have no cause for activity', and went on to ask, given that God was a human invention, why we couldn't dispense with such an outmoded belief altogether.[4]

Freud was greatly influenced by Feuerbach, the philosopher he 'revered and admired above all others'. He added what he called a 'psychological foundation' to Feuerbach's work, using his by-now accumulated experience of psychoanalysis. This of course revealed the connection between the father complex and belief in God, and from this Freud was able to explain religion as 'basically a distorted form of an obsessional neurosis'.[5]

Marx's criticism of religion was much more radical and its result much more profound. Where Feuerbach had argued that religion was the projection of human needs, Marx asserted that religion came from the 'sorrow and injustice' evident in the social situation of individuals within existing social structures. Feuerbach had fallen into error because he had not taken this social dimension properly into account.[6] As Marx put it:

> *Feuerbach resolves the religious essence into the human essence. But the essence of man is no abstraction inhering in each single individual. In its actuality it is the ensemble of social relationships. Feuerbach, who does not go into the criticism of this actual essence, is hence compelled:*
>
> *1. To abstract from the historical process and to establish religious feeling as something self-contained, and to presuppose an abstract — isolated — human individual;*
> *2. To view the essence of man merely as 'species', as an internal, dumb generality which unites the many individuals naturally.*[7]

If religion were the direct outcome of unjust social conditions, there was no need to engage in intellectual inquiry with any of its specific ideas:[8] 'All social life is essentially practical. All mysteries which lead theory to mysticism find their rational solution in human practice and in the comprehension of this practice.'[9] Religion is merely the 'halo' of the real world, and it is this real world, with its real oppression — not religion — that needs to be the subject of philosophical scrutiny and criticism. 'The abolition of religion as the illusory happiness of the people is the demand for their real happiness. To call on them to give up their illusions about their condition is to call on them to give up a condition that requires illusions.'[10]

The condition that required the illusion of religion was the socioeconomic condition that workers found themselves in under a system called capitalism. Marx would devote the rest of his life to the analysis of capitalism and he bade farewell to Feuerbach and classical philosophy with the famous words: 'The philosophers have only interpreted the world, in various ways; the point is to change it.'[11]

And change it Marx most certainly did, even though Volume 1 of his epic work *Das Kapital* was greeted more with silence and indifference than critical acclaim when it first appeared in 1867.[12] But rapid industrialisation throughout the Western world from that time on led to an enormous increase in what Marx had earlier described as the 'grave-diggers of capitalism', the industrial proletariat or working class. Mass socialist parties that relied on his revolutionary ideology, although somewhat thin on the ground at the time of his death in 1883, except in Germany, began to emerge after it, and by the outbreak of World War I in 1914 they were a formidable part of the political landscape across Europe and in the United States.[13] An influential minority were convinced by Marx's work that scientific socialism would inevitably replace capitalist exploitation, and for an increasing number of them the prospect of a new life on earth was more certain than the conditional promise of an afterlife somewhere else. Socialism became the new religion for those constructing the social New Jerusalem.[14]

The country where socialist revolution was least likely to occur, at least on Marx's analysis, was the place where, in 1917, it did occur. Backward tsarist Russia, where serfdom had finally been abolished less than 60 years previously, provided the unlikely setting for the event that was described by John Reed, a US journalist who watched it unfold, as *Ten Days That Shook the World*.[15] It wasn't that revolution was totally unexpected: a revolution had already taken place in 1905 following the disastrous Russo-Japanese War of 1904–05, and now World War I, with the 'flower of Russian manhood' buried beneath the mud of its many battlefronts, was proceeding in an equally disastrous way.[16] The tsarist regime was terminally ill and lurching towards its end, but who would dig its grave?

According to Marx, a proletarian socialist revolution required an advanced industrial working class of the sort that Russia had yet to develop, despite the fact that workers had organised themselves in councils known as 'soviets' in the 1905 revolution.[17] At best, in Marx's view, a revolution in Russia might act as an illustration, to the industrially more developed countries in Europe, of what could be achieved. It could provide a precedent for them to immediately follow by beginning their own revolutions.[18] This was a widely held Marxist view. The official language of the successor organisation to Marx's International Workingmen's Association (first set up in 1864), the Third or Communist International of 1919, was German. Although this organisation was located in Moscow, Vladimir Ilyich Lenin (1870–1924), the most important figure of the 1917 revolution, hoped that it would soon be able to relocate to Berlin.[19] The prospect of being buttressed by revolutionary socialist governments rather than isolated and surrounded by antagonistic capitalist states was part of the 'gamble' that Lenin took when the Bolsheviks seized power and set about the socialist transformation of Russia.[20] As one of Lenin's comrades wrote in the May Day proclamation of 1917: 'under the thunder of the Russian Revolution the workers in the West, too, rise from their slumber.'[21]

For a short time at least, it actually seemed something of a possibility. From a German prison cell Rosa Luxemburg (1871–1919), the Polish-born revolutionary, wrote: 'Unless it receives backing from an international proletarian revolution in time, the dictatorship of the proletariat in Russia is doomed to a stunning defeat, compared to which the fate of the Paris Commune will probably seem like child's play.'[22] Convinced that a German revolution would come, and come soon, she was concerned that it wouldn't come soon enough to save the Russian Revolution.[23]

It came on 9 November 1918, when a republic was proclaimed in Berlin. The previous day she had been released from prison, and at 11am on 11 November, World War I came to an end. It was not, however, a socialist revolution, even though a republic in that name was afterwards proclaimed in Bavaria and an even more revolutionary-sounding Soviet Republic was set up in Munich in early 1919.[24] For the revolutionary socialists who thought for a moment that they might claim Berlin (these included Lenin) it was all over rather quickly, and on the night of 15 January 1919, Rosa Luxemburg and her fellow Communist Party leader Karl Liebknecht were murdered.[25] The Russian Revolution would have to look after itself.

It did so with remarkable resilience, led by Lenin and ably assisted by the commissar for war Lev Davidovich Bronstein, better known as Leon Trotsky (1879–1940). It survived foreign intervention and the Civil War of 1918–20, although by this time the economy was in tatters. Industrial output had declined by over 80 per cent and steel production stood at a mere 5 per cent of pre-war levels. Workers were paid in kind, and thereafter obliged to barter for bread on the black market. The tens of thousands of destitute children who soon emerged, sniffing up to five grams of cocaine a day to ward off hunger and give them the courage to carry out their criminal activities, were among Moscow's more visible victims. Trotsky's solution was the militarisation of labour. Dressed up as war communism, this bore little resemblance to the promised workers' paradise, and the insurgents at Kronstadt who rose up to demand something better in March of 1921 well expressed what some workers, at least, thought of as economic and political oppression.[26]

After the Kronstadt rising, war communism was replaced by Lenin's New Economic Policy (NEP). The NEP was an attempt at establishing a mixed economy, one that effectively reintroduced the market while still being controlled by the state. State capitalism, Lenin called it, as Russia's revolutionary leadership struggled to construct a socialist economy, hampered by the lack of a practical example of how it might actually be achieved. Given his 'habitual realism', just how Lenin's long-term economic policies may have evolved can only be a matter of conjecture.[27] In May 1922 he suffered the first of a series of strokes; he was mostly incapacitated from this time until his death in January 1924. His successor abandoned the NEP in favour of a series of Five-Year Plans, the so-called planned economy, more properly called a command economy, driven by a particularly brutal politics.[28]

Joseph Vissarionovich Djugashvili (1879–1953) more commonly known as Josef Stalin (man of steel) was an uncommonly cruel man. His chief rival to succeed Lenin, Trotsky, was expelled from the Communist Party in 1927, expelled from Russia two years later, tried in absentia and sentenced to death. By the time the sentence was carried out, by an assassin with an icepick in Mexico in 1940, all Trotsky's children had died in mysterious circumstances.[29] Stalin's socialism was rule by terror: close to 10 million peasants died through either execution or famine in 1932–33 alone. His program of rapid industrialisation relied on a prison labour force that may have numbered as many as 13 million.[30]

When the Bolshevik conference of July 1917 was debating the likely fate of a revolution in one country, Russia, in the absence of revolutions in the West, Stalin argued that it was eminently possible to begin building socialism in Russia in such circumstances. When asked about the apparent contradiction between this view and that of Marx (as well as most Marxists), Stalin replied, 'There exists a dogmatic Marxism and a creative one. I am opting for the latter.' Lenin and Trotsky, on the other hand, insisted that while Russia could begin to build socialism before the more advanced countries, she couldn't, alone, carry it very far. Its success would ultimately depend on socialist revolution in the West.[31]

After Lenin's death, Stalin solved the problem in the autumn of 1924, when he developed the idea of 'socialism in one country'; this was despite the fact that he had earlier in the same year been a part of the consensus that held a contrary view, and written that it was not possible to establish a socialist economy in one country. The new dogma wasn't so much subject to critical debate as imposed as a loyalty test to the party and the state that Stalin would control for the next 30 years.[32] It rested on a truce between communism and capitalism, made in the belief that revolution was confined to Russia.[33] It meant that the tension between the USSR, which coexisted with other countries, and the communist movement, whose aim was to overthrow the governments of those countries, was resolved in favour of the USSR, as run by Stalin. Any revolution that might occur elsewhere had to be compatible with the USSR's interests and Soviet controlled.[34]

In the absence of supportive socialist revolutions in the West, what then would happen to the lone Russian Revolution? According to Trotsky, it would either succumb to a conservative Europe or defeat itself by becoming 'corroded in its economically and culturally primitive Russian environment'.[35] For Luxemburg, socialism entailed a broadening of democracy, and the consequence for any revolution which denied this would be 'a dictatorship, to be sure, but not the dictatorship of the proletariat: rather the dictatorship of a handful of politicians, ie, a dictatorship in the bourgeois sense, in the sense of a Jacobin rule ... every long-lasting regime based on martial law leads without fail to arbitrariness, and all arbitrary power tends to deprave society'.[36]

And so it came to be. Under Stalin, control would be exercised over not only people's lives, but their thoughts as well. Whatever else it was, it wasn't the Marxism which envisaged freedom from wage slavery and exploitation, total liberation and individual self-fulfilment.[37] It was certainly a far cry from the vision of Marx and Engels:

> *In communist society, where nobody has one exclusive area of activity and each can train himself in any branch he wishes, society regulates the general production, making it possible for me to do one thing today and another tomorrow, to hunt in the morning, fish in the afternoon, breed cattle in the evening, criticise after dinner, just as I like, without ever becoming a hunter, a fisherman, a herdsman, or a critic.*[38]

The decline of Marx and Engel's communist vision can be dated from the rise of Stalin. When Soviet tanks rolled into Budapest in 1956 they signalled not just the end of a Hungarian revolt, but the beginning of the end of Soviet communism.

Is historical materialism history?

Can what happened in practice be separated from what, according to Marx's theory, should have happened: the replacement of a class-antagonistic bourgeois society with 'an association in which the free development of each is the condition for the free development of all'?[39] Marx had, after all, continued the work of Adam Smith and David Ricardo. His doctrine has been described as the 'legitimate successor' to not only the best of English political economy but to German philosophy and French socialism as well.[40] But even allowing this assessment is correct, it is nevertheless the successor to the best of political economy, philosophy and politics in the latter part of the 19th century. Could the goal of a classless society rest on such foundations?

According to the dialectical approach taken by Marx and Engels, as the contradictions that come from the historical movement of the material forces of production are resolved, they give rise to new material arrangements that also bring with them generic conflicts. The final resolution which would bring communism to the world wouldn't, on one view at least, entirely remove all contradictions from the material powers that structure it. Change would still be governed by the dialectical process.[41] In this way, Marx's own work provides an explanation for the collapse of what purported to be communist states. More than 140 years before the event, he wrote that a social revolution of the sort that occurred in the USSR and eastern Europe from the late 1980s came from the inevitable conflict that turns the existing relations of production from forms of development into their fetters.[42]

It need hardly be said that there was no real development of the theory of historical materialism from the 1920s in the USSR or in those European countries that became part of the communist camp following World War II. Nor in China, where Mao Tse-tung's knowledge of Marxism was mediated by Stalinism; it rested almost entirely on his reading of *The History of the Communist Party of the Soviet Union*, a publication authorised by the Central Committee of the Party in 1938. According to its introduction, a study of such history 'helps us to master Bolshevism and sharpens our political vigilance'.[43]

Marx's historical materialism was a theory for interpreting the world that would eventually change it.[44] Capitalism didn't stand still with the publication of Marx's *Capital* or the Bolshevik Revolution, or with Stalinist domination of the world communist movement. It went through a series of what Engels might have termed evolutions that, beginning from the Stalinist ascendancy in 1924, stretched through the Great Depression and all the way to the domination of free-market ideology. Along the way, its death was prematurely announced on more than one occasion. Marx's more immediate successors, from the 1920s, largely failed to analyse these changes because the straitjacket of Stalinism, which extended far beyond the USSR, meant that any important critique of capitalist development was the exclusive domain of the Communist International in Moscow.[45] Honourable exceptions who had the courage to free themselves from such constraints, the Hungarian George Lukacs and Karl Korsch in Germany, were treated as heretics. They were either excommunicated (Korsch) or threatened with excommunication and thereafter marginalised (Lukacs). The most outstanding of them, Antonio Gramsci in Italy, only managed to escape a confrontation with Stalinism because of his decade-long isolation in an Italian prison cell, which resulted in his death in 1937.[46]

In these circumstances, Western Marxism managed to turn Marx's own movement — from philosophy to politics to economics — into a circular one that found itself firmly back in the discipline of philosophy.[47] Marxist theory, philosophically rummaging rather than practically changing, became separated from working-class struggle which it then struggled to understand from its eventual vantage point in the academy. Workers too would struggle to even follow the language of this academic discourse, politely described as a 'highly technical idiom'.[48]

Following World War II, Paris became the capital city of philosophy, just as it had earlier become the medical capital of the world, and if any one person was responsible for popularising the discipline it was Jean-Paul Sartre (1905–80). Philosopher, novelist and convert to Marxism, he edited an influential journal that, in tribute to Charlie Chaplin, was called *Modern Times*. Although a Marxist, he pointedly refused to join a communist party of France, which was still suffering from, but receiving no treatment for, the cancer of Stalinism. An exaggerated example of his wide influence was the fact that sections of the right-wing press in France held him personally responsible for the student-led revolt that convulsed the country in 1968.

This mass revolt, which was indeed outside of the control of the French Communist Party, was followed in the next five years by massive labour unrest in Italy, the United Kingdom and Japan, culminating in yet another crisis of capitalism, the worldwide recession of 1974.[49] It was also contemporaneous with the end of the original Western Marxist tradition that lived in the shadow of Stalin; a period when Marxists of the calibre of Ernest Mandel, Harry Braverman, Eric Hobsbawm and E P Thompson had come to dominate the left flank of the landscape.[50] By any measure it was a period of sharpening class struggle. But the synthesis of Marxist theory and practice failed to occur, even though conditions were now favourable to both. Though the 'poverty of theory' had been rectified, there still, it seems, remained significant problems of strategy. By 1977 *Time* magazine declared that Marx was finally dead and Sartre had renounced Marxism. Much more ominously, Michel Foucault proclaimed the 'end of politics'.[51] Marxism was defiantly called to battle with structuralism and its offspring, post-structuralism, both of them early strands of a philosophy that came to be known as postmodernism.

Structuralism had somewhat unusual origins: in the linguistic work of Ferdinand de Saussure (1857–1913). His enormous influence is based on a work that he neither saw nor wrote. The seminal text on which structuralism relies, Saussure's *Course in General Linguistics*, was published in 1916, three years after his death. It was put together from students' notes of the lectures that he delivered at the University of Geneva between 1907 and 1911, synthesised by two of Saussure's university colleagues who never themselves attended any of his lectures.[52] Nevertheless Saussure's work in linguistics was revolutionary, and pioneered the general science of signs known as semiotics. In order to uncover how language reveals meaning he looked at language as a system separate from speech (or writing) and examined its structure. Noise counts as language only when it expresses or communicates ideas, and the way in which language does this is by a system of signs. A sign is the union of a signifier (the word 'dog', for example) and a signified (dog), and these two exist only as components of the sign.[53] The relationship between the two is arbitrary, with the association of sound to its referent the result of custom and usage in collectively accepted social practice.[54] In this arbitrary process the signified associated with the signifier can take any form without having to possess an essential core of meaning.[55] Understood in these terms, meaning itself is the product of the relationship between two components of a sign that are themselves meaningless.

From this, through a tortuous route that employed an even more tortuous language, postmodernism was eventually able to question the certainty of meaning. If it didn't go so far as to declare that 'there is no meaning', it did insist that meaning was 'scattered'. At best this made it difficult to find and opened up what might be found to individual whim. At worst it made meaning impossible to discern.

The difficulty that structuralism and post-structuralism increasingly posed for Marxism was that there was no coherent idea in Marxism about the nature of the relationship between structure and subject. The relationship between the structural reality of historical change and the subjective forces contending for control of them was never clear.[56] *The Communist Manifesto* declared that the practical application of the principles laid down in it depended, 'everywhere and at all times', on the existing historical conditions. They also seemed to be dependent on the exhortation that 'working men of all countries unite'.[57] But how were they to unite? If the gravediggers aren't in some way organised, it is surely difficult to arrange any burial.

The endeavour to rethink the relations between structure and subject was initially undertaken in France by Sartre and others, but it was the application of Saussure's structural linguistics to anthropology (an improper application, on Saussure's own authority) that radically challenged the notion of the subject.[58] It did so by effectively dissolving it. According to the anthropologist Claude Levi-Strauss (b. 1908), the human subject was 'the spoilt brat of philosophy' and the ultimate goal of the human sciences was 'not to constitute man but to dissolve him'.[59] The post-structuralists Jacques Derrida (1930–2004) and Michel Foucault (1926–84) continued the process of dissolving the subject; given its interdependence with structure, structure too was inevitably subverted.[60]

Postmodernism then didn't so much engage with Marxism as attempt to erase the 'text' that surrounded it. Its most obvious virtue lies in the space it opened up for those groups otherwise subsumed by the Marxist notion of class: feminists and ethnic and other minorities now more able to proclaim their own identity politics. But for all its celebration of the 'other', postmodernism was the antithesis of Marxism. Neo-conservative rather than revolutionary, it seemed to deny the possibility of change. Derrida's notion of 'textual undecidability' did in fact decide something: it reinforced the preservation of the status quo by prohibiting an interrogation of truth.[61] Derridan deconstruction could be seen to 'function as the restoration of tradition and authority'. As Foucault pointed out, 'This pedagogy [which teaches the pupil that there is nothing outside the text] gives the teacher's voice that unlimited sovereignty which allows it to repeat the text indefinitely.'[62] Foucault's own work, particularly his critique of history as seen through the prism of power relationships, held much more promise until it too finally petered out, unable to explain, in the absence of a constant human subject in history, who was struggling against whom. Power is everywhere, he wrote, and is finally analysed as itself having such unlimited authority that when we are not fighting each other we are fighting something within ourselves.[63]

By the mid-1990s, postmodernism had largely gone out of fashion. As it expanded its reach in the redoubt of the academy, it had elsewhere contracted to a term of abuse.[64] Its reputation suffered somewhat at the hands of the physicist Alan Sokal, who in 1996 published an article entitled 'Transgressing the Boundaries: Towards a Transformative Hermeneutics of Quantum Gravity' in the journal *Social Text*, which had acquired something of a reputation for postmodernist scepticism towards science. The article, warmly received by many, purported to establish links between quantum mechanics and elements of postmodern philosophy. It was, however, a hoax, aimed at exposing scientific ignorance and postmodernist posturing. Sokal and a colleague later elaborated this critique in a book published in 1998 called *Fashionable Nonsense: Postmodernist Intellectuals' Abuse of Science*.[65]

At the same time there was a revival of interest in Marx's work in a place that most would never have predicted: Wall Street. Twenty years after he was finally declared dead he rose again, Lazarus-like, when a special issue of the *New Yorker* in late 1997 hailed Karl Marx as 'the next big thinker'. The insights that come from his study of capitalism had apparently convinced certain of those in the investment banking community that he was right after all and has much to teach us about global markets, alienation, the tendency to monopoly and political corruption.[66] It remains to be seen, of course, whether the post-structuralist view that society is now post-Marxist is correct.[67] The ultimate test of Marx is likely to be in his proposition that 'new superior relations of production never replace older ones before the material conditions of their existence have matured within the framework of the old society. Mankind thus inevitably sets itself only such tasks as it is able to solve'.[68]

Whatever the existing relations of production might be, their logic rests on the profit that comes from consumption. The broad political consensus that today encourages economic growth leads to an increasing rate of material goods production, production that is dependent on the exploitation of finite physical resources.[69] The task that most now recognise as increasingly necessary is to reduce production and consumption to sustainable levels, while somehow also taking into account the legitimate aspiration to higher levels of consumption in advancing economies. The size of this latter problem can be gauged by glimpsing the rapidly advancing Chinese economy. If the number of motor vehicles per head matched that of the United States, it would use 99 million barrels of oil a day. The world currently produces only 84 million barrels a day, and at present levels of consumption alone, oil will become scarce by mid-century.[70] To continue to put the finishing touch to production by consuming at ever-increasing rates, we would need to emulate the charlatans of the East India Company by once more being cleverer than the alchemists, producing all material goods, not just gold, out of nothing.

The revenge of religion

In 1961, when Yuri Gagarin became the first man to be rocketed beyond earth into the heavens, something like half the population of the world was, nominally at least, atheist. Over the next few years the movement away from religious belief, the logical extension of Marx's argument that improved social conditions would allow for the illusion of religion to be dispensed with, gained momentum. By late 1965 *Time* magazine was questioning, on its front cover: 'Is God dead?'[71] By the next decade the answer was clearly 'no', as religion made a comeback in the United States. Mind you, it never quite went away anywhere, not even in the Soviet collective.[72]

From the 1970s in the United States a Christian lifestyle industry emerged that allowed conspicuous consumption to be sanctified as serving a higher purpose.[73] Religion was back with an in-your-face boldness reminiscent of the radicalism of the previous decade. Scripture Candy and Testamints could now be munched on while watching a religious film or television program or listening to a religious radio station. By 1998 Christian music was outselling jazz and classical music put together, capturing 6 per cent of US sales, a figure that increased to 7 per cent by 2001. The previous year, Christian bookstore sales totalled US$4 billion and evangelical Christians, for whom the Bible is the infallible word of God, now make up a proportion of the population that has been estimated at as high as 40 per cent.[74] The number of atheists or non-believers throughout the world is now said to be in the range of 8–14 per cent.[75]

Slowly but surely religion has extracted its revenge on Marx, first by declaring consumption of opium, which he first wrote about in 1844, a sin, and then by convincing secular authorities to criminalise its use. It was a religious figure, in the person of Charles Henry Brent, bishop of the Philippines, who denied the people of that country their opium at the turn of the 20th century in the belief that they would then be more amenable to Protestant religious conversion. Brent was then instrumental in forging the international drug laws that added cocaine and cannabis to the opium that was to be denied to people around the world seeking secular solace in these substances rather than religion. His successors have succeeded in keeping the faith. As science has expanded the pharmacopoeia, they've extended the reach of prohibition.

The struggles that have dominated the early years of the 21st century, after the collapse of godless communism, have been in the name of religion rather than class. They were preceded by a bombing campaign by the Irish Republican Army, begun in the 1970s, that tore the United Kingdom apart. The campaign had its immediate origins in the late 1960s, when a struggle erupted over civil rights denied to a Catholic minority by a Protestant majority in Northern Ireland.

The religious fanatics who have terrorised cities around the world since September 2001 have done so using the technique of suicide warfare, which developed in an earlier religion-based struggle between Israelis and Palestinians. A war on religion-fuelled terror has replaced the class war of Marx, and its dominant leader, George W Bush, and many of his dogged supporters are themselves sustained by a conservative Christian faith.

Religion clearly continues to provide illusory happiness in adverse social conditions. But irrespective of social conditions, opiates and other drugs continue to be a necessary part of life for many. If religion remains the soul of soulless conditions and the heart of a heartless world, it continues to have a soul mate in the drug consumption of the oppressed. In an irony that Marx, whose drug taking seems to have been limited to tobacco and alcohol, might have appreciated, there are now four million opiate users in Europe. Two-thirds of them reside in the east and the Russian Federation is now Europe's largest heroin market.

Endnotes

Introduction

1   Karl Marx's description of religion as the opium of the people first appeared in
    an article entitled 'A Contribution to the Critique of Hegel's Philosophy of Right:
    Introduction'. It was published in Paris in 1844 in the first and only edition of the
    German-French Yearbook (Deutsch-Französische Jahrbucher). See *Karl Marx.: Early Writings*
    (Penguin. London. 1992), pp 28, 243–57, 435. In an introduction to these early
    writings Lucio Colletti makes the observation that Marx's theoretical communism
    was developed while he was writing his critiques of Hegel's philosophy in 1843 and
    early 1844; pp 45, 243.

2   Virginia Berridge, *Opium And The People* (Free Association Books. London and
    New York. 1999), p 37.

3   ibid., p294, extracted from Table 2: Imported Home Consumption of Opium,
    1827–60.

4   Richard Davenport-Hines, *The Pursuit of Oblivion* (Weidenfeld & Nicolson. London.
    2001), p 36.

5   Berridge, 1999, op. cit., pp 292–93, extracted from Table 1: The Source and
    Quantities (in pounds) of England's Opium Imports 1827–1900. Opium was of
    course exported from, as well as imported into, England.

6   Friedrich Engels, *The Condition of the Working Class in England* (Progress Publishers.
    Moscow. 1984; Elecbook. London. 1998), pp 177–79.

7   Berridge, 1999, op. cit., p 31.

8   ibid., p 49.

9   Thomas De Quincey, *Confessions of an English Opium-Eater* (Wordsworth Classics.
    Hertfordshire. 1994), Introduction.

10 John and Dorothy Colmer, *Mainly Modern* (Rigby. Adelaide. 1978), p 83.

11 Colin N Crisswell, *The Taipans: Hong Kong's Merchant Princes* (Oxford University Press.
    Hong Kong. 1981), pp 3–4.

12 Carl A Trocki, *Opium, Empire and the Global Political Economy* (Routledge. London.
    1999), p 107.

13 Crisswell, 1981, op. cit., p 33.

14 ibid., pp 57, 66.

15 Alfred W. McCoy, *The Politics of Heroin: CIA Complicity in the Global Drug Trade*
    (Lawrence Hill Books. New York. 1991), pp 53–63.

16 Trocki, 1999, op. cit., p 167. Davenport-Hines, 2001, op. cit., p ix.

Chapter 1

1   Davenport-Hines, 2001, op. cit., p 203.

2   Alfred W McCoy, *Drug Traffic, Narcotics and Organised Crime in Australia*
    (Harper & Row. Sydney. 1980), pp 54, 69. The term 'patent medicine' comes from

the English practice of patenting compound medicines, which boomed in the 18th century. Patent medicines sold in England at the time attracted a duty and carried a government stamp. Since most 'patent' medicines came to be neither patented nor patentable, they are more properly referred to as 'proprietary' medicines. See Christine MacLeod, *Inventing the Industrial Revolution: The English Patent System 1600–1800* (Cambridge University Press. Cambridge. 1988), pp 84–85; T R Nevett, *Advertising in Britain* (Heinemann. London. 1982), p 24.

3   Berridge, 1999, op. cit., p 131.

4   Martin H Levinson, *The Drug Problem* (Praeger. Westport CT. 2002), p 12.

5   *Sears and Roebuck 1897 Catalogue*, WA State Library collection.

6   Davenport-Hines, 2001, op. cit., p 178.

7   ibid., p 204.

8   Berridge, 1999, op. cit., p 241.

9   Davenport-Hines, 2001, op. cit., pp 90, 160.

10   Levinson, 2002, op. cit., p 14.

11   Davenport-Hines, 2001, op. cit., p 185.

12   World heroin production fell from 20,000 pounds in 1926 to 2,200 pounds in 1931. Opium production, which stood at 41,600 tonnes in 1906, was down to 7,600 tonnes in 1934. See Alfred W. McCoy, 1991, op. cit., p 10.

13   David. T Courtwright, 'The Road to H: The Emergence of the American Heroin Complex, 1898–1956', in David F Musto (ed), *One Hundred Years of Heroin* (Auburn House. Westport CT. 2002). In Australia, heroin was prohibited for medical purposes in 1953 (see Chapter 2).

14   Berridge, 1999, op. cit., p 76.

15   Levinson, 2002, op. cit., p 11.

16   Jill Jonnes, *Hep-cats, Narcs and Pipe Dreams* (Scribner. New York. 1996), pp 18, 25.

17   Davenport-Hines, 2001, op. cit., p 81.

18   Caroline Jean Acker, 'From All Purpose Anodyne to Marker of Deviance: Physicians' Attitudes Towards Opiates in the US from 1890 to 1940', in Roy Porter and Mikulas Teich (eds), *Drugs and Narcotics in History* (Cambridge University Press. Cambridge. 1995).

19   ibid.

20   Joseph F Spillane, *Cocaine: From Medical Marvel to Modern Menace in the United States, 1884–1920* (Johns Hopkins University Press. Baltimore MD. 2000), p 91.

21   Courtwright, 2002, op. cit., p 4.

22   ibid., pp 8–9.

23   See Acker, 1995, op. cit., p 124.

24   ibid., p 123.

25   William L White, 'Trick or Treat? A Century of American Responses to Heroin Addiction', in Musto (ed), 2002, op. cit.

26   Desmond Manderson, *From Mr Sin to Mr Big: A History of Australian Drug Laws* (Oxford Unitversity Press. Melbourne. 1993), pp 106, 133.

27   ibid., pp 105–06.
28   Davenport-Hines, 2001, op. cit., p 297.
29   Michel Foucault, *The Birth of the Clinic: An Archaelogy of Medical Perception* (Routledge. London and New York. 2003), p xii.
30   Nevett, op. cit., p 35.
31   Acker, 1995, op. cit., p 115.
32   Lois N. Magner, *A History of Medicine* (Marcel Dekker Inc. New York. 1992), p 2. Roy Porter, *The Greatest Benefit to Mankind: A Medical History of Humanity* (W W Norton & Company. New York and London. 1997), p 18.
33   Porter, 1997, op. cit., pp 18–20.
34   ibid., p 31.
35   ibid. See also Guenter B Risse, 'Medical Care', in W F Bynum and Roy Porter (eds), *Companion Encyclopedia of the History of Medicine* (Routledge. London and New York. 1994).
36   Risse, 1994, op. cit.
37   Roderick E McGrew, *Encyclopedia of Medical History* (McGraw-Hill Book Company. New York. 1985), pp 142–43.
38   Porter, 1997, op. cit., p 82.
39   Magner, 1992, op. cit., p 82.
40   Toby Gelfand, 'The History of the Medical Profession', in Bynum and Porter, 1994, op. cit.
41   ibid.
42   Roy Porter (ed), *The Cambridge Illustrated History of Medicine* (Cambridge University Press. Cambridge. 1996), pp 97–98.
43   Harold J Cook, 'Physical Methods', in Bynum and Porter, 1994, op. cit.
44   McGrew, 1985, op. cit., pp 30–31.
45   ibid.
46   Gelfand, 1994, op. cit.
47   ibid.
48   See Gelfand, 1994, op. cit.
49   Roger Scruton, *A Dictionary of Political Thought* (Pan Books. London. 1983), p 354.
50   See Risse, 1994, op. cit.
51   Adam Smith, *An Inquiry into the Nature and Causes of the Wealth of Nations* (George Bell & Sons. London and New York. 1896), vol. 1, pp 62–63, 115.
52   Gelfand, 1994, op. cit.
53   See Foucault, 2003, op. cit., pp36–39.
54   ibid., pp 68–69. Gelfand, 1994, op. cit.
55   Foucault, 2003, op. cit., pp82–83.
56   Risse, 1994, op. cit.
57   Paul Rabinow (ed), *The Foucault Reader* (Penguin Books. London. 1991), pp 277–78.
58   Foucault, 2003, op. cit., pp 18, 77, 89.
59   See Risse, 1994, op. cit. Also Ivan Illich, *Limits to Medicine: Medical Nemesis: The Expropriation of Health* (Marion Boyars. London. 2002), pp155–57.

60 Foucault, 2003, op. cit., p xxi.
61 See Risse, 1994, op. cit.
62 ibid.
63 Maurice B Strauss (ed), *Familiar Medical Quotations* (J & A Churchill Ltd. London. 1968), p 394.
64 See Risse, 1994, op. cit., Illich, 2002, op. cit., pp156–57.
65 See Arthur L Caplan, 'The Concepts of Health, Illness and Disease', in Bynum and Porter, 1994, op. cit.
66 Porter, 1997, op. cit., p 360.
67 Robert. E Adler, *Medical Firsts: From Hippocrates to the Human Genome* (John Wiley & Sons, Inc. Hoboken NJ. 2004), p 84.
68 See Magner, 1992, op. cit., p 280.
69 ibid. McGrew, 1985, op. cit., p14.
70 Ulrich Trohler, 'Surgery (Modern)', in Bynum and Porter, 1994, op. cit.
71 Ross Patrick, *Horsewhip the Doctor: Tales from our Medical Past* (University of Queensland Press. Brisbane. 1985), p 18.
72 Adler, 2004, op. cit., p 92.
73 McGrew, 1985, op. cit., p 17.
74 ibid.
75 Stephen Lehrer, *Explorers of the Body* (Doubleday & Company, Inc., New York. 1979), pp 62–63.
76 See Risse, 1994, op. cit., Gelfand, 1994, op. cit.
77 Berridge, 1999, op. cit., p 114.
78 Porter, 1997, op. cit., p 351. Philippa Martyr, *Paradise of Quacks: An Alternative History of Medicine in Australia* (Macleay Press. Sydney. 2002), p 11.
79 See Porter, 1997, op. cit., p 351.
80 ibid., p 354.
81 ibid.
82 Martyr, 2002, op. cit., pp 194, 299.
83 See Evan Willis, *Medical Dominance: The Division of Labour in Australian Health Care* (Allen & Unwin. Sydney. 1989), pp 2–3. See also Manderson, 1993, op. cit., p 81.
84 Porter, 1997, op. cit., pp 355–56.
85 Manderson, 1993, op. cit., p 6.
86 Catherine Crawford, 'Medicine and the Law', in Bynum and Porter, 1994, op. cit.
87 Martyr, 2002, op. cit., pp 57–58.
88 ibid., See also pp 113–16.
89 Willis, 1989, op. cit., pp 41, 55.
90 Martyr, 2002, op. cit., p 162.
91 Willis, 1989, op. cit., p 85.
92 ibid., p 54, quoting K Russell, *The Melbourne Medical School. 1862–1972* (Melbourne University Press. Melbourne. 1977), p 214.
93 Willis, 1989, op. cit., p 85. J H Portus, *Australian Compulsory Arbitration 1900–1970* (Hick Smith & Sons. Sydney. 1971), p 25.

94 Willis, 1989, op. cit., pp 84–86.

95 Simon Marginson, *Markets in Education* (Allen and Unwin. Sydney. 1997), pp 131–32, 145.

96 Department of Education, *Science and Training. Students 2003. Selected Higher Education Statistics*. Appendix 2.1, p 186; CDAMS 2004, *Medical Students Statistics*. Committee of Deans of Australia Medical Schools. Private Correspondence 23 February 2005.

97 *The Sydney Morning Herald*, 3 May 2004, citing Rodney Tiffen and Ross Gittins, *How Australia Compares* (Cambridge University Press. Melbourne. 2004).

98 Porter, 1997, op. cit., p 281.

99 Edward Shorter, 'The Doctor–Patient Relationship', in Bynum and Porter, 1994, op. cit.

100 See Rene Dubois, *Pasteur and Modern Science* (Science Tech Publishers. Madison WI. 1988), pp 116–21.

101 ibid.

102 Ann G Carmichael, 'Diphtheria', in Kenneth F Kipple (ed), *The Cambridge World History of Human Disease* (Cambridge University Press. Cambridge. 1995) pp 680–83.

103 Shorter, 1994, op. cit.

104 Theodore L Sourkes, *Nobel Prize Winners in Medicine and Physiology 1901–1965* (Abelard-Schuman. London. 1967), pp 3–9.

105 See Shorter, 1994, op. cit.

106 Roy Porter and W F Bynum, 'The Art and Science of Medicine', in Bynum and Porter, 1994, op. cit.

107 Porter, 1997, op. cit., p 11.

108 Brian Inglis, *The Diseases of Civilisation* (Hodder & Stoughton. London. 1981), p vii.

109 Porter, 1997, op. cit., p 410.

110 Deborah Cadbury, *Seven Wonders of the Industrial World* (Fourth Estate. London and New York. 2003), ch 4.

111 W A Sinclair, 'Economic Growth and Wellbeing, Melbourne 1870–1914', *Economic Record* 51: 153–73, 1975, cited in Willis, 1989, op. cit.

112 Thomas McKeown, *The Role of Medicine: Dream, Mirage or Nemesis?* (Blackwell Pubishers. Oxford. 1979), cited in Inglis, 1981, op. cit., p x.

113 Gelfand, 1994, op. cit.

114 ibid.

115 See Gelfand, 1994, op. cit.

116 ibid.

117 Edward Shorter, *A History of Psychiatry* (John Wiley & Sons Inc. New York. 1997), pp 90–91, citing Rosemary Stevens, *American Medicine and the Public Interest* (Yale University Press. New Haven CT. 1971), p 60, n. 13.

118 Jan Goldstein, 'Psychiatry', in Bynum and Porter, 1994, op. cit., Shorter, 1997, op. cit., p 17.

119 Porter, 1997, op. cit., p 495.

120 ibid.
121 ibid., p 496.
122 ibid.
123 ibid.
124 *The Oxford Textbook on Psychiatry*, third edition (Oxford University Press. Oxford. 1996), states that in 1772, William Cullen published a classification of mental disorders grouped together as part of a broad class of 'neuroses'. In 1845 Feuchterleben first suggested the category of psychosis.
125 See Goldstein, 1994, op. cit.
126 ibid.
127 ibid.
128 Shorter, 1997, op. cit., p 130.
129 ibid.
130 Gelfand, 1994, op. cit.
131 See Shorter, 1997, op. cit., ch 2 passim.
132 ibid., pp 113, 119, 131–32.
133 ibid., pp 113, 145, 160–61.
134 ibid., pp 143, 181.
135 ibid., p 145.
136 ibid., p 146.
137 Goldstein, 1994, op. cit., Shorter, 1997, op. cit., p 146.
138 Porter, 1997, op. cit., p 503.
139 See Shorter, 1997, op. cit., pp 225–29.
140 McGrew, 1985, op. cit., p 283.
141 Goldstein, 1994, op. cit., Shorter, 1997, op. cit., pp 255–29, n 64, p 399.
142 Shorter, 1997, op. cit., p 252.
143 D.L. Rosenhan, 'On Being Sane in Insane Places', *Science* 179: 250 58, 1973, cited in Illich, 2002, op. cit., p 166, n. 29.
144 Graham Meadows and Bruce Singh (eds), *Mental Health in Australia: Collaborative Community Practice* (Oxford University Press. Melbourne. 2001), pp 52, 66, 70–72.
145 *Medical Journal of Australia* 181: 10, November 2003, pp 544–48.
146 Dorothy Porter, 'Public Health', in Bynum and Porter, 1994, op. cit.
147 Crawford, 1994, op. cit.
148 Daniel M Fox, 'Medical Institutions and the State', in Bynum and Porter, 1994, op. cit.
149 ibid. See also Inglis, 1981, op. cit., p viii.
150 In Inglis, 1981, op. cit., p x.
151 Illich, 2002, op. cit.
152 See Inglis, 1981, op. cit., p viii.
153 Porter, 1997, op. cit., p 687.
154 *The Australian*, 18 August 2003. The number of deaths said to be preventable ranged from 4,500 to 12,000.
155 *The Weekend Australian*, 22–23 October 2005.

156 Porter, 1997, op. cit., p 688.

157 Andrea Mant, *Thinking About Prescribing* (McGraw-Hill. Sydney NSW. 1999), p 18.

158 Illich, 2002, op. cit., pp 41–42.

159 Richard C. Hollinger and Dean A. Dabney, 'Social factors associated with pharmacists' unauthorised use of mind-altering prescription medications', *Journal of Drug Issues*, vol. 32, no. 1, Winter 2002, pp 231–64

Chapter 2

1   Davenport-Hines, 2001, op. cit., p 207.

2   Manderson, 1993, op. cit., pp 110–13. Although Australia had agreed to ratify the 1936 Convention, World War II intervened.

3   ibid., pp 125–31.

4   ibid., pp 95–98.

5   Andrew Campbell, *The Australian Illicit Drug Guide* (Black Inc. Melbourne. 2001), p 74.

6   Miles Weatherall, 'Drug Therapies', in Bynum and Porter, 1994, op. cit.

7   *Chambers Biographical Dictionary*. Magnus Magnusson (ed) (Chambers. Edinburgh. 1996), pp 867–68.

8   Foucault, 2003, op. cit., p 161.

9   Porter (ed), 1996, op. cit., p 260.

10 Weatherall, 1994, op. cit.

11 ibid.

12 ibid.

13 Martin Booth, *Opium: A History* (Simon & Schuster. London. 1996), pp 68–70.

14 Weatherall, 1994, op. cit.

15 Erika Hickel, 'Das Kaiserliche Gesundheitsamt (Imperial health Office) and the German Chemical Industry in Germany during the Second Empire: Partners or Adversaries?', in Porter and Teich, 1995, op. cit.

16 Arthur W Slater, 'Fine Chemicals', in Charles Singer, E J Holmyard, A R Hall and Trevor I Williams (eds), *A History of Technology* (Oxford University Press. Oxford. 1958), vol. V, p 299.

17 Porter (ed), 1996, op. cit., p 261.

18 Eric Hobsbawm, *The Age of Capital* (Abacus. London. 2001), p 58.

19 Weatherall, 1994, op. cit.

20 ibid. Porter (ed), 1996, op. cit., pp 261–62.

21 In Porter (ed), 1996, op. cit., p 260.

22 Judy Slinn, 'Research and Development in the UK Pharmaceutical Industry from the Nineteenth Century to the 1960s', in Porter and Teich, 1995, op. cit.

23 J D Bernal, *Science in History* (C A Watts & Co. Ltd. London. 1969), vol. 2, pp 562, 569, 631–32.

24 Weatherall, 1994, op. cit.

25 Edward Thomas and M Arthur Auslander (eds), *Chemical Inventions and Chemical*

Patents (Clark Boardman Company Ltd. New York. 1964), pp 151, 226. Michael Bliss, *The Discovery of Insulin* (University of Chicago Press. Chicago. 1982), p 275, n.62.

26   Weatherall, 1994, op. cit. The exclusion lasted until 1941.

27   Susan Quinn, *Marie Curie: A Life* (Simon & Schuster. New York. 1995), p 418.

28   Bliss, 1982, op. cit., p 133.

29   ibid., p 240. See also Lehrer, 1979, op. cit., p 432.

30   Bernal, 1969, op. cit., vol. 3, pp 926–27. Magner, 1992, op. cit., pp 353–54.

31   See Matthew Richardson, *Imagination: 100 years of Bright Ideas in Australia* (IP Australia. Woden ACT. 2004), p 61.

32   Magner, 1992, op. cit., p 354.

33   See Allan M Brandt, 'Sexually Transmitted Diseases', in Bynum and Porter, 1994, op. cit., where it is noted that while there is 'considerable evidence' that syphilis was brought back from the Americas by Columbus's crew in 1493, others have argued that venereal infections had been present in Europe long before this time but had not been distinguished from leprosy.

34   ibid.

35   ibid.

36   Magner, 1992, op. cit., pp 346–47.

37   Brandt, 1994, op. cit.

38   Weatherall, 1994, op. cit.

39   Magner, 1992, op. cit., p 348.

40   ibid. See also Weatherall, 1994, op. cit.

41   Magner, 1992, op. cit., p 349. Brandt, op. cit.

42   This section on the German Imperial Health Office is sourced from Hickel, 1995, op. cit.

43   ibid.

44   See Porter (ed), 1996, op. cit., p 135. Weatherall, 1994, op. cit. Eduard Farber, *The Evolution of Chemistry: A History of its Ideas, Methods, and Materials*, second edition (The Ronald Press Company. New York. 1969), p 183.

45   Davenport-Hines, 2001, op. cit., p 99.

46   Australian Academy of Technological Science and Engineering, *Technology in Australia* (Melbourne. 1988), p 652.

47   Porter (ed), 1996, op. cit., p 135.

48   B Travers and F L Freiman (eds), *Medical Discoveries* (UXL Detroit. 1997), vol. I, p 75. *Barbiturates* (The Drug Education Centre, WA Alcohol and Drug Authority. Perth. 1986).

49   WA Alcohol and Drug Authority, 1986, op. cit.

50   Davenport-Hines, 2001, op. cit., pp 190–1. Charles F Levinthal, *Drugs, Behaviour and Modern Society*, third edition (Allyn & Bacon. Boston MA. 2002), p 30.

51   Davenport-Hines, 2001, op. cit., p 250.

52   Mant, 1999, op. cit., p 14.

53   WA Alcohol and Drug Authority, 1986, op. cit.

54   McCoy, 1991, op. cit., p 6.

55 Nevett, 1982, op. cit., p 24. See also Berridge, 1999, op. cit., pp 21–24.

56 Manderson, 1993, op. cit., p 52.

57 Nevett, 1982, op. cit., p 113. McCoy, 1980, op. cit., pp 63, 65.

58 Manderson, 1993, op. cit., p 52.

59 ibid., p 50. McCoy, 1980, op. cit., pp 63–68.

60 Eric Hobsbawm, *The Age of Empire: 1875–1914* (Abacus. London. 2001), pp 237–38.

61 David Weatherall, *David Ricardo: A Biography* (Martinus Nijhoff. The Hague. 1976), p 123.

62 Brian Inglis, *The Opium War* (Coronet Books. Great Britain. 1979), p 93. See also *The Works and Correspondence of David Ricardo, Volume V* (Cambridge University Press, for the Royal Economic Society. Cambridge. 1952). *Beer Duties Bill*, 13 June 1823, p 322.

63 See Nevett, 1982, op. cit., p 35, 113.

64 James B Twitchell, *20 Ads that Shook the World* (Crown Publishers. New York. 2000), p 28.

65 ibid., p 31.

66 McCoy, 1980, op. cit., p 53.

67 Michael Schudson, *Advertising:The Uneasy Persuasion* (Basic Books, Inc. New York. 1984), p 162.

68 McCoy, 1980, op. cit., p 53.

69 Manderson, 1993, op. cit., p 54.

70 Mitford M Mathews (ed), *A Dictionary of Americanisms on Historical Principles* (University of Chicago Press. Chicago IL. 1951), vol. II, p 1186. See also Illich, 2002, op. cit., pp 133–54, where there is a discussion of the history and meaning of pain, and Roy Porter, *Pain and Suffering*, in Bynum and Porter, 1994, op. cit., both of which are sources for this section on pain.

71 *Technology in Australia*, 1988, op. cit., p 652.

72 McCoy, 1980, op. cit., p 54.

73 ibid., p 42.

74 Manderson, 1993, op. cit., p 53.

75 McCoy, 1980, op. cit., p 54. Davenport-Hines, 2001, op. cit., p 239.

76 Manderson, 1993, op. cit., p 136.

77 Eileen Hennessey, *A Cup of Tea, a Bex and a Good Lie Down* (Department of History & Politics, James Cook University. Townsville Qld. 1993), pp 6, 28.

78 ibid., p 26.

79 Davenport-Hines, 2001, op. cit., p 239.

80 Hennessey, 1993, op. cit., pp 49, 50.

81 ibid.

82 Davenport-Hines, 2001, op. cit., p 237.

83 McCoy, 1980, op. cit., p 266.

84 ibid., p 25.

85 *The Weekend Australian*, 26–27 July 2003.

86 Richard Isralowitz, *Drug Use, Policy and Management* (Auburn House. Westport CT.

2002), p 8, citing N Saunders, *E for Ecstasy* (N Saunders. London. 1991).

87   Jeffrey Robinson, *Prescription Games* (Simon & Schuster. London. 2001), p 12.

88   Australian Bureau of Statistics. *National Health Survey. Summary of Results*. cat. no. 4364. 0. 2001 (2001).

89   M Miller and G Draper, *Statistics on Drug Use in Australia 2000*, AIHW cat. no. PHE 30 (AIHW [Drug Statistics Series no. 8]. Canberra. 2001). *The Australian*, 22 June 2006.

90   Campbell, 2001, op. cit., pp 10, 55, 80, 106, 135, citing *Global Illicit Drug Trends 2000* (UN Office on Drugs and Crime. Vienna. 2001).

91   Harry Braverman, *Labour and Monopoly Capital* (Monthly Review Press. New York and London. 1974), p 161.

92   Slinn, 1995, op. cit.

93   Beatrice Faust, *Benzo Junkie* (Viking. Melbourne Vic. 1993).

94   ibid., pp 23, 29, 27, 88.

95   Porter (ed), 1996, op. cit., p 276.

96   Faust, 1993, op. cit., p 75.

97   Jay S. Cohen MD, *Overdose: The Case Against the Drug Companies* (Tarcher Putnam Inc. New York, 2001), p 2, citing a case study published in the *Journal of the American Medical Association*, 1998.

98   ibid., p 5.

99   Robinson, 2001, op. cit., pp 35–36.

100 Cohen, 2001, op. cit., p 8: 46 per cent of Americans purchased prescriptions in 1999, and the total number they purchased was 2,587,575,000.

101 Robinson, 2001, op. cit., p 10.

102 *The Guardian Weekly*, 5–11 June 2003. *New Internationalist*, November 2003, citing Pharmaceutical Executive, May 2003.

103 *Le Monde Diplomatique*, November 2003.

104 *The Guardian Weekly*, 17–23 July 2003.

105 Robinson, 2001, op. cit., p 9. *New Internationalist*, November 2003. *The Australian*, 4 August 2006.

106 Robinson, 2001, op. cit., p 12.

107 *New Internationalist*, November, 2003.

108 *Medical Journal of Australia* 183(2): 73–74, 18 July 2005, citing M Angell, 'Excess in the pharmaceutical industry' *Canadian Medical Association Journal* (*CMAJ*) 171: 1451–53, 2004.

109 Mant, 1999, op. cit., Foreword, by Richard Day MD FRACP, Professor of Clinical Pharmacology, St Vincents Hospital, University of New South Wales.

110 *The Weekend Australian*, 29–30 March 2003 quoting Associate Professor Leon Slack, Flinders University School of Psychology.

111 *The Australian*, 30 November 2005, 1 December 2005.

112 Robinson, 2001, op. cit., pp 257, 265.

113 Cohen, 2001, op. cit., pp 144–47. Robinson, 2001, op. cit., pp 255–85.

114 Cohen, 2001, op. cit., p 145. Robinson, 2001, op. cit., p 265.

115 Robinson, 2001, op. cit., p 282.

116 *Washington Post*, 21 June 2003.

117 *Le Monde Diplomatique*, November 2003.

118 Robinson, 2001, op. cit., p 230.

119 *The Australian*, 3 December 2004.

120 Robinson, 2001, op. cit., p 232.

121 *New York Times*, 21 November 2001.

122 *The Guardian Weekly*, 20–26 March 2003. *The Australian*, 15 October 2003.

123 *The West Australian*, 17 October 2003.

124 *The West Australian*, 15 December 2003.

125 *New Internationalist*, November 2003. *The Guardian Weekly*, 24–30 March 2006.

126 *The Age*, 25 July 2003.

127 *New Internationalist*, November 2003.

128 *The Guardian Weekly*, 9–15 January 2002.

129 *Direct to Consumer Advertising of Prescription Drugs in New Zealand.* Report to Minister of Health supporting the case for a ban on DTCA, February 2003 (www.healthyskepticism.org).

130 *The New York Times*, 21 November 2001.

131 Robinson, 2001, op. cit., p 246.

132 *The Weekend Australian*, 18–19 September 2004. *The Australian*, 6 June 2005.

133 *The Weekend Australian*, 21–22 February 2004.

134 *The Australian*, 4 October 2004.

135 *The Australian*, 3 November 2004.

136 *The West Australian*, 5 January 2005.

137 *The Weekend Australian*, 19–20 April 2005.

138 *The Guardian Weekly*, 20–26 May 2004.

139 *The Guardian Weekly*, 24–30 September 2004.

140 *The West Australian*, 23 October, 2004.

141 *The Weekend Australian*, 11–12 June 2005.

142 Allen Roses, senior executive with GlaxoSmithKline, reported in *The Australian*, 9 December 2003. See also *The Guardian Weekly*, 24–30 September 2004.

143 Douglas Husak, *Legalise This! The Case for Decriminalising Drugs* (Verso. London and New York. 2002), p 61.

Chapter 3

1   See Porter, 1997, op. cit., p 102. Porter (ed), 1996, op. cit., pp 66–68.

2   See S W F Holloway, 'The Regulation and Supply of Drugs in Britain Before 1868', in Porter and Teich, 1995, op. cit.

3   See John Parascandola, 'The Drug Habit: The Association of the Word "Drug" with Abuse in American History', in Porter and Teich, 1995, op. cit.

4   ibid.

5   The US National Commission on Marihuana [sic] and Drug Abuse omits food from its definition of drugs: 'a drug is any substance other than food which by its chemical nature affects the structure and function of the living organism' (*Drug Use in America: Problem in Perspective*, Second Report of the NCMDA. US

Government Printing Office. Washington DC. 1973), p 9. See Isralowitz, 2002, op. cit., p 3. Both the *US Food and Drug Act* and the *Controlled Substances Act* contain the above definition and, as well, define drugs as those listed in the official US Pharmacopeia or those used in the treatment or prevention of disease in humans or animals. These definitions serve the licit/illicit divide of drugs. On the above construction a drug can't be a food and a food (however else it might be defined) can't be a drug even though it is a psychoactive stimulant (as coffee and chocolate are). See Husak, 2002, op. cit., pp 27–33.

6   Stuart Walton, *Out of It: A Cultural History of Intoxication* (Penguin. London. 2002), p ix.

7   Terence McKenna, *Food of the Gods. The Search for the Original Tree of Knowledge: A Radical History of Plants, Drugs and Human Evolution* (Rider. London. 1992), pp 20, 42, 49, ch 3 and 4 passim.

8   Richard Sennett, *The Corrosion of Character* (W W Norton & Company. New York. 1998), pp 22, 27.

9   Rudi Mathee, 'Exotic Substances: The Introduction and Global Spread of Tobacco, Coffee, Cocoa, Tea and Distilled Liquor, Sixteenth to Eighteenth Century', in Porter and Teich, 1995, op. cit.

10 Ian McAllister, Rhonda Moore and Tani Makkai, *Drugs in Australian Society* (Longman Cheshire. Melbourne. 1991), p 94. n. 6, citing Robin Walker in *Under Fire: A History of Tobacco Smoking in Australia* (Melbourne University Press. Melbourne. 1984).

11 Mathee, 1995, op. cit.

12 Kenneth F Kipple and Kriemhild Conee Ornelas (eds), *The Cambridge World History of Food* (Cambridge University Press. Cambridge. 2000), vol. 1, p 643.

13 Mathee, 1995, op. cit. Kipple and Ornelas, 2000, op. cit., p 639.

14 John Burnett, *Liquid Pleasures: A Social History of Drinks in Modern Britain* (Routledge. London. 1999), pp 52–56.

15 Engels, 1984, op. cit., pp 140–41. Also the source of all of the quotes in this paragraph; see pp 371–72 for pauperism in agricultural districts, and p 247 for the effects of working conditions on premature death.

16 Burnett, 1999, op. cit., pp 57–58, 61, 67, 110. Burnett also points out that there was an actual decline in the consumption of both tea and sugar between 1810 and 1841. Low wages are the obvious reason.

17 Robin Walker and Dave Roberts, *From Scarcity to Surfeit: A History of Food and Nutrition in New South Wales* (UNSW Press. Sydney. 1988), pp 22–24.

18 ibid., pp 25, 133.

19 ibid., p 22.

20 Peter Macinnis, *Bittersweet: The Story of Sugar* (Allen & Unwin. Sydney. 2002), p 111 and passim.

21 C M H Clark, *A History of Australia* (Melbourne University Press. Melbourne, 1981), vol. V, pp 132, 200–03.

22 Walker and Roberts, 1988, op. cit., p 92.

23 ibid., p 133.

24 *Apparent Consumption of Foodstuffs Australia*. ABS cat. no. 4306. 0, October 2000. Figures are for 1998–99.

25 *New Internationalist*, December 2003. According to a US survey, teenagers drinking one can of sugary drink a day are likely to be up to 6.4 kg heavier than those drinking unsweetened drinks. *The Australian*, 7 March 2006.

26 Burnett, 1999, op. cit., pp 55, 110, 189.

27 Isralowitz, 2002, op cit., p 12. Michael Wood, *Conquistadors* (BBC Worldwide Limited. London. 2000), pp 16–17.

28 Mathee, 1995, op. cit.

29 ibid.

30 ibid.

31 Robin Walker, *Under Fire: A History of Tobacco Smoking in Australia* (Melbourne University Press. Melbourne. 1984), p 3.

32 See Mathee, 1995, op. cit.

33 Richard Kluger, *Ashes to Ashes* (Alfred A Knopf. New York. 1996) is the main source of this account of the history and development of cigarette manufacturing. See ch 1 passim.

34 Walter Adams and James W Brock, 'Tobacco: Predation and Persistent Market Power', in David I Rosenbaum (ed), *Market Dominance: How Firms Gain, Hold, or Lose It and the Impact on Economic Performance* (Praeger. Westport CT. 1998).

35 Kluger, 1996, op. cit., pp 41–43.

36 Walker, 1984, op. cit., pp 45–46.

37 Ian Tyrrell, *Deadly Enemies: Tobacco and its Opponents in Australia* (UNSW Press. Sydney. 1999), pp 8–13.

38 ibid., p 13.

39 Robert Caldwell, *The Gold Era of Victoria* (James Blundell & Co. Melbourne. 1855), p 129.

40 Walker, 1984, op. cit., pp 32–33.

41 Tyrrell, 1999, op. cit., pp 113, 208.

42 *Statistics on Drug Use in Australia 2002*. AIHW cat. no. PHE 43 (Drug Statistics Series no. 11), 2003.

43 Tyrrell, 1999, op. cit., p 115. Walker, 1984, op. cit., pp 65, 72, 85.

44 Levinthal, 2002, op. cit., p 239.

45 Isralowitz, 2002, op. cit., p 13.

46 Levinthal, 2002, op. cit., p 241.

47 A total of 34.6 per cent of volunteers were rejected: Burnett, 1999, op. cit., p 37. For the pattern of volunteers see Eric Hobsbawm, *The Age of Empire*, 2001, op. cit., pp 160–61.

48 Walker, 1984, op. cit., p 7. Tyrrell, 1999, op. cit., pp 21–23.

49 Philip J Hilts, *Smokescreen: The Truth Behind the Tobacco Industry Cover-Up* (Addison-Wesley Publishing Company, Inc. Reading MA. 1996), p 2.

50 Tyrrell, 1999, op. cit., p 162.

51 Hilts, 1996, op. cit., pp 25–31, ch 3 passim.

52 Tyrrell, 1999, op. cit., p 172.

53 Hilts, 1996, op. cit., p 12.

54 ibid., pp 30, 64, 88, 201, 219.

55 Tyrrell, 1999, op. cit., pp 177, 201, 206.

56 Just how big the tobacco companies are can be seen by their 1999 sales figures. The three largest transnational companies had sales of almost US$100 billion — Philip Morris $47.1 billion; British American Tobacco $31.1 billion; Japan Tobacco International $21.6 billion: *The Tobacco Atlas* (World Health Organization. London. 2002).

57 Isralowitz, 2002, op. cit., pp 16–18.

58 Hilts, 1996, op. cit., p 65.

59 Isralowitz, 2002, op. cit., p x., citing D Kessler and M Myers, 'Beyond the Tobacco Settlement', *New England Journal of Medicine* 345(7): 535, 16 August 2001. *The West Australian*, 20 June 2003. Levinthal, 2002, op. cit., p 247.

60 Isralowitz, 2002, op. cit., p 88.

61 ibid., p 88, citing B Hafne, *Alcohol: The Crutch that Cripples* (West Publishing, St Paul MN. 1977), pp 1–2.

62 Levinthal, 2002, op. cit., pp 187–88.

63 David G Mandelbaum, 'Alcohol and Culture', in Mac Marshall (ed), *Belief, Behaviour and Alcoholic Beverages* (University of Michigan Press. Ann Arbor MI. 1979).

64 ibid.

65 Jean-Charles Sournia, *A History of Alcoholism* (Basil Blackwell Ltd. Oxford. 1990), pp 5, 6, 11.

66 ibid., Introduction, by Roy Porter.

67 Levinthal, 2002, op. cit., pp 186–87, 190.

68 Walton, 2002, op. cit., p 130.

69 Levinthal, 2002, op. cit., p 187.

70 Patrick Dillon, *The Much-Lamented Death of Madam Geneva: The Eighteenth Century Gin Craze* (Review. London. 2002), pp 7–10, 83.

71 ibid., pp 4, 17, 37, 112.

72 ibid., p 219. Some sources put the production of gin in England during this period at 11 million gallons, but Dillon contends that production was overstated by the inclusion of 'low wines', the first run-off from the distilling process, which was then distilled a second time to make proof spirits: see pp 9, 278.

73 ibid., pp 265–79.

74 Sournia, 1990, op. cit., p 22. Sournia also makes the point that no records were kept of the alcohol such as beer and rum that was consumed in place of gin.

75 Dillon, 2002, op. cit., pp 291–93.

76 Sournia, 1990, op. cit., p 21.

77 ibid., p 35.

78 ibid., p 103. Hobsbawm, *The Age of Capital*, 2001, op. cit., pp 200–02.

79 Sournia, 1990, op. cit., p 142.

80 Clark, 1981, op. cit. vol. I, pp 87–88.

81 Andrew Wells, *Constructing Capitalism: An Economic History of Eastern Australia 1788–1901* (Allen and Unwin. Sydney. 1989), p 13.

82 H V Evatt, *Rum Rebellion* (Times House. Sydney. 1984), pp x, 26–33.

83 Clark, 1981, op. cit., vol. I, pp 219–21, 265, 269.

84 ibid., passim.

85 McAllister, Moore and Makkai, 1991, op. cit., p 36.

86 A J P Taylor, *The First World War: An Illustrated History* (Penguin. London. 1966), pp 68–70, 82–83, 107, 159.

87 McCoy, 1980, op. cit., p 84. Six o'clock closing was introduced in New South Wales, South Australia, Tasmania and Victoria. In Western Australia it was 9 pm, with 11 pm in the goldfields. Queensland had longer hours until 1923, when 8 pm closing was introduced: Richard Waterhouse, *Private Pleasures, Public Leisure: A History of Australian Popular Culture since 1788* (Longman. Melbourne. 1995), pp 159–62.

88 Manderson, 1993, op. cit., p 51.

89 McCoy, 1980, op. cit., p 28 and passim.

90 ibid., p 18.

91 *The Australian*, 17 July 2003, 23 July 2003. A breakdown of the per capita consumption of the 9.32 litres of alcohol consumed in 200/01 shows: medium and full-strength beer 42.1 per cent : low alcohol content beer 10.2 per cent : wine 28.7 per cent and spirits (both neat and premixed) 18.8 per cent. See T Chikritzhs et al., *Australian Alcohol Indicators, 1990–2001 Patterns of Alcohol Use and Related Harms for Australian States and Territories* (National Drug Research Institute. Perth WA. 2003).

92 Edward Shann, *An Economic History of Australia* (Cambridge University Press. London. 1930), p 37, uses the imperial measurements of 5 gallons 3 quarts and 2 gallons 3 quarts respectively.

93 *Weekend Australian*, 21–22 June 2003, *The Australian*, 22 July 2003.

94 *Reuters Health*, 25 February 2003, citing Professor Juergen Rehm, Director Addiction Research Institute, Switzerland.

95 Elizabeth Unwin and Jim Codde, *Comparison of Deaths Due to Alcohol, Tobacco and Other Drugs in Western Australia and Australia* (Epidemiology and Analytical Services, Health Information Centre, Health Department of Western Australia. Perth. 1998).

96 *The West Australian*, 25 February 2003, citing David Collins, Professor of Economics, Macquarie University, from an analysis presented to the International Research Symposium on Preventing Substance Abuse, Fremantle WA.

97 *The West Australian*, 17 July 2003, *The Australian*, 21 June 2004. Miller and Draper, 2001, op. cit. The 2005–6 Federal Budget increased the amount spent on anti-smoking campaigns to $25 million. *The Australian*, 14 June 2005.

Chapter 4

1 Joseph Kennedy, *Coca Exotica* (Fairleigh Dickinson University Press. Rutherford NJ. 1985), p 13.

2   ibid. Levinthal, 2002, op. cit., p 78.
3   Edmundo Morales, *Cocaine: White Gold Rush in Peru* (University of Arizona Press. Tuscon AZ 1989), p 51. Walton, 2002, op. cit., pp 104–05.
4   Kennedy, 1985, op. cit., pp 26–28.
5   Wood, 2000, op. cit., p 17.
6   ibid.
7   Kennedy, 1985, op. cit., pp 48–49.
8   Levinthal, 2002, op. cit., p 82.
9   Kennedy, 1985, op. cit., pp 84–86. Walton, 2002, op. cit., p 107.
10   Levinthal, 2002, op. cit., p 79.
11   Kennedy, 1985, op. cit., p 86.
12   Davenport-Hines, 2001, op. cit., pp 112–13.
13   Spillane, 2000, op. cit., p 123.
14   The Stepan Company of New Jersey is contracted to the Coca-Cola Company to produce 'decocanized flavour essence' each year from 175,000 kilograms of coca leaves which, in turn, produces 1,750 kilograms of cocaine. The resultant cocaine is then sold on the legitimate medical market: Michael W Miller, 'Quality Stuff: Firm is Peddling Cocaine, and Deals are Legit', *Wall Street Journal*, 17 October 1994, cited in Levinthal, 2002, op. cit., p 80.
15   Davenport-Hines, 2001, op. cit., p 113.
16   Porter, 1997, op. cit., p 351.
17   Walton, 2002, op. cit., p 138.
18   Davenport-Hines, 2001, op. cit., p 117.
19   ibid., Spillane, 2000, op. cit., pp 48–49.
20   Spillane, 2000, op. cit., pp 44–47.
21   See Hobsbawm, *Age of Empire, 2001*, op. cit., pp 35, 342–45, and Eric Hobsbawm, *Age of Extremes* (Abacus. London. 2000), p 97.
22   *Chambers Biographical Dictionary*, 1996, op. cit., p 463.
23   See Spillane, 2000, op. cit., p 2.
24   ibid., pp 72, 56. Spillane notes at p 68 that most of the 5,398 listed drug manufacturers in the United States at the end of the 19th century were in the proprietary medicine business. The earlier quoted sales pitch is in Jonnes, 1996, op. cit., p 20, cited in Levinson, 2002, op. cit., p 12.
25   Spillane, 2000, op. cit., p 85.
26   ibid., pp 86–88.
27   George Beard, *A Practical Treatise on Nervous Exhaustion (Neurasthenia): Its Symptoms, Nature, Sequences, Treatment* (William Wood. New York. 1880), cited in Spillane, 2000, op. cit., p 17.
28   Hobsbawm, *Age of Capital*, 2001, op. cit., p 57.
29   *Chambers Biographical Dictionary*, 1996, op. cit., p 1436.
30   See Davenport-Hines, 2001, op. cit., p 126.
31   *British Medical Journal: Volume II*, 29 November 1902, p 1729.
32   Spillane, 2000, op. cit., pp 92–93.
33   Richard O Boyer and Herbert M Morais, *Labor's Untold Story* (United Electrical,

Radio and Machine Workers of America. Pittsburgh PA. 2003), p 144.

34   Spillane, 2000, op. cit., pp 93, 184, n. 20.

35   ibid, p 39.

36   Trohler, 1994, op. cit.

37   E M Thornton, *The Freudian Fallacy: Freud and Cocaine* (Palladin Grafton Books. London. 1986), p 176.

38   The promotional claims of Vin Mariani appear in Kennedy, 1985, op. cit., p 63, and those of Pemberton's French Wine Cola in Davenport-Hines, 2001, op. cit., pp 112–13.

39   Thornton, 1986, op. cit., p 43. Robert Byck (ed), *Cocaine Papers: Sigmund Freud* (Stonehill. New York. 1974), p 15.

40   Thornton, 1986, op. cit., pp 30, 33–34, 37–38.

41   Byck, 1974, op. cit., pp 5–6.

42   ibid.

43   ibid., pp 6–8.

44   See E Merck, *Cocaine and its Salts*, November 1884. *Chicago Medical Journal and Examiner*, February 1885. *The Saint Louis Medical and Surgical Journal*, December 1885. *Vienna Medical Press*, August 1885. Parke-Davis and Company promotional Brochure, *Coca Erythroxylon and its Derivatives*, 1885: in Byck, 1974, op. cit.

45   Byck, 1974, op. cit., pp 27, 49–73, 388–91.

46   ibid, pp 14–19.

47   Spillane, 2000, op. cit., pp 68–71.

48   Thornton, 1986, op. cit., pp 45–46. Byck, 1974, op. cit., p 71.

49   Thornton, 1986, op. cit., p 46. Byck, 1974, op. cit., p 71.

50   Thornton, 1986, op. cit., pp 49–51. Byck, 1974, op. cit., pp 112–18.

51   Byck, 1974, op. cit., pp xxv, xxvi, 122–3.

52   Spillane, 2000, op. cit., p 68.

53   Thornton, 1986, op. cit., pp 50–51.

54   ibid.

55   Davenport-Hines, 2001, op. cit., p 117.

56   Madelon Sprengnether, 'Reading Freud's Life', in Anthony Elliott (ed), *Freud 2000* (Melbourne University Press. Melbourne. 1998), pp 143–44.

57   Byck, 1974, op. cit., p 369.

58   Thornton, 1986, op. cit., pp 9, 307.

59   ibid, p 317.

60   Weatherall, 1994, op. cit.

61   McCoy, 1980, op. cit., pp 84–5.

62   ibid. Davenport-Hines, 2001, op. cit., pp 169–70.

63   Spillane, 2000, op. cit., p 91.

64   'Lumpen proletariat' is an expression used in the 1848 German edition of *The Communist Manifesto*. In the 1888 English translation it is replaced by 'social scum', described as 'that passively rotting mass thrown off by the lowest layers of old society'. The lumpen proletariat are the most miserable members of the working

class, such as petty thieves and prostitutes, who can't even be relied on by the rest of the working class — they are wretched, purposeless, unprincipled.

65 Spillane, 2000, op. cit., pp 91, 119–20

66 Byck, 1974, op. cit., p xxviii, citing David F Musto, *The American Disease: Origins of Narcotic Control* (Yale University Press. New Haven CT. 1973), p 7.

67 Spillane, 2000, op. cit., p 132.

68 McCoy, 1980, op. cit., p 140.

69 ibid., p 123. Manderson, op. cit., pp 95–98. See also Desmond Manderson, 'History of Australian Law: Conventional Wisdom', in Russell Fox and Ian Mathews, *Drugs Policy: Fact, Fiction and the Future* (The Federation Press. Sydney. 1992).

70 David T Courtwright, 'The Rise and Fall and Rise of Cocaine in the United States', in Jordan Goodman, Paul E Lovejoy and Andrew Sherratt, *Consuming Habits* (Routledge. London and New York. 1995).

71 Davenport-Hines, 2001, op. cit., pp 349–51: he also notes of Chile that, from the late 1920s, it was the port of Valparaiso that was the commercial centre of America's opium trade, p 223. Pinochet's alleged involvement in cocaine trafficking was reported in *The Guardian Weekly* of 14–20 December 2000, where two books are cited in support of the allegation: Hugh O'Shaughnessy, *Pinochet: The Politics of Torture* and Rodrigo de Castro and Juan Gasparini, *The Thin White Line*. See also *The Guardian Weekly*, 21–27 July 2006.

72 *The Guardian*, 21 May 2001.

73 US General Accounting Office, Washington DC, 8 January 2003. Correspondence to the Honourable Charles H Taylor, House of Representatives. GAO-03-319R. Coca Estimates in Colombia.

74 *The Guardian Weekly*, 8–14 July 2005.

75 The term 'post-industrial society', encompassing a rise in service sector employment and a decline in manufacturing industry employment, was first used by Daniel Bell in a lecture in Boston in 1962. Thomas Moutner (ed), *The Penguin Dictionary of Philosophy* (Penguin. London. 2000), p 302. Hobsbawm, in *Age of Extremes*, 2000, op. cit., p 302, points out that manufacturing employment began to decline in the United States from 1965.

76 The first Options contracts were traded in Chicago on 26 April 1973 and the first financial futures contracts that covered foreign exchange were introduced on 16 May 1972: Sarkis J Khoury, *The Deregulation of the World Financial Markets: Myths, Realities and Impact* (Pinter Publishers. London. 1990), p 18. The Eurodollar market (which includes other currencies) grew from $7 billion in 1963 to $65 billion in 1970 and had grown to $755 billion a decade later: Julian Walmsley, *Macmillan Dictionary of International Finance*, second edition (Macmillan. London. 1985), p 79. See also Hobsbawm, *Age of Extremes*, 2000, op. cit., p 278.

77 Spillane, 2000, op. cit., p 96.

78 Levinthal, 2002, op. cit., p 84.

79 Davenport-Hines, 2001, op. cit., p 353.

80 ibid.

81 Courtwright, 1995, op. cit.
82 Davenport-Hines, 2001, op. cit., p 356.
83 *The Guardian Weekly*, 17–23 April 2003.
84 Davenport-Hines, 2001, op. cit., p 357, citing Amnesty International 1999.
85 Michael Moore, *Stupid White Men* (Regan Books. New York. 2001), pp 4–8.
86 Francis Pisani, 'How to Fight the Terror Networks', *Le Monde Diplomatique*, June 2002.
87 *The Guardian Weekly*, 30 January–5 February 2003. *The Weekend Australian Financial Review*, 17–21 April 2003.
88 *World Drug Report*, 2005.
89 *The Guardian Weekly*, 3–9 December 2004, 16–22 September 2005, 23–29 September 2005.
90 *The Weekend Australian*, 6–7 August 2005.
91 *The Australian*, 26 June 2003, *The West Australian*, 27 June 2003, *The Guardian Weekly*, 22–28 July 2005.
92 *The Australian*, 27 July 2005.
93 *The Sydney Morning Herald*, 7 November 2005.
94 See Porter (ed), 1996, op. cit., p 261.
95 Ian McAllister, Rhonda Moore and Toni Makkai, *Drugs in Australian Society* (Longman Cheshire. Melbourne. 1991), p 163. John Caldwell (ed), *Amphetamines and Related Stimulants: Chemical, Biological, Clinical and Sociological Aspects* (CRC Press, Inc. Boca Raton FL. 1980), p 2. Hillary Klee (ed), *Amphetamine Misuse: International Perspectives on Current Trends* (Harwood Academic Publishers. Amsterdam. 1997), p 200.
96 Caldwell, 1980, op. cit. William H Brock, *The Fontana History of Chemistry* (Fontana Press. London. 1992), p 601.
97 Kee Chang Huang, *The Pharmacology of Chinese Herbs*, second edition (CRC Press. Boca Raton FL. 1999), pp 3, 7.
98 Walter Sneader, *Drug Discovery: The Evolution of Modern Medicine* (John Wiley & Sons. New York. 1986), pp 100–101.
99 Caldwell, 1980, op. cit. Klee, op. cit., p 6.
100 Klee, 1997, op. cit., p 5. It is also noted, at p 200, that Nagai synthesised methamphetamine from ephedrine in 1893.
101 ibid. Caldwell, 1980, op. cit., p 102.
102 Klee, 1997, op. cit., p 2. The term 'ATS-amphetamine type stimulant' is also used.
103 Klee, 1997, op. cit., p 114, citing Lester Grinspoon and Peter Hedblom, *Speed Culture: Amphetamine Use and Abuse in America* (Harvard University Press. Cambridge MA. 1975) See also Courtwright, 2002, op. cit., Davenport-Hines, 2001, op. cit., p 243, Walton, 2002, op. cit., p 102.
104 See McAllister et al., 1991, op. cit., p 164.
105 Robert Kaplan, 'Doctor to Dictator: The Career of Theodor Morell, Personal Physician to Adolf Hitler', in *Australasian Psychiatry* 10(4): 389–92, 2002. See also Walton, 2002, op. cit., p 102.
106 Walton, 2002, op. cit., p 101. Davenport-Hines, 2001, op. cit., pp 243–44. Fox and

Mathews, 1992, op. cit., p 15.

107 Davenport-Hines, 2001, op. cit., p 243.
108 *The West Australian*, 16 January 2003.
109 Walton, 2002, op. cit., p 243.
110 Daniel M Perrine, *The Chemistry of Mind-Altering Drugs: History, Pharmacology and Cultural Context* (American Chemical Society. Washington DC. 1996), p 195.
111 *Chambers Biographical Dictionary*, 1996, op. cit., p 77. Davenport-Hines, 2001, op. cit., p 243.
112 Caldwell, 1980, op. cit., p 8.
113 Klee, 1997, op. cit., p 216.
114 Perrine, 1996, op. cit., p 194.
115 Klee, 1997, op. cit., pp 6, 70.
116 ibid., pp 201–02.
117 ibid. *Illicit Psychostimulant Use in Australia* (Australian Government Printing Service. Canberra. 1993), p 59, citing Grinspoon and Hedblom, 1975, op. cit.
118 *Illicit Psychostimulant Use in Australia*, 1993, op. cit.
119 Klee, 1997, op. cit., pp 70, 114, 216.
120 *Illicit Psychostimulant Use in Australia*, 1993, op. cit.
121 Caldwell, 1980, op. cit., p 176. Klee, 1997, op. cit., p 115, citing Grinspoon and Hedblom, 1975, op. cit.
122 Caldwell, 1980, op. cit., pp 8–9. *Illicit Psychostimulant Use in Australia*, 1993, op. cit., p 60.
123 Klee, 1997, op. cit., pp 7–8.
124 Caldwell, 1980, op. cit., p 176. Klee, 1997, op. cit., p 115, citing Grinspoon and Hedblom, 1975, op. cit.
125 Klee, 1997, op. cit., p 217.
126 ibid., pp 116, 136.
127 ibid.
128 *The Australian*, 8 March 2005.
129 *The Weekend Australian*, 17–18 May 2008.
130 Klee, 1997, op. cit., p 138. Perrine, 1996, op. cit., p 196.
131 *The Guardian Weekly*, 19–25 June 2003.
132 *The Guardian Weekly*, 19–25 August 2005.
133 *World Drug Report*, 2005.
134 In April 2003 the captain and 29 crew of the North Korean ship *Pong So* were arrested over their alleged involvement in dumping $80 million worth of high-grade heroin off the NSW coast. As well as heroin, methamphetamines are also exported, with thousands of kilograms from North Korea seized in China and Japan. Japanese police claim that 44 per cent of the Japanese illicit drug market is serviced by North Korea. The director of the Japan-Korea Economic Research Centre, Yoichi Mabe, maintains that the North Korean government raises international currency through drug trafficking. The US State Department has a 'strong suspicion' that the North Korean government is involved in drug exports and the Japanese government has asked the United Nations to confront

Pyongyang about the illicit trade in amphetamines: *The Australian*, 2 April 2003.

135   Bertil Lintner, *Blood Brothers* (Allen and Unwin. Sydney. 2002), pp 157–58.

136   *The Australian*, 2 April 2003.

137   *2001 National Drug Strategy Household Survey: Detailed Findings*, AIHW cat. no. PHE 41 (AIHW [Drug Statistics Series No. 11]. Canberra ACT. 2002). *The Australian*, 28 October 2005, also cites the figure of one in ten Australians having used ice or its variants.

138   *The Australian*, 22 July 2003, 30 July 2003.

139   Professor John Edwards from Flinders University's Department of Environmental Health, in *The Australian*, 31 August 2005.

140   *The Age*, 23 July 2003, *The Australian* 24 July 2003, 31 August 2005.

141   Perrine, 1996, op. cit., pp 196–97.

142   Mark A Stewart, MD and Sally Wendkos Olds, *Raising a Hyperactive Child* (Harper & Row. New York. 1973), p 236.

143   *The Australian*, 19 September 2005.

144   *The Sydney Morning Herald*, 13 March 2003.

145   *The Age*, 18 November 2002.

146   *The West Australian*, 14 April 2002.

147   *The Weekend Australian* Magazine, 8–9 February 2003.

148   *The West Australian*, 24 September 2002, 18 February 2005, *The Australian*, 13 April 2004.

149   *The West Australian*, 16 February 2005.

150   *The Australian*, 19 September 2005, 28 March 2006, *The Age*, 28 March 2006.

151   *The Weekend Australian* Magazine, 8–9 February 2003.

152   *The Weekend Australian*, 8–9 January 2005.

Chapter 5

1   Kee Chang Huang, 1999, op. cit., p 236. Rowan Robinson, *The Great Book of Hemp* (Park Street Press. Rochester VT. 1996), pp 45, 75. Lester Grinspoon and James B Bakalar, *Marihuana, the Forbidden Medicine* (Yale University Press. New Haven and London. 1993), p 3.

2   Robinson, 1996, op. cit., p 116.

3   Grinspoon and Bakalar, 1993, op. cit., p 3.

4   ibid., p 1. Leslie L Iversen, *The Science of Marijuana* (Oxford University Press. Oxford. 2000), p 5.

5   Grinspoon and Bakalar, 1993, op. cit., p 1.

6   Iversen, 2000, op. cit., p 12. Dr Ivan Bosca and Michael Karus, *The Cultivation of Hemp: Botany, Varieties, Cultivation and Harvesting* (Hemptech. Sebastopol CA. 1998), pp 4–5.

7   Robinson, 1996, op. cit., p 126.

8   ibid., p viii. Iversen, 2000, op. cit., p 12.

9   See Grinspoon and Bakalar, 1993, op. cit., p 3. Iversen, 2000, op. cit., p 122. *Chambers Biographical Dictionary*, 1996, op. cit., p 371.

10   Iversen, 2000, op. cit., pp 19–20. Davenport-Hines, 2001, op. cit., p 3.

11 Iversen, 2000, op. cit., pp 20–23.

12 Bosca and Karus, 1998, op. cit., pp 17–18, who note that the earliest written reference to hemp in Europe dates from the 8th century.

13 Iversen, 2000, op. cit., pp 23–24. Davenport-Hines, 2001, op. cit., pp 59–66.

14 ibid.

15 Iversen, 2000, op. cit., pp 123–25. Chris Conrad, *Hemp: Lifeline to the Future* (Creative Xpressions Publications. Los Angeles CA. 1994), pp 13–14.

16 ibid.

17 Grinspoon and Bakalar, 1993, op. cit., p 4. Conrad, 1994, op. cit., p 15.

18 Iversen, 2000, op. cit., p 126.

19 Grinspoon and Bakalar, 1993, op. cit., p 4.

20 Robinson, 1996, op. cit., p 47. Conrad, 1994, op. cit., p 14. Iversen, 2000, op. cit., p 27, 130.

21 Robinson, 1996, op. cit., p 53. Conrad, 1994, op. cit., p 15.

22 Iversen, 2000, op. cit., pp 129–30. Grinspoon and Bakalar, 1993, op. cit., pp 7–8 where, in relation to the dangers of aspirin, which might not seem immediately apparent, it is pointed out that between 500 and 1000 people die each year in the United States from aspirin-induced bleeding.

23 Iversen, 2000, op. cit., pp 26, 236. Noel Deerr, *The History of Sugar: Volume 2* (Chapman & Hall Ltd. London. 1950), p 398.

24 See Davenport-Hines, 2001, op. cit., pp 153, 185.

25 Iversen, 2000, op. cit., p 26.

26 Davenport-Hines, 2001, op. cit., pp 185–86. Robinson, 1996, op. cit., pp 81, 145.

27 Robinson, 1996, op. cit., p 81.

28 ibid., pp 144–45.

29 Davenport-Hines, 2001, op. cit., p 189.

30 Robinson, 1996, op. cit., pp 145–50.

31 Davenport-Hines, 2001, op. cit., pp 177, 195.

32 ibid., p 195. Robinson, 1996, op. cit., p 152.

33 Alexander Cockburn and Jeffrey St Clair, *Whiteout: The CIA, Drugs and the Press* (Verso. London and New York. 1999), p 72.

34 ibid. Davenport-Hines, 2001, op. cit., p 290.

35 Sally Denton and Roger Morris, *The Money and the Power* (Alfred A Knopf. New York. 2001), p 26.

36 Davenport-Hines, 2001, op. cit., p 275.

37 Denton and Morris, 2001, op. cit., p 25.

38 Robinson, 1996, op. cit., p 153.

39 Conrad, 1994, op. cit., p 41, Robinson, 1996, op. cit., p 149.

40 Robinson, 1996, op. cit., p 153.

41 Cockburn and St Clair, 1999, op. cit., p 72.

42 Robinson, 1996, op. cit., p 135. The others cited are James Madison, James Monroe, Andrew Jackson, Zachary Taylor and Franklin Pierce.

43 See Levinson, 2002, op. cit., p 151. Davenport-Hines, 2001, op. cit., p 277.

44 Conrad, 1994, op. cit., p 46. Citing Committee on Ways and Means, House of

Representatives, 'Hearing Transcript' 75c1s HR6385, 27–30 April and 4 May 1937.

45   See Conrad, 1994, op. cit., pp 35–54, passim. Jack Herer, *The Emperor Wears No Clothes* (AH HA Publishing. Van Nuys CA. 1998).

46   Robinson, 1996, op. cit., pp 149–50.

47   ibid., citing Herer, 1998, op. cit.

48   Conrad, 1994, op. cit., pp 44–45.

49   ibid., p 53.

50   Robinson, 1996, op. cit., pp 160–64.

51   ibid., p 148. Davenport-Hines, 2001, op. cit., p 278.

52   Robinson, 1996, op. cit., p 157.

53   Cockburn and St Clair, 1999, op. cit., p 72. Jerome L Himmelstein, *The Strange Career of Marijuana: Politics and Ideology of Drug Control in America* (Greenwood Press. Westport CT. 1983), p 62.

54   *Chambers Biographical Dictionary*, 1996, op. cit., p 934. It was the fact that he was a serving judge that made McCarthy's election as a senator contrary to the constitution.

55   Lillian Hellman, *Scoundrel Time* (Quartet Books. London. 1978), p 157, commentary by Gary Wills.

56   ibid., Introduction by James Cameron, pp 15–16.

57   Conrad, 1994, op. cit., p 226. Citing H Anslinger and F Ourswler, *The Murderers* (Farrar, Strauss & Cudahy. New York. 1961). See also Eric Schlosser, *Reefer Madness* (Houghton Mifflin Co. Boston and New York. 2003), p 22. Herer, 1998, op. cit., p 38, citing Dean Latimer and Jeff Goldberg, *Flowers in the Blood: The Story of Opium* (F Watts. New York. 1981).

58   Denton and Morris, 2001, op. cit., pp 251–53.

59   Davenport-Hines, 2001, op. cit., p 275.

60   ibid., p 340.

61   McCoy, 1991, op. cit., p 220.

62   Davenport-Hines, 2001, op. cit., p 340.

63   Himmelstein, 1983, op. cit., p 4.

64   Davenport-Hines, 2001, op. cit., p 343.

65   Himmelstein, 1983, op. cit., p 4.

66   Herer, 1998, op. cit., p 105.

67   Schlosser, 2003, op. cit., p 25.

68   ibid., pp 71, 27. Iversen, 2000, op. cit., p 266.

69   Davenport-Hines, 2001, op. cit., p 354.

70   Herer, 1998, op. cit., p 95. Schlosser, 2003, op. cit., p 14.

71   Schlosser, 2003, op. cit., p 14.

72   See Iversen, 2000, op. cit., p 215.

73   Davenport-Hines, 2001, op. cit., p 338.

74   Herer, 1998, op. cit., pp 75, 217, citing Kitty Kelley, *Nancy Reagan: The Unauthorized Biography* (Doubleday Co. New York, 1991).

75   ibid., citing *The Dallas Observer*, 23 August 1990.

76   Conrad, 1994, op. cit., p 228, citing *The New York Times*, 30 March 1992.

77   J H Hatfield, *Fortunate Son* (Soft Skull Press. New York. 2001), p 48. Kitty Kelley, *The Family* (Bantam Press. London. 2004), pp xxvi, 266, 304, 575, 578–80.

78   See John Gascoigne, *Science in the Service of Empire: Joseph Banks, the British State and the Uses of Science in the Age of Revolution* (Cambridge University Press. Cambridge. 1998), p 186.

79   ibid., p 186–87. Clark, 1981, op. cit., vol. I, p 61.

80   Gascoigne, 1998, op. cit., p 105–06, 118–19. *Marijuana Australiana (The Marijuana Australiana* Project. Kent Town SA. 2001), p 16.

81   *Marijuana Australiana*, 2001, op. cit.

82   T A Coghlan, *Labour and Industry in Australia from the First Settlement in 1788 to the Establishment of the Commonwealth in 1901* (Oxford University Press. London. 1918), vol. 1, p 130.

83   *Marijuana Australiana*, 2001, op. cit., p 17. Clark, 1981, op. cit., vol. IV, pp 230–32. Marcus Clarke, *For the Term of his Natural Life* (Times House. Sydney NSW. 1992), Introduction, by Hilary Lofting.

84   'Cannabis Indica', *Colonial Monthly* 1, no. 6, February 1868, in Michael Wilding, *Marcus Clarke* (University of Queensland Press. Brisbane. 1976), pp 541–55.

85   Wilding, 1976, op. cit., Introduction, p xiv.

86   'The Chinese Quarter', *Argus*, 9 March 1868, in L T Hergenham (ed), *A Colonial City: High and Low Life: Selected Journalism of Marcus Clarke* (University of Queensland Press. Brisbane. 1972), pp 113–25.

87   Wilding, 1976, op. cit., pp xi, xiii, xxvi.

88   'Corpses for Dissection; Social and Religious Laws at Variance: Medical Education for Women; Futuristic Food and Medicine', *Australasian*, 12 July 1873, in Hergenham, 1972, op. cit., pp 275–81.

89   McCoy, 1980, op. cit., p 65. *Marijuana Australiana*, 2001, op. cit., p 10.

90   *Marijuana Australiana*, 2001, op. cit., p 11.

91   Christine Stevens, *Tin Mosques and Ghantowns: A History of Afghan Cameldrivers in Australia* (Oxford University Press. Melbourne. 1989), p 1.

92   ibid., pp 24–26.

93   ibid., pp 72–73, 248.

94   Personal interview. WMW. Wombarra NSW, July 2004.

95   *Marijuana Australiana*, 2001, op. cit., pp 7–8, 12–13.

96   ibid.

97   Manderson, 1993, op. cit., pp 125, 143–44.

98   *Marijuana Australiana*, 2001, op. cit., pp 14–16.

99   See Manderson, 1993, op. cit., pp 141–49.

100 Official Yearbook of the Commonwealth of Australia. Drug Offences, Nos 58–87 (Commonwealth [later Australian] Bureau of Census and Statistics. Canberra. 1972–2005).

101 *Marijuana Australiana*, 2001, op. cit., p 77.

102 In the National Drug Survey of 2004, 33. 6 per cent of Australians were reported as having tried cannabis. The question asked in the survey changed in 2001 from

'have you ever tried' to 'have you ever used' a particular drug. Had the previous question been asked in 2004 it is estimated that the self-reporting rate would have been 43. 6 per cent. Given that self-reporting is likely to underestimate drug use, the likely figure is closer to 50 per cent. *The Weekend Australian*, 29–30 October 2005, 5–6 November 2005.

103 2001 National Drug Strategy Household Survey: detailed findings, AIHW cat. no. PHE 41. (AIHW [Drug Statistics Series No 11]. Canberra. 2002).

104 Reported in *The Australian*, 21 October 2005.

105 Iversen, 2000, op. cit., pp 207–08.

106 ibid., p 145. Levinson, 2002, op. cit., p 160. Grinspoon and Bakalar, 1993, op. cit., p 19.

107 Iversen, 2000, op. cit., pp 241–47, 253.

108 ibid., pp 187, 242.

109 ibid., pp 189–90. *The Lancet* 8574: 1483–85, 26 December 1987.

110 ibid., p 190

111 *The Australian*, 13 April–2005, *The Age*, 1 December 2005, *The Guardian Weekly*, 20–26 January 2006.

112 *The Guardian Weekly*, 6–12 November 2003.

113 Iversen, 2000, op. cit., p 250.

114 Schlosser, 2003, op. cit., p 69.

115 Walton, 2002, op. cit., p 120.

116 ibid., pp 38–41. Kenneth F Kipple, 'The Ecology of Disease', in Bynum and Porter, 1994, op. cit. R C Cooke, *Fungi, Man and his Environment* (Longman. London and New York. 1977), pp 104–08. C J Alexander, C W Mims and M Blackwell, *Introductory Mycology* (John Wiley & Sons, Inc. New York. 1996), p 8. However, it was reported in 2006 that DNA-based evidence from human remains found in a mass grave dating from the time of the Athens plague led scientists to believe that it may have been typhoid fever rather than ergotism that was its cause. See *The Guardian Weekly*, 3–9 February 2006.

117 Weatherall, 1994, op. cit. Cooke, 1977, op. cit.

118 Martin A Lee and Bruce Shlain, *Acid Dreams: The Complete Social History of LSD: The CIA, the Sixties and Beyond* (Pan Books. London. 2001), p xviii.

119 ibid., pp xviii, xix.

120 ibid., pp 12–13, 26.

121 John Ranelagh, *The Agency: The Rise and Decline of the CIA* (Weidenfeld & Nicolson. London. 1986), p 203.

122 ibid., p 211. The British Secret Intelligence Service, MI6, was also involved in carrying out clandestine LSD experiments on servicemen without their consent, for which they later paid compensation. *The Guardian Weekly*, 3–9 March 2006.

123 ibid., p 207.

124 ibid., p 205. Lee and Shlain, 2001, op. cit., pp 28–29. Davenport-Hines, 2001, op. cit., p 262.

125 Lee and Shlain, 2001, op. cit., pp 32–33, 35, 40.

126 ibid., pp 26–27.

127 ibid., pp 55–56.

128 ibid., pp 57, 61–2. See also Walton, 2002, op. cit., p 121. Davenport-Hines, 2001, op. cit., p 265.

129 Lee and Shlain, 2001, op. cit., pp 44–45, 50–51.

130 In 'The Marriage of Heaven and Hell' (1791), Blake writes, 'If the doors of perception were cleansed everything would appear to man as it is, infinite.'

131 Lee and Shlain, 2001, op. cit., p 54.

132 Walton, 2002, op. cit., p 123. Davenport-Hines, 2001, op. cit., p 265.

133 Lee and Shlain, 2001, op. cit., pp 58, 119. Davenport-Hines, 2001, op. cit., p 262.

134 Lee and Shlain, 2001, op. cit., pp 179, 211.

135 ibid., pp 196, 229.

136 ibid., pp 186, 191.

137 Davenport-Hines, 2001, op. cit., p 266. Lee and Shlain, 2001, op. cit., p 163. Jill Jonnes, 'Hip to be High: Heroin and Popular Culture in the Twentieth Century', in Musto (ed), 2002, op. cit.

138 Material on 1960s African-American history is sourced from Manning Marable and Leith Mullings, *Freedom: A Photographic History of the African American Struggle, Part IV: 1954–1975: We Shall Overcome* (Phaidon Press. London and New York. 2002).

139 Hatfield, 2001, op. cit., pp 37–48. Kelley, 2004, op. cit., pp 294–95.

140 Lee and Shlain, 2001, op. cit., pp 209–10.

141 ibid., p 71.

142 ibid., pp 147, 241–43, 248–51.

143 ibid., pp 288–89.

144 Manderson, 1993, op. cit., p 148. **WHICH ONE?**

145 AIHW 2002. *2001 National Drug Strategy Household Survey: Detailed Findings*, AIHW cat. no PHE 41. (AIHW [Drug Statistics Series No 11]. Canberra ACT. 2002). *2004 National Drug Household Survey: First Results*, AIHW cat. no. PHE 57. (AIHW [Drug Statistics Series No 13]. Canberra ACT. 2005).

146 Campbell, 2001, op. cit., p 172. Jennifer Stafford et al., *Australian Trends in Ecstasy and Related Drug Markets 2004: Party Drugs: Initiative Findings.* National Drug and Alcohol Research Centre Monograph no. 57, p 117.

147 Push and Mireille Silcott, *the book of e* (Omnibus Press. London. 2000), p 7. Campbell, 2001, op. cit., p 100.

148 Push and Mireille Silcott, 2000, op. cit., pp 22–23.

149 ibid., pp 25–26.

150 ibid., pp 7, 27–29. Walton, 2002, op. cit., pp 116–17.

151 Push and Mireille Silcott, 2000, op. cit., pp 29–31. The ecstasy experience is described as: EUPHORIGENIC — euphoria-inducing or providing unique feelings of 'connectedness' with oneself, significant others and strangers, in which the routines and roles of everyday life are temporarily forgotten or transcended; NOETIC — providing an experience of 'seeing the world for the first time' — a child-like vision; ENTACTOGENIC — providing a feeling of 'communicating with an inner self' or a 'touching within'; EMPATHOGENIC — creating and

sustaining empathy. Campbell, 2001, op. cit., p 111.

152 Push and Mireille Silcott, 2000, op. cit., pp 27, 31.

153 Walton, 2002, op. cit., p 117.

154 Spillane, 2000, op. cit., p 94.

155 Push and Mireille Silcott, 2000, op. cit., p 19, Chapter 3 passim.

156 ibid.

157 Push and Mireille Silcott, 2000, op. cit., pp 56, 130.

158 Campbell, 2001, op. cit., pp 110–13.

159 ibid.

160 *New Scientist*, 25 January 1997. In Push and Mireille Silcott, 2000, op. cit., pp 137–38.

161 Campbell, 2001, op. cit., pp 102.

162 *Australian Trends in Ecstasy and Related Drug Markets. 2004*, op. cit., p 23. 2004 National Drug Household Survey, op. cit.

163 Engels, 1984, op. cit., p 207.

Chapter 6

1   Walton, 2002, op. cit., p 111.

2   Trocki, 1999, op. cit., p xiii. Trocki concedes that this is difficult to prove; the challenge he poses is to explain how the projects of Empire might have been financed once you extract the total influence of opium from the fiscal balance sheets of the time.

3   Booth, 1996, op. cit., pp 1–2.

4   Berridge, 1999, op. cit., p xxii.

5   Booth, 1996, op. cit., pp 21–22.

6   Berridge, 1999, op. cit., pp xxii-xxiii.

7   McCoy, 1991, op. cit., p 3.

8   Berridge, 1999, op. cit., p xxiii.

9   Davenport-Hines, 2001, op. cit., p 24.

10   Berridge, 1999, op. cit., pp 32–33.

11   Booth, 1996, op. cit., p 2.

12   Some 950 Tasmanian farmers had 13,000 hectares of opium poppies under cultivation in 2004, a reduction of about 5,000 hectares on the 2003 figures, due to market fluctuations. *The Mercury.* 7 January 2004.

13   Davenport-Hines, 2001, op. cit., p 12.

14   Inglis, 1979, op. cit., p 13.

15   Booth, 1996, op. cit., p 105.

16   ibid.

17   McCoy, 1991, op. cit., p 79.

18   Trocki, 1999, op. cit., p 36.

19   Booth, 1996, op. cit., p 109.

20   ibid.

21   ibid., pp 107, 109.

22   Karl Marx, 'The East India Company — Its History and Results', *New York Daily*

Tribune, 11 July 1853. In *Karl Marx and Friedrich Engels: Articles on Britain* (Progress Publishers. Moscow. 1975).

23   Inglis, 1979, op. cit., p 17.

24   Karl Marx, *New York Daily Tribune*, 11 July 1853, op. cit.

25   A description by Lord Grenville to the parliamentary committee set up in 1813 to consider the extension of the East India Company charter: in Inglis, 1979, op. cit., p 52.

26   ibid., p 35.

27   ibid., p 51. See also 'Karl Marx', *New York Daily Tribune*, 11 July 1853, op. cit.

28   Inglis, 1979, op. cit., p 20.

29   McCoy, 1991, op. cit., p 4.

30   ibid., pp 83–84.

31   ibid., p 82.

32   Karl Marx, *Capital: Volume 1* (Penguin Books. London. 1990), p 917. A note was added to this passage by the author in the following terms: 'In the year 1866 more than a million Hindus died of hunger in the province of Orissa alone. Nevertheless, an attempt was made to enrich the Indian treasury by the price at which the means of subsistence were sold to the starving people.' Hastings was president of the East India Company Council, and from 1773 was governor-general of Bengal. He was impeached by the House of Lords in 1788 for crimes allegedly committed in India. Acquitted after a trial that lasted more than seven years, he thereafter passed his life as a country gentleman, generously provided for by the East India Company.

33   Booth, 1996, op. cit., pp 109–10.

34   ibid., p 109. Inglis, 1979, op. cit., p 206.

35   Inglis, 1979, op. cit., p 206.

36   ibid.

37   Parliamentary address of Sir James Graham in 1840, in Inglis, 1979, op. cit., p 158.

38   See Inglis, 1979, op. cit., pp 93–95.

39   Karl Marx, *New York Daily Tribune*, 11 July 1853, op. cit. See also 'Free Trade and Monopoly', written for the *New York Daily Tribune*, 25 September 1858.

40   McCoy, 1991, op. cit., p 84. Booth, 1996, op. cit., p 128.

41   Booth, 1996, op. cit., p 121.

42   McCoy, 1991, op. cit., p 82.

43   A 'chest' of opium consisted of 40 opium 'balls', each weighing about 1.5 kilograms. More than 7,000 of the chests handed over belonged to Jardine Matheson, and according to Lin, some 6,000 chests belonged to their principal competitor, Launcelot Dent; 1,500 chests were the property of American merchants. Booth, 1996, op. cit., pp 9–10. Inglis, 1979, op. cit., pp 132, 134, 165.

44   In Inglis, 1979, op. cit., p 133.

45   ibid., pp 169–70.

46   ibid., p 139.

47   Eric Hobsbawm, *The Age of Revolution. 1798–1848* (Abacus. London. 2001), p 365.

48   Inglis, 1979, op. cit., p 172.

49   McCoy, 1991, op. cit., p 86.
50   ibid., p 88.
51   In Trocki, 1999, op. cit., p 98.
52   Karl Marx, 'The Opium Trade', *New York Daily Tribune*, 20 September 1858, in *Karl Marx and Friedrich Engels: Articles on Britain*, op. cit. The treaty here referred to is the 1858 Treaty of Tientsin, in spite of which the war continued until eventually settled by the 1860 Convention of Peking. See Booth, 1996, op. cit., p 145. 'Habitual insight' is an expression used by Eric Hobsbawm in describing Marx's analysis of the relationship between Napoleon III and the French peasantry. See Hobsbawm, *The Age of Capital*, 2001, op. cit., p 126.
53   Eric Hobsbawm, *Industry and Empire: An Economic History of Britain Since 1750* (Weidenfeld & Nicolson. London. 1968), p 89.
54   J Y Wong, *Deadly Dreams: Opium and the Arrow War (1856–1860) in China* (Cambridge University Press. Cambridge. 1998), pp 444–46.
     In 1870, half of China's imports still consisted of opium (a) and the trade was the subject of agreements between India and China as late as 1907 and 1911 that restricted imports into China. (b) The percentage of British trade with 'India and the Far East' decreased by 1.6 per cent between 1844 and 1889 and rose by 4 per cent between 1889 and 1913. (c) British control over China's trade is another matter. The Englishman Robert Hart, from his formal position as inspector general of Chinese customs (1863–1909), effectively ran the Chinese economy (d) which was dominated by foreign shipping (e).
     (a) Hobsbawm, *Industry and Empire*, 1968, op. cit.
     (b) *The Cambridge Economic History of India*, vol. 2, c.1757–c.1970 (Cambridge University Press. Cambridge. 1983).
     (c) Wilfred Smith, *An Economic Geography of Great Britain* (Methuen & Co. Ltd. London. 1951).
     (d) Hobsbawm, *The Age of Capital*, 2001, op. cit.
     (e) *Cambridge Economic History of Europe: Volume VI: Part II* (Cambridge University Press. Cambridge. 1965).
     'Habitual insight' is an expression used by Eric Hobsbawm in describing Marx's analysis of the relationship between Napoleon III and the French peasantry (see Hobsbawm, *The Age of Capital*, 2001, op. cit., p 126.
55   McCoy, 1991, op. cit., p 4. Trocki, 1999, op. cit., p 91 cites the figure of 40 million opium smokers in China in 1890 as a conservative one.
56   Booth, 1996, op. cit., pp 168–69. McCoy, 1991, op. cit., p 123.
57   Berridge, 1999, op. cit., p 24.
58   See Manderson, 1993, op. cit., p 6.
59   Geoffrey Blainey, *Black Kettle and Full Moon: Daily Life in a Vanished Australia* (Penguin Books. Melbourne. 2003), p 330.
60   Eric Rolls, *Sojourners* (University of Queensland Press. Brisbane Qld. 1992), p 402. David Day, *Smugglers and Sailors: The Customs History of Australia 1788–1901* (Australian Government Printing Service. Canberra ACT. 1992), pp 299–300.

61 Day, 1992, op. cit., pp 298–99.
62 T A Coghlan, *A Statistical Account of the Seven Colonies of Australasia* (Government Printer. Sydney. 1892), p 57.
63 McCoy, 1980, op. cit., p 79.
64 ibid., p 48.
65 *The Sydney Morning Herald*, 11 March 1844.
66 Rolls, 1992, op. cit., p 399.
67 ibid.
68 ibid., p 401. Manderson, 1993, op. cit., p 22.
69 Manderson, 1993, op. cit., p 30.
70 Rolls, 1992, op. cit., pp 128–38.
71 ibid., pp 464–76.
72 In Manderson, 1993, op. cit., p 18.
73 ibid., p 36.
74 ibid., pp 32–33.
75 Rolls, 1992, op. cit., p 405.

Chapter 7
1   McCoy, 1991, op. cit., p 8, citing Musto, 1973, op. cit.
2   Hobsbawm, *The Age of Capital*, 2001, op. cit., p 80.
3   ibid., p 81. Rolls, 1992, op. cit., p 104.
4   Rolls, 1992, op. cit., p 104.
5   Davenport-Hines, 2001, op. cit., p 90.
6   ibid.
7   Walter LaFeber, *The Cambridge History of American Foreign Relations: Volume II* (Cambridge University Press. Cambridge. 1993), p 52. Rolls, 1992, op. cit., p 471–73.
8   McCoy, 1991, op. cit., p 93.
9   A description of the war by John Hay, US ambassador to the Court of St James and secretary of state from 1898, in LaFeber, 1993, op. cit., p 145.
10 ibid, p 165. McCoy, 1991, op. cit., p 91 (n. 55 p 508), citing Arnold H Taylor, *American Diplomacy and the Narcotics Traffic, 1900–1939: A Study in International Humanitarian Reform* (Duke University Press. Durham NC. 1969).
11 LaFeber, 1993, op. cit., pp 101, 142.
12 Davenport-Hines, 2001, op. cit., p 156.
13 ibid., p 157. McCoy, 1991, op. cit., p 98.
14 McCoy, 1991, op. cit., p 98.
15 Davenport-Hines, 2001, op. cit., pp 159–60.
16 McCoy, 1991, op. cit., p 99.
17 Davenport-Hines, 2001, op. cit., pp 160–61.
18 ibid., pp 174, 202.
19 Manderson, 1993, op. cit., pp 62–63.
20 ibid., pp 71–72.
21 ibid., p 62. Berridge, 1999, op. cit., p 241.

22 Dillon, 2002, op. cit., p 299.
23 World opium production stood at 41,600 tons in 1906, and by 1934 it had significantly reduced to a still substantial 7,600 tons. McCoy, 1991, op. cit., p 10.
24 Rolls, 1992, op. cit., pp 381, 409.
25 ibid., p 400. Booth, 1996, op. cit., p 51 records Indian opium with a morphine content of 4–6 per cent and Turkish opium at 10–13 per cent.
26 Booth, 1996, op. cit., p 70.
27 ibid., p 78. Booth has the name 'heroin' derived from the German 'heroish' meaning 'mighty or heroic' (p. 77). Berridge has the German word as meaning 'large or powerful' in medical terminology (p. xx) and Musto has it as 'strong' (p. xv).
28 Booth, 1996, op. cit., p 70.
29 See Davenport-Hines, 2001, op. cit., pp 83–85.
30 ibid.
31 Rolls, 1992, op. cit., p 410.
32 Musto (ed), 2002, op. cit., p xiii.
33 Booth, 1996, op. cit., pp 78, 91.
34 Musto (ed), 2002, op. cit., p xvi, attributing the phrase to the New York City health commissioner of the time.
35 See Courtwright, 2002, op. cit., p 7.
36 Stephen Fox, *Blood and Power: Organised Crime in Twentieth Century America* (William Morrow & Company, Inc. New York. 1989), p 26.
37 Denton and Morris, 2001, op. cit., pp 21–22.
38 Cockburn and St Clair, 1999, op. cit., p 121.
39 Denton and Morris, 2001, op. cit., p 22.
40 ibid., pp 22–23.
41 ibid., pp 23–24.
42 Cockburn and St Clair, 1999, op. cit., p 122.
43 ibid.
44 Courtwright, 2002, op. cit., p 10.
45 ibid. McCoy, 1991, op. cit., pp 24, 27. Davenport-Hines, 2001, op. cit., pp 197, 206–07, 211–14.
46 Courtwright, 2002, op. cit., p 10.
47 McCoy, 1991, op. cit., p 29.
48 Denton and Morris, 2001, op. cit., p 50. Cockburn and St Clair, 1999, op. cit., p 122.
49 McCoy, 1991, op. cit., pp 10, 29.
50 ibid., pp 29–30.
51 Denton and Morris, 2001, op. cit., p 5.
52 McCoy, 1991, op. cit., pp 18, 25.

Chapter 8

1   Isaac Deutscher, *Stalin: A Political Biography* (Penguin Books. Middlesex. 1986), p 485. Deutscher notes the contribution of allied war supplies, particularly clothing,

food and transport vehicles, at p 499.

2   ibid., p 485–86. Walker notes that until the US and British troops invaded Italy in 1943, they were facing only four German divisions, while the Red Army was facing more than two hundred. Martin Walker, *The Cold War and the Making of the Modern World* (Fourth Estate. London. 1993), p 29.

3   Deutscher, 1986, op. cit., p 497.

4   Walker, 1993, op. cit., p 11. See also Deutscher, 1986, op. cit., p 503.

5   Deutscher, 1986, op. cit., p 529.

6   Walker, 1993, op. cit., pp 41–42.

7   See Deutscher, 1986, op. cit., pp 557–58, 576.

8   ibid., p 527.

9   Walker, 1993, op. cit., p 30.

10   ELAS — Ethnikon Laikos Apeleftherikos Stratos (National Popular Liberation Army).

11   Deutscher, 1986, op. cit., p 566.

12   ibid., pp 515, 576.

13   Walker, 1993, op. cit., p 29.

14   Fox, 1989, op. cit., p 141.

15   Cockburn and St Clair, 1999, op. cit., pp 125–26. The extent to which labour problems on the New York waterfront were sabotaging the war effort may well have been exaggerated. The *Normandie* fire was most likely accidental and the extent of labour unrest can be gauged by the fact that there were no significant waterfront strikes in New York between 1919 and 1945: see Fox, 1989, op. cit., p 196. On the west coast during the prewar period there were complaints of sabotage from the German consul when a German ship on her maiden voyage sank alongside an Oakland wharf. In a centennial retrospective published by the Harry Bridges Institute in 2001, Bridges describes the sinking as a 'complete accident'.

16   ibid., ch 5 passim.

17   McCoy, 1991, op. cit., p 38–39.

18   ibid., p 44.

19   ibid., p 38.

20   ibid., p 44–45.

21   R T Naylor, *Hot Money and the Politics of Debt* (Black Rose Books. Montreal. 1994), p 21.

22   ibid.

23   ibid., p 51.

24   Denton and Morris, 2001, op. cit., pp 103–04.

25   McCoy, 1991, op. cit., pp 52–63.

26   Fred L Block, *The Origins of International Economic Disorder* (University of California Press. Berkeley CA. 1977), pp 88–91.

27   Cockburn and St Clair, 1999, op. cit., pp 139–40, state that US$1 million each year was given to the anti-communist unions from the late 1940s to the early 1950s.

28   See Walker, 1993, op. cit., pp 54–55.

29   Deutscher, 1986, op. cit., p 571.

30 Tariq Ali, *The Clash of Fundamentalisms* (Verso. London. 2002), p 80.

31 McCoy, 1991, op. cit., pp 61–63.

32 ibid., p 196.

33 ibid., pp 113–15.

34 ibid., pp 19, 128.

35 Cockburn and St Clair, op. cit., p 217, citing figures for 1997.

36 *The Guardian Weekly*, 22–28 January 2004.

37 Kathryn Meyer, 'From British India to the Taliban: Lessons from the History of the Heroin Market', in Musto (ed), 2002, op. cit.

38 McCoy, 1991, op. cit., pp 263–64.

39 Cockburn and St Clair, 1999, op. cit., pp 219–21.

40 ibid.

41 William Blum, *The CIA: A Forgotten History* (Zed Books Ltd. London and New Jersey. 1986), pp 16–17.

42 Lintner, 2002, op. cit., p 16.

43 Booth, 1996, op. cit., p 279.

44 Cockburn and St Clair, 1999, op. cit., pp 225–30.

45 ibid.

46 John Pilger, *Hidden Agendas* (Vintage. Great Britain. 1998), p 553.

47 John Pilger, *Heroes* (Pan Books. London and Sydney. 1986), pp 180–81.

48 'Dissident communist' is a description of the partisan leader and later communist president of the Yugoslav Federal Republic, Marshal Tito (Josif Broz), who severed relations with Stalin in 1948 and became leader of the non-aligned movement. Hobsbawm, *Age of Extremes*, 2000, op. cit., p 358.

49 Pilger, 1986, op. cit., p 179.

50 ibid., p 181.

51 ibid. McCoy, 1991, op. cit., pp 149–50.

52 The Binh Xuyen were a criminal gang originally formed in the 1920s by ill-treated contract labourers who fled from the slave labour conditions of the rubber plantations south of Saigon. They established themselves in the piracy and extortion business along the Cholon canals of Saigon's Chinese twin city, from where urban criminals were recruited to their ranks. For a brief period in 1945 they were allied with the Vietminh; they sided with the French in 1946. McCoy, 1991, op. cit., pp 148, 151–53.

53 McCoy, 1991, op. cit., pp 141–43.

54 Pilger, 1986, op. cit., p 183.

55 ibid., p 184.

56 Blum, 1986, op. cit., p 139.

57 McCoy, 1991, op. cit., p 197.

58 ibid.

59 ibid., pp 222–23, 258.

60 Booth, 1996, op. cit., p 237.

61 Cockburn and St Clair, 1999, op. cit., pp 249–51.

62 Ali, 2002, op. cit., p 189.

63   Cockburn and St Clair, 1999, op. cit., p 263.
64   Ali, 2002, op. cit., p 195. Cockburn and St Clair, 1999, op. cit., p 270.
65   Cockburn and St Clair, 1999, op. cit., p 260.
66   ibid., p 264.
67   McCoy, 1991 op. cit., pp 449–450.
68   Ali, 2002, op. cit., pp 195–97.
69   ibid., pp 210–11, 215.
70   ibid.
71   *The Guardian Weekly*, 26 November–2 December 2004, 4–10 March 2005.
72   Cockburn and St Clair, 1999, op. cit., pp 8–9.
73   *The Australian*, 7 June 2004. *The Guardian Weekly*, 7–13 April 2006.
74   Cockburn and St Clair, 1999, op. cit., p 9.
75   ibid.
76   ibid., pp 4–5.
77   ibid., p 281. *The Guardian Weekly*, 25 February–3 March 2005.
78   For a detailed account of the cocaine and crack operation see Gary Webb, *Dark Alliance* (Seven Stories Press. New York. 1999).
79   McCoy, 1991, op. cit., p 482.
80   ibid., pp 478–84.
81   Cockburn and St Clair, 1999, op. cit., p 279.
82   ibid., pp 303–04.
83   ibid., p 14.
84   ibid., p 17.
85   Jeffrey Robinson, *The Laundrymen* (Simon & Schuster. London. 1994), pp 287–90.
86   McCoy, 1991, op. cit., p 478. Cockburn and St Clair, 1999, op. cit., p 309.
87   Cockburn and St Clair, 1999, op. cit., p 309.
88   *The Guardian Weekly*, 16–22 July 2004.

Chapter 9
1   Booth, 1996, op. cit., pp 286–87. McCoy, 1980, op. cit., pp 261–64.
2   McCoy, 1980, op. cit., pp 258–59.
3   ibid.
4   ibid., p 261.
5   ibid., pp 291, 345–47.
6   Evan Whitton, *Can of Worms* (The Fairfax Library. Sydney NSW. 1986), pp 320–22.
7   McCoy, 1980, op. cit., pp 243, 251, 282.
8   ibid., p 292.
9   Whitton, 1986, op. cit., p 45.
10   ibid., p 333.
11   ibid., pp 45, 306–7.
12   Davenport-Hines, 2001, op. cit., p 345.
13   McCoy, 1980, op. cit., pp 24, 345, 347.
14   Whitton, 1986, op. cit., pp 47, 269–70, 333.

15   McCoy, 1980, op. cit., p 309.
16   Davenport-Hines, 2001, op. cit., p 340, quoting the Haight-Ashbury drug expert Dr David Smith.
17   McCoy, 1980, op. cit., p 271.
18   John Langmore and John Quiggin, *Work for All Full Employment in the Nineties* (Melbourne University Press. Melbourne Vic. 1994), p 18.
19   McCoy, 1980, op. cit., pp 40, 311.
20   *Royal Commission of Inquiry into the Activities of the Nugan Hand Group* (Australian Government Publishing Service. Canberra ACT. 1985), p 387.
21   ibid., p 383.
22   ibid., pp 100, 92–95.
23   ibid., Appendix C, pp 1175–77.
24   ibid., p 291.
25   ibid., personal profiles of Black, Manor and Cocke, pp 115–17, 212–14, 128–30.
26   ibid., pp 216–19. Robinson, 1994, op. cit., p 266.
27   ibid., pp 130–32.
28   McCoy, 1991, op. cit., pp 473–74. *Commonwealth–New South Wales Joint Task Force on Drug Trafficking*, vol. 4, p 773 (Australian Government Printing Service. Canberra ACT. 1983).
29   *Royal Commission of Inquiry into the Activities of the Nugan Hand Group Report, 1985*, op. cit., pp 81, 130–32.
30   Robinson, 1994, op. cit., p266.
31   McCoy, 1991, op. cit., p 472.
32   ibid., p 477. *Royal Commission of Inquiry into the Activities of the Nugan Hand Group Report, 1985*, op. cit., p 192.
33   *Royal Commission of Inquiry into the Activities of the Nugan Hand Group Report, 1985*, op. cit., pp 409–11, 743.
34   ibid., p 397.
35   ibid., p 409.
36   ibid., p 397.
37   ibid., p 149. *Commonwealth–New South Wales Joint Task Force on Drug Trafficking*, vol. 2, pp 319–20 (Australian Government Printing Service. Canberra ACT. 1982).
38   ibid., p 190.
39   McCoy, 1991, op. cit., p 463.
40   *Royal Commission of Inquiry into the Activities of the Nugan Hand Group Report, 1985*, op. cit., p 190.
41   ibid.
42   ibid., p 191.
43   ibid., pp 65, 191.
44   McCoy, 1991, op. cit., p 463.
45   *Royal Commission of Inquiry into the Activities of the Nugan Hand Group Report, 1985*, op. cit., pp 291–92.
46   Whitton, 1986, op. cit., p 43.
47   *Royal Commission of Inquiry into the Activities of the Nugan Hand Group Report, 1985*, op.

cit., pp 191–92.

48   McCoy, 1991, op. cit., p 471.

49   ibid., p 462. *Royal Commission of Inquiry into the Activities of the Nugan Hand Group Report, 1985*, op. cit., pp 63–64.

50   *Royal Commission of Inquiry into the Activities of the Nugan Hand Group Report, 1985*, op. cit., p 64.

51   McCoy, 1991, op. cit., p 322.

52   ibid, p 462. Booth, 1996, op. cit., p 258.

53   *Royal Commission of Inquiry into the Activities of the Nugan Hand Group Report, 1985*, op. cit., pp 95, 104.

54   ibid., pp 65–66.

55   ibid., p 67.

56   McCoy, 1991, op. cit., pp 463–64.

57   ibid., p 466.

58   *Royal Commission of Inquiry into the Activities of the Nugan Hand Group Report, 1985*, op. cit., pp 668–69.

59   ibid., pp 865–66.

60   ibid., pp 881–82.

61   *Commonwealth–New South Wales Joint Task Force on Drug Trafficking*, vol. 3, pp 484–86 (Australian Government Printing Service. Canberra ACT. 1983).

62   ibid., vol. 4, pp 747–48.

63   ibid., p 830.

64   *Royal Commission of Inquiry into the Activities of the Nugan Hand Group Report, 1985*, op. cit., pp 74–75.

65   ibid., p 294.

66   ibid., p 372.

67   ibid., pp 397–98.

68   ibid., p 45.

69   Whitton, 1986, op. cit., p 40.

70   ibid., p 172.

71   ibid., p 59.

72   Marian Wilkinson, *The Fixer: The Untold Story of Graham Richardson* (William Heinemann. Australia. 1996), pp 90–92.

73   *Royal Commission of Inquiry into the Activities of the Nugan Hand Group Report, 1985*, op. cit., p 45.

74   ibid., pp 397–98.

75   ibid., p 478.

76   ibid., p 233.

77   ibid., p 51.

78   ibid., pp 232–33.

79   The figures on world illicit drug consumption cited in this section are sourced from UNODC (United Nations Office on Drugs and Crime), *World Drug Report 2004*, *World Drug Report 2005*.

80   Lintner, 2002, op. cit., p 308.

81 Paul Dietze, Ann-Marie Laslett and Greg Rumbold, 'The Epidemiology of Australian Drug Use', in Margaret Hamilton, Trevor King and Alison Ritter (eds), *Drug Use in Australia* (Oxford University Press. Melbourne. 2004).

82 Wayne Hall, 'Heroin and Other Opioid Overdose Deaths in Australia', in *Heroin Crisis* (Bookman. Melbourne. 1999).

83 Wayne Hall, Joanne F. Ross, Michael T Lynskey, Mathew G Law and Louisa J Degenhardt, 'How Many Dependent Heroin Users are There in Australia?', *Medical Journal of Australia* 173: 528–31, 20 November 2000.

84 ibid.

85 Lintner, 2002, op. cit., p 212.

86 ibid., p 323.

87 For a more detailed account of the 'boat people' see Pilger, 1986, op. cit., pp 244–53.

88 See Lintner, 2002, op. cit., p 309.

89 ibid.

90 *Royal Commission of Inquiry into the New South Wales Police Service. First Interim Report 1996.* Final Report 1997, vol. I: Corruption, pp 3, 161.

91 ibid., vol. I: Corruption, pp 16, 97, 100.

92 ibid., p 133.

93 Whitton, 1986, op. cit., p 276.

94 Lintner, 2002, op. cit., p 308.

95 ibid., pp 334–35.

96 Peter Chalk, 'The Global Heroin and Cocaine Trade', in Geoffrey Stokes, Peter Chalk and Karen Gillen (eds), *Drugs and Democracy: In Search of New Directions* (Melbourne University Press. Melbourne Vic. 2000).

97 Lintner, 2002, op. cit., p 333.

98 *The Australian*, 3 May 2005. Campbell, 2001, op. cit., p 129. Seizure rates in the United Kingdom in 2005 were reported as higher, but still less than 20 per cent: *The Guardian Weekly*, 8–14 July 2005. In 2006 a leaked report to the British prime minister estimated that 15 per cent of worldwide heroin production and 23 per cent of cocaine production was seized: *The Australian*, 23 February 2006. In the United States in 2006, despite all the resources devoted to the war on terror, only one in 20 sea containers were being checked: *The Guardian Weekly*, 3–9 March 2006.

Chapter 10

1 Karl Marx and Friedrich Engels, *Manifesto of the Communist Party* (Foreign Language Press. Peking. 1970). A reproduction of the translation made by Samuel Moore in 1888 from the original German text of 1848 and including the prefaces to the German editions of 1872, 1883 and 1890, the Russian edition of 1882, the English edition of 1888, the Polish edition of 1892 and the Italian edition of 1893.

2 Francis Fukuyama, *Trust: The Social Virtues and the Creation of Prosperity* (Free Press. New York. 1995), p 3, citing Francis Fukuyama, *The End of History and the Last Man* (Free Press. New York. 1992).

3   See Pilger, 1998, op. cit., pp 566–70. *The Guardian Weekly*, 16–22 December 2005.

4   By 1949 the USSR had exploded its first nuclear bomb. The United States tested its first hydrogen bomb in 1952; the USSR followed in 1953. In 1956 the United States exploded the first airborne hydrogen bomb. In 1957 the USSR tested its first inter-continental ballistic missile (ICBM) and in the same year launched its first Sputnik satellite. In April of 1961 the USSR launched the first man into space; the United States followed suit a month later.

(a) In 1962 the United States had 3,267 nuclear warheads and 1,653 launchers; the USSR had 481 warheads and 235 launchers. By 1980 the United States had 2,022 launchers and 10,608 nuclear warheads; the USSR had more launchers by this time (2,545) and had closed the gap on nuclear warheads with 7,480. (b) At the conclusion of the Cold War, the number of nuclear warheads stockpiled around the world, almost 70,000, (c) had an explosive power of something like 1.5 million Hiroshima bombs. (d)

(a) Richard Alan Schwartz, *The Cold War Reference Guide* (McFarland & Company, Inc. Jefferson NC. 1997), pp 41, 87, 91, 97.

(b) Walker, 1993, op. cit., p 214.

(c) Paul Rogers, *Losing Control: Global Security in the Twenty-first Century* (Pluto Press. London. 2000), p 40.

(d) *Armament & Disarmament Questions and Answers* (Department for Disarmament Affairs, Co-ordination and World Disarmament Campaign Section. United Nations. New York. 1985).

5   See Walker, 1993, op. cit., pp 234–35.

6   ibid., p 215.

7   See Hobsbawm, *Age of Extremes*, 2000, op. cit., pp 471–72.

8   ibid., pp 473–74.

9   The hard currency export earnings of the USSR after 1980 were somewhere between $27 and $32 billion a year; its subsidies to other countries alone amounted to between $15 and $20 billion. See Walker, 1993, op. cit., p 280.

10   ibid., pp 268–69.

11   Gary Wills, *Reagan's America: Innocents at Home* (Heinemann. London. 1988), p 246.

12   ibid., pp 245–47.

13   ibid., pp 249–50, 253. Schwartz, 1997, op. cit., p 226.

14   See Walker, 1993, op. cit., p 264.

15   ibid., pp 226, 330–31.

16   Milton Friedman, *Capitalism and Freedom* (University of Chicago Press. Chicago. 1962), p 8, cited in Elton Raynack, *Not So Free: The Political Economy of Milton Friedman and Ronald Reagan* (Praeger. New York. 1987), p 9.

17   Milton and Rose Friedman, *Free to Choose a Personal Statement* (Harcourt Brace Jovanovich. New York. 1979), p 64.

18   Eamonn Butler, *Milton Friedman: A Guide to his Economic Thought* (Gower/ Maurice Temple Smith. Aldershot, England. 1985), p 207.

19   See Andrew Gamble, *Hayek: The Iron Cage of Liberty* (Westview Press. Boulder

CO. 1996), p 2. Hayek did see a role for the state. As he put it, 'In no system that could be rationally defended would the state just do nothing. An effective competitive system needs an intelligently designed and continuously adjusted legal framework as much as any other.' State planning, though, would be limited to 'planning for competition': F A Hayek, *The Road to Serfdom* (Dymock's Book Arcade Ltd. Sydney. 1944), pp 42–43.

20 See Gamble, 1996, op. cit., p 69, citing the 'bleak conclusion' that Janos Kornai came to that there is 'no Third Way' available between capitalism and socialism, in *The Socialist System* (Clarendon Press. Oxford. 1992), ch. 21. Hayek, 1944, op. cit., also refers to there being no 'Middle Way' between "atomistic" competition and central direction'.

21 Gamble, 1996, op. cit., pp 128–33.

22 Although Hayek and Friedman had similar views on free enterprise, they nevertheless disagreed on other issues, such as monetarism which holds that the supply of money is critical to the control of inflation. See Gamble, 1996, op.cit., pp 52, 168.

23 Milton Friedman, in an article in *Newsweek* (25 January 1982) described Chile (as a result of its support for a fully free-market economy since the overthrow of its elected president Salvador Allende in 1973) as an economic and political miracle. The military dictatorship of General Augusto Pinochet, under which thousands of Chilean citizens were imprisoned, tortured and murdered and tens of thousands forced into exile, is difficult to reconcile with any notion of freedom. The Chilean economy had also fallen a little short of miraculous when Friedman's article appeared and as Rayack (op. cit., at p 62) has observed, 'Rather than free markets being a necessary condition for political freedom, it seems that in the Chilean case at least, the suppression of political freedom may be a necessary condition for imposing free markets.' On the link between political and economic freedom, Friedman modified his position somewhat in the light of the Chilean experience and criticism of the role that he played in it. In the *Newsweek* article, while not retreating from the generalisation that 'economic freedom is a necessary but not sufficient condition for political freedom', he said that it now had to be accompanied by the proposition that 'political freedom in turn is a necessary condition for the long-term maintenance of economic freedom'. Raynack attributes this change to 'protecting the sacred validity of his free-market economic model'. See pp 70–71.

24 Walker, 1993, op. cit., p 261 quotes Ronald Reagan as saying, 'People will stay free when enterprise remains free', citing *Public Papers of the Presidency*, 1981, 26 February 1981, p 170.

25 Smith, 1896, op. cit., vol. I, pp 455–56.

26 Gamble, 1996, op. cit., pp 109–10, citing the works of Murray Rothbard: *Power and Markets* (Sheed Andrews and McNeel. Kansas. 1977) and *For a New Liberty: The Libertarian Manifesto* (Collier-Macmillan. New York. 1978)

27 See *The Australian*, 31 July 2003.

28 Smith, 1896, op. cit., vol. I, p 15 puts the nature of the exchange this way: 'Whoever offers to another a bargain of any kind, proposes to do this: give me that which I

want, and you shall have this which you want, is the meaning of every such offer; and it is in this manner that we obtain from one another the far greater part of those good offices which we stand in need of. It is not from the benevolence of the butcher, the brewer, or the baker that we expect our dinner, but from their regard to their own interest. We address ourselves, not to their humanity but to their self-love, and never talk to them of our own necessities but of their advantages.'

29 See Alan Haworth, *Anti-Libertarianism: Markets, Philosophy and Myth* (Routledge. London. 1994), p 3.

30 See Philip Bean, *Drugs and Crime* (Willan Publishing. Devon. 2002), p 124.

31 Inglis, 1976, op. cit., pp 204–11, writing in the context of the first opium war, offers a somewhat different view of illicit drug markets. He argues that with illegal drugs it is often the availability of supply that creates demand. This arises because high profit margins allow producers to 'push' their products in a way that they would be unable to do if profit margins were small.

32 Vincenzo Ruggerio and Nigel South, *Eurodrugs: Drug Use, Markets and Trafficking in Europe* (UCL Press. London. 1995), p 3.

33 Kenneth W Clements, *Pricing and Packaging: The Case of Marijuana*, Economics Program, Discussion Paper 0403, University of Western Australia.

34 R T Naylor, *Wages of Crime Black Markets, Illegal Finance, and the Underworld Economy* (Cornell University Press. Ithaca and London. 2004), pp 11, 15.

35 As to the difficulty in measuring the size of both the illicit drug market and illicit markets generally, Naylor says, 'The reality is that no one has a clue how much illegal money is earned or saved or laundered or moved around the world, or how it is distributed among a host of malefactors': ibid., p 8. At pp 33–34 he discusses the estimates of the annual turnover of the worldwide illegal drug business.

36 See Naylor, 2004, op. cit., p 11.

37 In Husak, 1992, op. cit., p 54, citing Mark Deninger, 'The Economics of Heroin: Key to Optimising the Legal Response', *Georgia Law Review* 10: 565, 583, 1976. Mark Kleiman and Aaron Saiger, 'Drug Legalisation: The Importance of Asking the Right Question', *Hofstra Law Review* 18: 527, 542, 1990.

38 *The Weekend Australian*, 2–3 July 2005.

39 In *Karl Marx and Friedrich Engels: Collected Works* (Lawrence & Wishart. London. 1983), vol. 39, p 165. See also Hobsbawm, *The Age of Capital*, 2001, op. cit., p 79.

40 *Marx and Engels: Collected Works*, 1983, op. cit., vol. 38, p 461.

41 Naylor, 2004, op. cit., p 16.

42 In Robinson, 1996, op. cit., p 192.

43 ibid., p 191.

44 ibid.

45 ibid., p 194–95.

46 *The Sydney Morning Herald*, 14 October 2004. *The Weekend Australian*, 1–2 October 2005.

47 *The Australian*, 19 August 2005.

48 *The Weekend Australian*, 28–29 May 2005.

49   *The Age*, 19 May 2005.
50   *The Health Report*, ABC Radio National, 1 August 2005. *The West Australian*, 20 July 2005.
51   *The Health Report*, op. cit.
52   *The Australian*, 22 September 2005.
53   *The Weekend Australian*, 4–5 June 2005. *The Australian*, 8 June 2005.
54   See Raynack, 1987, op. cit., p 2. Butler, op. cit., pp 7–8.
55   Milton and Rose Friedman, 1979, op. cit., pp 66, 305.
56   Illicitly used prescription drugs, together with non-prescription analgesics, are the second most commonly used illicit drugs after cannabis: *2004 National Household Survey: First Results*, AIHW cat. No. PHE 57 (AIHW]Drug Statistic Series No. 13]. Canberra. 2005).
57   Royal Commission into whether there has been Corrupt or Criminal Conduct by any Western Australian Police Officer, vol. I, parts II, III and IV, January 2004. *The Weekend Australian*, 19–20 June 2004.
58   *The Australian*, 10 March 2004, 28 May 2004.
59   *The Australian*, 20 May 2005, 13 May 2005, 2 June 2005.
60   *The Weekend Australian*, 10–11 December 2005.
61   Berridge, 1999, op. cit., pp xxx, 105–09.
62   Husak, 1992, op. cit. Husak, 2002, op. cit. Although confined to the United States, these studies have more than general application elsewhere given the US hegemony over international drug policy.
63   Husak, 2002, op. cit., pp 10–18.
64   ibid., p 64.
65   ibid., pp 82–93.
66   ibid., pp 94–98.
67   ibid., pp 77–79.
68   Of the 25,000 deaths from illicit drugs recorded by the National Institute on Drug Abuse in the United States, 14,300 are due to hepatitis and Aids mostly caused by the dirty needles that heroin addicts tend to share. About 2,500 deaths are caused intentionally and 1,460 are due to injuries inflicted accidentally or purposely: ibid., pp 101, 137.
69   Husak, 2002, op. cit., pp 101–07.
70   Husak, 1992, op. cit., p 105 adopts a broad definition which lists seven factors that characterise addiction or 'dependence syndrome':
     1. A subjective awareness of compulsion to use a drug or drugs, usually during attempts to stop or moderate drug use.
     2. A desire to stop drug use in the face of continued use.
     3. A relatively stereotyped pattern of drug-taking behaviour.
     4. Evidence of neuroadaption (that is, tolerance and withdrawal symptoms).
     5. Use of the drug to relieve or avoid withdrawal symptoms.
     6. The salience of drug-seeking behaviour relative to other important priorities.
     7. Rapid reinstatement of the syndrome after a period of abstinence.
71   See Husak, 1992, op. cit., pp 102–05.

72 ibid., pp 123–24.
73 Husak, 2002, op. cit., pp 97, 106.
74 Husak, 1992, op. cit., p 208.
75 David Musto, *The American Disease: Origins of Narcotic Control* (Oxford University Press. New York. 1987), p 260, cited in Husak, 1992, op. cit., p 36.
76 See Husak, 1992, op. cit., p 95. Husak, 2002, op. cit., pp 163–64.
77 Kenneth W Clements and Mert Daryal, *The Economics of Marijuana Consumption*, Department of Economics, Discussion Paper 99.20, University of Western Australia, September 1999; *Exogenous Shocks and Related Goods: Drinking and the Legalisation of Marijuana*, Discussion Paper 05.14, Revised, Business School. University of Western Australia, 23 February 2005.
78 Iversen, 2000, op. cit., pp 250–51.
79 William Bennett, *National Drug Control Strategy* (Office of the National Drug Control Policy. Washington DC. 1989), p 7, cited in Husak, 1992, op. cit., p 71.
80 John Lawn, 'The Issue of Legalising Illicit Drugs', *Hofstra Law Review* 18: 703, 715, 1990, cited in Husak, 1992, op. cit., p 61.
81 Husak, 2002, op. cit., pp 109–14.
82 William Bennett, 'The Plea to Legalise Drugs is a Siren Call to Surrender', in Michael Lyman and Gary Potter (eds), *Drugs in Society* (Anderson Publishing Co. Cincinnati. 1991), pp 336, 339, cited in Husak, 1992, op. cit., p 78.
83 *Drug Problems in Australia: An Intoxicated Society? Report from the Senate Standing Committee on Social Welfare* (Australian Government Printing Service. Canberra ACT. 1977), p 15.
84 Husak, 1992, op. cit., p 7.
85 *The Australian Financial Review*, 17–21 April 2003. *The Guardian Weekly*, 2–8 December 2005.
86 See Husak, 2002, op. cit., pp 120–23.
87 See Husak, 1992, op. cit., p 80.
88 Husak, 2002, op. cit., p 190. Decriminalisation is taken to mean that no form of punishment should be imposed on people simply because they use a drug for recreational purposes, p 51.
89 Ronald K Seigel, *Intoxication: Life in Pursuit of Artificial Paradise* (E P Dutton & Co. New York. 1989), pp 308, 313, cited in Husak, 1992, op. cit., p 48.
90 *The Guardian Weekly*, 4–10 November 2005.
91 *2004 National Drug Strategy Household Survey: First Results*, AIHW Cat. No. PHE 57 (AIHW [Drug Statistics Series no. 13]. Canberra. 2005). *The Bulletin*, 27 January 2004. *The Australian*, 3 September 2004.
92 *The Australian*, 26 July, 19 November 2004.
93 *The Australian*, 7 February 2006.
94 Andrew Weil, *The Natural Mind*, second edition (Houghton Mifflin Co. Boston. 1986), cited in Husak, 1992, op. cit., p 47. Husak, 2002, op. cit., p 128.
95 Walton, 2002, op. cit., pp 9–10, also citing Weil, 1986, op. cit.
96 Levinthal, 2002, op. cit., pp 276–77.
97 ibid., p 280. *2001 National Drug Household Survey: Detailed Findings*, AIHW

Cat. No. PHE 41 (AIHW (Drug Statistics Series No. 11]. Canberra ACT. 2002).

98   See Walton, 2002, op. cit., pp 10–11.

99   Husak, 1992, op. cit., pp 11–12. Schlosser, 2003, op. cit., p 27.

100 Bean, 2002, op. cit., p 121.

101 *Official Yearbook of the Commonwealth of Australia 2006, Drug Offences* (Australian Bureau of Statistics. Canberra ACT. 2006), pp 329, 331. Official yearbook of the Commonwealth of Australia 2008.

102 *The Weekend Australian*, 28–29 January 2006.

103 AIHW 2005 (Drug Statistics Series No. 13), op. cit.

104 *The West Australian*, 5 July 2004.

105 AIHW 2005 (Drug Statistics Series No. 13), op. cit.

106 D Kessler and M Myers, 'Beyond the Tobacco Settlement', *New England Journal of Medicine* 345(7): 535, 16 August 2001. Also cited in Isralowitz, 2002, op. cit., p x.

107 *The Age*, 5 October 2004.

108 *The Australian*, 8 February 2006.

109 *The Age*, 5 October 2004.

110 *The Australian*, 27 December 2005.

111 *The Guardian Weekly*, 11–17 February 2005. *The Australian*, 19 October 2005.

112 *New Internationalist*, June 2004.

113 *The Australian*, 26 January 2004.

114 *The Guardian Weekly*, 14–20 January 2005. *The Australian*, 25 November 2004. *ABC World Today*, 5 September 2005.

115 *The Guardian Weekly*, 24 December 2004–6 January 2005.

116 Australian Tax Office, Press Release, Canberra ACT, 12 August 2003. *The Australian*, 25 November 2004.

117 T Chikritzhs, P Catalano, T Stockwell, S Donath, H Ngo, D Young and S Matthews, *Australian Alcohol Indicators, 1990–2001: Patterns of Alcohol Use and Related Harms for Australian States and Territories* (National Drug Research Institute. Canberra ACT. 2003). The report notes that in 2001 the number of lives saved by alcohol actually outweighed the number of deaths caused by the drug. However, in terms of premature loss of life the net outcome was markedly negative, because the lives lost involved many young people with long life expectancies while the deaths prevented almost always involved older people with much shorter life expectancies.

118 ibid.

119 *The Australian*, 31 December 2004.

120 Levinthal, 2002, op. cit., pp 200–201. *The Guardian Weekly*, 26 November–2 December 2004.

121 See the statement in these terms by the executive director of the Australian Hotels Association, reported in *The Australian*, 3 June 2005. The statement followed the prosecution of a bar worker and hotel manager for supplying liquor to a drunken person who subsequently fell to her death.

122 Chikritzhs et al., 2003, op. cit., pp x, 42.

123 Jerome H Jaffe (Editor in Chief), *Encyclopedia of Drugs and Alcohol* (Simon &

Schuster Macmillan. New York.1995) vol I, pp 85–91, 97–100. Porter, 1997, op. cit., pp 510, 704. Saner Gilman, 'Psychotherapy', in Bynum and Roy Porter, 1994, op. cit.

124 *The Sydney Morning Herald*, Weekend Edition, 31 May–1 June 2008.

Epilogue

1 Alistair McGrath, *The Twilight of Atheism: The Rise and Fall of Disbelief in the Modern World* (Doubleday. New York. 2004), pp 1, 21, 47.

2 See ibid., p 56–57. *Chambers Biographical Dictionary*, 1996, op. cit., p 512. Ludwig Feuerbach, *The Essence of Christianity*, trans. Marian Evans, second edition (Trubner & Co. London. 1881), p 193.

3 See McGrath, 2004, op. cit. and Feuerbach, 1881, op. cit., pp xiii, 204. McGrath at p 25 quotes Voltaire in full:
   'If the heavens, stripped of their noble imprint,
   Could ever cease to reveal him,
   If God did not exist, it would be necessary to invent him,
   Whom the sage proclaims, and whom Kings adore.'
   He goes on to assert that Voltaire defended the notion of a supreme being while criticising religion in general and warring Christian sects in particular.

4 Feuerbach, 1881, op. cit., p 301. McGrath, 2004, op. cit., p 58.

5 See McGrath, 2004, op. cit., pp 68–74.

6 See ibid., p 63.

7 Karl Marx, *Theses on Feuerbach*, in Loyd D. Easton and Kurt H. Guddat (trans, eds), *Writings of the Young Marx on Philosophy and Society* (Anchor Books. New York. 1967), pp 400–02.

8 See McGrath, 2004, op. cit., p 64.

9 Marx, *Theses on Feuerbach*, in Easton and Guddat (eds), 1967, op. cit.

10 Marx, *A Contribution to the Critique of Hegel's Philosophy of Right Introduction*, in Easton and Guddat (eds), 1967, op. cit., pp 243–44.

11 Marx, *Theses on Feuerbach*, in Easton and Guddat (eds), 1967, op. cit.

12 Francis Wheen, *Karl Marx* (Fourth Estate. London. 1999), pp 310–13.

13 See Hobsbawm, *Age of Empire*, 2001, op. cit., pp 112–18.

14 See ibid., pp 132–35.

15 *Ten Days That Shook the World*, by the American journalist John Reed (1887–1920), is a first-hand account of the Bolshevik insurrection in Petrograd.

16 See Deutscher, 1986, op. cit., p 138.

17 Hobsbawm, *Age of Empire*, 2001, op. cit., p 297.

18 See Hobsbawm, *Age of Extremes*, 2000, op. cit., pp 57–58. See also *Manifesto of the Communist Party*, 1970, op. cit., Preface to the Russian edition of 1882.

19 ibid., p 376. Lenin was formerly Ulyanov.

20 ibid.

21 Deutscher, 1986, op. cit., p 150. The proclamation was written by Joseph Stalin.

22 Paul Frolich, *Rosa Luxemburg* (Pluto Press and Bookmarks. London. 1994), trans. Joanna Hoormweg, p 241.

23   ibid., p 261.

24   Hobsbawm, *Age of Extremes*, 2000, op. cit., p 68.

25   Frolich, 1994, op. cit., pp 301–02. Lenin, on 10 November, wrote of the beginning of a victorious revolution in Germany with power having already passed into the hands of the Soviets of Workers' and Soldiers' Deputies in Kiel and other northern towns and ports as well as Berlin. See Paul M Sweezy, *Modern Capitalism and Other Essays* (Monthly Review Press. New York. 1972), p 174, citing Lenin's work *The Proletarian Revolution and the Renegade Kautsky*.

26   Deutscher, 1986, op. cit., pp 222–26. The cocaine sniffing among the 50,000 'waifs and strays' in Moscow was reported in the 1926 despatches of the British diplomat Sir Robert Hodgson. See Davenport-Hines, 2001, op. cit., pp 224–25.

27   ibid. See also Hobsbawm, *Age of Extremes*, 2000, op. cit., p 378.

28   See ibid., p 386.

29   Deutscher, 1986, op. cit., pp 312, 317, 381–82.

30   *Chambers Biographical Dictionary*, 1996, op. cit., p 1385. Hobsbawm, *Age of Extremes*, 2000, op. cit., p 381.

31   Deutscher, 1986, op. cit., pp 160–62.

32   See ibid., pp 283–84.

33   See ibid., p 388.

34   See Hobsbawm, *Age of Extremes*, 2000, op. cit., pp 71–72.

35   Deutscher, 1986, op. cit., p 285.

36   Paul Levi (ed), *The Russian Revolution: A Critical Appreciation from the Papers of Rosa Luxemburg* (Berlin. 1963), cited in Frolich, 1994, op. cit., p 255.

37   See Hobsbawm, *Age of Extremes*, 2000, op. cit., pp 387, 467.

38   Karl Marx and Friedrich Engels, *The German Ideology*, in Easton and Guddat (eds), 1967, op. cit., pp 424–25.

39   *Manifesto of the Communist Party*, 1970, op. cit.

40   V I Lenin, *Selected Works in Two Volumes* (Foreign Language Publishing House. Moscow. 1950), vol. I, part I, p 76.

41   See Scruton, 1983, op. cit., pp 126–27.

42   See Hobsbawm, *Age of Extremes*, 2000, op. cit., pp 496–97. In the preface to *A Contribution to the Critique of Political Economy* written in January 1859, Marx wrote, 'It is not the consciousness of men that determines their existence, but their social existence that determines their consciousness. At a certain stage of development, the material productive forces of society come into conflict with the existing relations of production or — this merely expresses the same thing in legal terms — with the property relations within the framework of which they have operated hitherto. From forms of development of the productive forces these relations turn into their fetters. Then begins an era of social revolution': *Karl Marx: Early Writings*, 1992, op. cit., pp 424–28.

43   See Hobsbawm, *Age of Extremes*, 2000, op. cit., p 467. *History of the Communist Party of the Soviet Union (Bolshevik) Short Course* (Foreign Language Publishing House. Moscow. 1950), p 2.

44   Ellen Meiksins Wood, *Democracy Against Capitalism* (Cambridge University

Press. Cambridge. 1997), p 19.

45   Perry Anderson, *Considerations on Western Marxism* (NLB. London. 1977), p 36.

46   ibid., pp 29–32.

47   ibid., p 52.

48   ibid., p 53. See also pp 92–93.

49   ibid., pp 95–96.

50   See Perry Anderson, *In the Tracks of Historical Materialism* (Verso. London. 1983), pp 21–25.

51   ibid., pp 26–30.

52   Jonathon Culler, *Saussure* (Fontana/Collins. London. 1976), pp 9, 16.

53   ibid., p 19.

54   See ibid., p 29.

55   See ibid., p 23.

56   See Anderson, 1983, op. cit., pp 33–4.

57   *Manifesto of the Communist Party*, 1970, op. cit., Preface to the German edition of 1872.

58   Anderson, 1983, op. cit., pp 35, 42.

59   Claude Levi-Strauss, *The Savage Mind* (Weidenfeld & Nicolson. London. 1966), cited in Anderson, 1983, op. cit., p 37. See also Madan Sarup, *An Introductory Guide to Post-Structuralism and Postmodernism* (University of Georgia Press. Athens GA. 1989), p 1.

60   See Anderson, 1983, op. cit., pp 51–54. Sarup, 1989, op. cit., p 2.

61   See Sarup, 1989, op. cit., p 60.

62   Didier Eribon, *Michel Foucault* (faber and faber. London. 1993), p 121.

63   See Sarup, 1989, op. cit., pp 89–90.

64   Steven Connor (ed), *The Cambridge Companion to Postmodernism* (Cambridge University Press. Cambridge. 2004), p 5.

65   ibid., pp 149, 164.

66   Wheen, 1999, op. cit., p 5.

67   See Sarup, 1989, op. cit., p 130.

68   Karl Marx, *A Contribution to the Critique of Political Economy Preface* (January 1859), in *Karl Marx: Early Writings*, 1992, op. cit., p 426.

69   The post-industrial economy that is said to be characterised by the production of knowledge rather than material goods is held to operate differently to the industrial economy (See Ursula K Heise, 'Science, technology and postmodernism', in Connor (ed), op. cit.) Leaving aside just how large a part of the world economy the knowledge economy is, its participants are nevertheless consumers of energy and material goods outside the world of work and continue to rely on energy and material goods such as mobile phones and computers for access to and dissemination of knowledge. According to a report in the United Kingdom, PCs on average are now discarded and replaced every three years, mobile phones every 18 months (*The Guardian Weekly*, 31 March–6 April 2006). As to energy resources, it is estimated that about 70 per cent of the earth's crude oil reserves have already been exhausted and, at the current usage rate, oil will become scarce

by mid-century. There are some 60 years of natural gas left and 50 years of known low-cost uranium. Coal, as well as being more polluting than most energy sources, is also more abundant, with between 165 and 285 years' supply left at current rates of use (*The Guardian Weekly*, 17–23 March 2006).

70 *The Guardian Weekly*, 17–23 March 2006.

71 McGrath, 2004, op. cit., pp xi, 144.

72 Irina Korovushkina Paert, 'Memory and Survival in Stalin's Russia: Old Believers in the Urals during the 1930s–50s', in Daniel Bertaux et al. (eds), *On Living Through Soviet Russia* (Routledge. London and New York. 2004).

73 Heather Hendershot, *Shaking the World for Jesus* (University of Chicago Press. Chicago. 2004), pp 4, 11.

74 ibid., pp 11, 31, 56.

75 There are no precise figures on the number of atheists or religious adherents around the world and the various surveys and other data that purport to measure the relevant statistics are the source of some controversy. Thus one figure has it that those considered religious account for 86 per cent of the world's population and the non-religious 14 per cent (see http://www.atheistempire.com/reference/stat). Another figure, based on data extracted from Michael Martin (ed), *The Cambridge Companion to Atheism* (Cambridge University Press. Cambridge. 2005), has the worldwide number of atheists, agnostics and non-believers in God at between 504,962,830 and 749,247,571 out of a total world population in 2005 of 6,437,993,942. From this it is then maintained that between 87.6 per cent and 92.2 per cent of the world's population professes belief in God, deities or similarly understood higher power (see http://www.adherents.com/adh_faq.html#god).

Bibliography

Adler, Robert E. *Medical Firsts: From Hippocrates to the Human Genome*. John Wiley & Sons, Inc. Hoboken. New Jersey. 2004.

AGPS. *Illicit Psychostimulant Use in Australia*. Canberra. 1993.

Alexander, C J with Mims, C W and Blackwell, M. *Introductory Mycology*. John Wiley & Sons, Inc. New York. 1996.

Ali, Tariq. *The Clash of Fundamentalisms*. Verso. London. 2002.

Anderson, Perry. *Considerations on Western Marxism*. NLB. London. 1977.

——. *In the Tracks of Historical Materialism*. Verso. London. 1983.

Australian Academy of Technological Science. *Technology in Australia*. Melbourne. 1988.

Australian Bureau of Statistics:

——. *Apparent Consumption of Foodstuffs in Australia*. Cat. no. 43060.0 October 2000.

——. *National Health Survey*. Cat. no. 4364.0 2001.

Australian Institute of Health and Welfare:

——. AIHW 2001. *Statistics on Drug Use in Australia 2000*. Cat. no. PHE 30 (Drug Statistics Series no. 8)

——. AIHW 2002. *2001 National Drug Strategy Household Survey: detailed findings*. Cat. no. PHE 41 (Drug Statistics Series no. 11)

——. AIHW 2003. *Statistics on Drug Use in Australia 2002*. Cat. no. PHE 43 (Drug Statistics Series no. 12)

——. AIHW 2005. *2004 National Drug Household Survey*. First Results. Cat. no. PHE 57 (Drug Statistics Series no.13)

Bean, Philip. *Drugs and Crime*. Willan Publishing. Devon. UK. 2002.

Bernal, J D. *Science in History*. C A Watts & Co Ltd. London. 1969.

Berridge, V. *Opium and the People*. Free Association Books. London and New York. 1999.

Bertaux, Daniel, with Thompson, Paul and Rotkirch, Anna (eds). *On Living Through Soviet Russia*. Routledge. London and New York. 2004.

Blainey, Geoffrey. *Black Kettle and Full Moon: Daily Life in a Vanished Australia*. Penguin Books. Australia. 2003.

Bliss, Michael. *The Discovery of Insulin*. The University of Chicago Press. Chicago. 1982.

Block, Fred. L. *The Origins of International Economic Disorder*. University of California Press. Berkeley. 1977.

Blum, William. *The CIA: A Forgotten History*. Zed Books Ltd. London and New Jersey. 1986.

Bosca, Ivan with Karus, Michael. *The Cultivation of Hemp: Botany, Varieties, Cultivation and Harvesting*. Hemptech. Sebastopol. California. 1998.

Boyer, Richard O with Morais, Herbert M. *Labor's Untold Story*. United Electrical, Radio and Machine Workers of America. Pittsburgh PA. 2003.

Braverman, Harry. *Labour and Monopoly Capital*. Monthly Review Press. New York and London. 1974.

Brock, William H. *The Fontana History of Chemistry*. Fontana Press. London. 1992.

Burnett, John. *Liquid Pleasures: A Social History of Drinks in Modern Britain*. Routledge. London. 1999.

Butler, Eamonn. *Milton Friedman: A Guide to his Economic Thought*. Gower/Maurice Temple Smith. Aldershot. England. 1985.

Byck, Robert (ed). *Cocaine Papers*. Sigmund Freud. Stonehill. New York. 1974.

Cadbury, Deborah. *Seven Wonders of the Industrial World*. Fourth Estate. London and New York. 2003.

Carstairs, Andrew McLaren. *A Short History of Electoral Systems in Western Europe*. George Allen & Unwin. London. 1980.

Caldwell, John. (ed) *Amphetamines and Related Stimulants: Chemical, Biological, Clinical and Sociological Aspects*. CRC Press, Inc. Boca Raton. Florida. 1980.

Caldwell, Robert. *The Gold Era of Victoria*. James Blundell & Co. Melbourne. 1855.

Cambridge Economic History of Europe. Cambridge. 1965.

Cambridge Economic History of India. Cambridge. 1983.

Campbell, Andrew. *The Australian Illicit Drug Guide*. Black Inc. Melbourne. 2001.

Carter, J W with Harland, D J. *Contract Law in Australia*. Fourth edition. Butterworths. Australia. 2002.

Chalk, Peter with Gillen, Karen. *Drugs and Democracy: In Search of New Directions*. Melbourne University Press. Melbourne. 2000.

Clark, C M H. *A History of Australia*. Melbourne University Press. Melbourne. 1981.

Clarke, Marcus. *For the Term of his Natural Life*. Times House. Sydney. 1992.

Clements, Kenneth W. *Pricing and Packaging: The Case of Marijuana*. The University of Western Australia (UWA). Discussion Paper 0403.

——. with Daryal, Mert. 'The Economics of Marijuana Consumption.' UWA Discussion Paper 99.20. September 1999.

——. 'Exogenous Shocks and Related Goods: Drinking and the legalisation of Marijuana.' Discussion Paper 05.14 revised 23 February 2005.

Cockburn, Alexander with St Clair, Jeffrey. *Whiteout: The CIA Drugs and the Press*. Verso. London and New York. 1999.

Coghlan, T A. *A Statistical Account of the Seven Colonies of Australia*. Government Printer. Sydney. 1892.

——. *Labour and Industry in Australia from the First Settlement in 1788 to the Establishment of the Commonwealth in 1901*. Oxford University Press. London. 1918.

Cohen, Jay S. *Overdose: The Case Against the Drug Companies*. Tarcher Putnam Inc. New York. 2001.

Colmes, John and Dorothy. *Mainly Modern*. Rigby. Adelaide. 1978.

Commonwealth of Australia. *Official Yearbooks 1972–2006*. Commonwealth Bureau of Census and Statistics (later ABS). Canberra.

Commonwealth–NSW Joint Task Force on Drug Trafficking. AGPS Canberra. 1982, 1983.

Connor, Steven (ed). *The Cambridge Companion to Postmodernism*. Cambridge University Press. Cambridge. 2004.

Conrad, Chris. *Hemp: Lifeline to the Future*. Creative Xpressions Publications. Los Angeles. California. 1994.

Cooke, R C. *Fungi, Man and his Environment.* Longman. London and New York. 1977.

Crisswell, Colin N. *The Taipans: Hong Kong's Merchant Princes.* Oxford University Press. Hong Kong. 1981.

Culler, Jonathon. *Suassure.* Fontana/Collins. Great Britain. 1976.

Davenport-Hines, Richard. *The Pursuit of Oblivion.* Wiedenfeld and Nicolson. London. 2001.

Day, David. *The Customs History of Australia 1788–1901.* AGPS. Canberra. 1992.

Deer, Noel. *The History of Sugar.* Chapman and Hall Ltd. London. 1950.

Denton, Sally with Morris, Roger. *The Money and the Power.* Alfred A Knopf. New York. 2001.

Department of Education. *Science and Training: Students 2003.* Selected Higher Education Statistics.

De Quincey, Thomas. *Confessions of an English Opium-Eater.* Wordsworth Classics. Hertfordshire. 1994.

Deutscher, Isaac. *Stalin: A Political Biography.* Penguin Books. Middlesex, England. 1986.

Dillon, Patrick. *The Much-Lamented Death of Madame Geneva: The Eighteenth Century Gin Craze.* Review. London. 2002.

Drug Education Centre. Western Australian Alcohol and Drug Authority. Information Booklet, Barbiturates.1986.

Dubois, Rene. *Pasteur and Modern Science.* Science Tech Publishers. Madison WI. 1988.

Easton, Loyd with Guddat, Kurt H (eds). *Writings of the Young Marx on Philosophy and Society.* Anchor books. New York. 1967.

Elliot, Anthony (ed). *Freud 2000.* Melbourne University Press. Melbourne. 1998.

Engels, Friedrich. *The Condition of the Working Class in England.* Elecbook. London. 1998.

Eribon, Didier. *Michel Foucault.* faber and faber . London. 1993.

Evatt, H V. *Rum Rebellion.* Times House. Silverwater, NSW. 1984.

Farber, Eduard. *The Evolution of Chemistry: A History of its Ideas, Methods, and Materials.* Second edition. The Ronald Press Company. New York. 1969.

Faust, Beatrice. *Benzo Junkie.* Viking. Burwood. Victoria. 1993.

Feuerbach, Ludwig. *The Essence of Christianity.* Translated by Marion Evans. Second edition. Trubner & Co. Ludgate Hill, London. 1881.

Foucault, Michel. *The Birth of the Clinic: An Archaeology of Medical Perception.* Routledge. London and New York. 2003.

Fox, Russell with Mathews, Ian. *Drugs Policy: Fact, Fiction and the Future.* The Federation Press. Sydney. 1992.

Fox, Stephen. *Blood and Power: Organised Crime in Twentieth Century America.* William Morrow and Company, Inc. New York. 1989.

Franklin, Bob (ed). *The Rights of Children.* Basil Blackwell. Oxford. 1986.

Frolich, Paul. *Rosa Luxemburg.* Pluto Press and Bookmarks. London. 1994.

Friedman, Milton and Rose. *Free to Choose: A Personal Statement.* Harcourt Brace Jovanovich. New York. 1979.

Fukuyama, Francis. *Trust: The Social Virtues and the Creation of Prosperity.* The Free Press. New York. 1995.

Gamble, Andrew. *Hayek: The Iron Cage of Liberty.* Westview Press. Boulder, Colorado. 1996.

Gascoigne, John. *Science in the Service of Empire: Joseph Banks, the British State and the uses of Science in the Age of Revolution.* Cambridge University Press. Cambridge. 1998.

Goodman, Lester with Lovejoy, Paul E and Sherratt, Andrew. *Consuming Habits.* Routledge. London and New York. 1995.

Grinspoon, Lester with Bakalar, James B. *Marihuana: The Forbidden Medicine.* Yale University Press. New Haven and London. 1993.

Gunningham, Neil. *Safeguarding the Worker: Job Hazards and the Rule of Law.* The Law Book Company Limited. North Ryde, NSW. 1984.

Hatfield, J H. *Fortunate Son.* Soft Skull Press. New York. 2001.

Hannan, June with Auchterlonie, Mitzi and Holden, Katherine. *International Encyclopaedia of Women's Suffrage.* ABC-CLIO. Santa Barbara. California. 2000.

Haworth, Alan. *Anti-Libertarianism: Markets, Philosophy and Myth.* Routledge. London. 1994.

Hayek, F A. *The Road to Serfdom.* Dymock's Book Arcade Ltd. Sydney. 1944.

Hellman, Lillian. *Scoundrel Time.* Quartet Books. London. 1978.

Hendershot, Heather. *Shaking The World for Jesus.* The University of Chicago Press. Chicago. 2004.

Hennessey, Eileen. *A Cup of Tea, a Bex and a Good Lie Down.* Department of History and Politics. James Cook University of North Queensland. 1993.

Herer, Jack. *The Emperor Wears No Clothes.* AH HA Publishing. Van Nuys. California. 1998.

Hergenham, L T (ed). *In a Colonial City: High and Low Life: Selected Journalism of Marcus Clarke.* University of Queensland Press. St. Lucia. 1972.

Heroin Crisis. (Foreword by Barry Jones). Bookman. Melbourne. 1999.

Hilts, Philip J. *Smokescreen. The Truth Behind the Tobacco Industry Cover-Up.* Addison-Wesley Publishing Company Inc. Reading, Massachusetts. 1996.

Himmelstein, Jerome L. *The Strange Career of Marijuana: Politics and Ideology of Drug Control in America.* Greenwood Press. Westport. Connecticut. 1983.

History of the Communist Party of the Soviet Union (Bolshevik): Short Course. Foreign Language Publishing House. Moscow. 1950.

Hobsbawm, Eric. *Industry and Empire: An Economic History of Britain Since 1750.* Wiedenfeld and Nicolson. London. 1991.

——. *The Age of Revolution. 1789–1848.* Abacus. London. 2001.

——. *The Age of Capital. 1848–1875.* Abacus. London. 2001.

——. *The Age of Empire. 1875–1914.* Abacus. London. 2001.

——. *Age of Extremes: The Short History of the Twentieth Century. 1914–1991.* Abacus. London. 2000.

Huang, Kee Chang. *The Pharmacology of Chinese Herbs.* Second edition. CRC Press. Boca Raton. 1999.

Husak, Douglas. *Drugs and Rights.* Cambridge University Press. Cambridge. 1992.

——. *Legalise This! The case for Decriminalising Drugs.* Verso. London. New York. 2002.

Illich, Ivan. *Limits to Medicine: Medical Nemesis: The Expropriation of Health.* Marion Boyars. London. 2002.

Inglis, Brian. *The Opium War.* Coronet Books. London. 1979.

——. *The Diseases of Civilisation.* Hodder and Staughton. London. 1981.

Isralowitz, Richard. *Drug Use, Policy and Management.* Auburn House. Westport, Connecticut.

2002.

Iverson, Leslie, L. *The Science of Marijuana.* Oxford University Press. Oxford. 2000.

Jaffe, Jerome H (editor in chief). *Encyclopaedia of Drugs and Alcohol.* Simon and Schuster Macmillan. New York. 1995.

Jonnes, Jill. *Hep-cats, Narcs and Pipe Dreams.* Scribner. New York 1996.

Kelley, Kitty. *The Family.* Bantam Press. London. 2004.

Kennedy, Joseph. *Coca Exotica.* Fairleigh Dickinson University Press. Rutherford. 1985.

Khoury, Sarkis J. *The Deregulation of the World Financial Markets: Myths, Realities and Impact.* Pinter Publishers. London. 1990.

King, Trevor with Ritter, Allison (eds). *Drug Use in Australia.* Oxford University Press. Melbourne. 2004.

Kinnear, Michael. *The British Voter: An Atlas and Survey Since 1885.* B T Batsford Ltd. London. 1968.

Kipple, Kenneth F (ed). *The Cambridge World History of Human Disease.* Cambridge University Press. Cambridge. 1995.

——. with Ornelas, Kriemhild C (eds). *The Cambridge World History of Food.* Cambridge University Press. Cambridge. 2000.

Klee, Hillary (ed). *Amphetamine Misuse: International Perspectives on Current Trends.* Harwood Academic Publishers. Amsterdam. 1997.

Kluger, Richard. *Ashes to Ashes.* Alfred A Knopf. New York. 1996.

LaFeber, Walter. *The Cambridge History of American Foreign Relations.* Cambridge University Press. Cambridge. 1993.

Langmore, John with Quiggin, John. *Work for All: Full Employment in the Nineties.* Melbourne University Press. Melbourne. 1994.

Lee, Martin A with Shlain, Bruce. *Acid Dreams: The Complete Social History of LSD: The CIA, the Sixties and Beyond.* Pan Books. London. 2001.

Lehrer, Stephen. *Explorers of the Body.* Doubleday & Company, Inc. New York. 1979.

Lenin, V I *Selected Works in Two Volumes.* Foreign Language Publishing House. Moscow. 1950.

Levinthal, Charles F. *Drugs, Behaviour and Modern Society.* Third edition. Allyn & Bacon. Boston. 2002.

Levinson, Martin H. *The Drug Problem.* Praeger. Westport, Connecticut. 2002.

Linter, Bertil. *Blood Brothers: Crime, Business and Politics in Asia.* Allen and Unwin. Sydney. 2002.

Macinnis, Peter. *Bittersweet: The Story of Sugar.* Allen and Unwin. Crows Nest, NSW. 2002.

MacLeod, Christine. *Inventing the Industrial Revolution: The English Patent System 1600–1800.* Cambridge University Press. Cambridge. 1988.

Magner, Lois N. *A History of Medicine.* Marcel Dekker Inc. New York. 1992.

Magnusson, Magnus (ed). *Chambers Biographical Dictionary.* Chambers. Edinburgh. 1996.

Manderson, Desmond. *From Mr Sin to Mr Big: A History of Australian Drug Laws.* Oxford University Press. Melbourne. 1993.

Mant, Andrea. *Thinking About Prescribing.* The McGraw-Hill Companies Inc. Sydney. 1999.

Marable, Manning with Mullins, Leith. *Freedom: A Photographic History of the African-American Struggle.* Phaidon Press. London and New York. 2002.

Marginson, Simon. *Markets in Education*. Allen and Unwin. St Leonards, NSW 1997.

Marijuana Australiana Project. Marijuana Australiana. Kent Town, SA 2001.

Marshall, Mac (ed). *Belief, Behaviour and Alcoholic Beverages*. University of Michigan Press. US. 1979.

Martyr, Philippa. *Paradise of Quacks: An Alternative History of Medicine in Australia*. Macleay Press. Sydney. 2002.

Marx, Karl. *Early Writings*. Penguin. London. 1992.

——. *Capital*. Vol. 1. Penguin Books. London 1990.

——. with Friedrich Engels. *Articles on Britain*. Progress Publishers. Moscow. 1975.

——. *Manifesto of the Communist Party*. Foreign Language Press. Peking. 1970.

——. *Collected Works*. Lawrence & Wishart. London.1983.

Mathews, Mitford M (ed). *A Dictionary of Americanism on Historical Principles*. University of Chicago Press. Chicago. 1951.

Mautner, Thomas (ed). *The Penguin Dictionary of Philosophy*. Penguin Books. London. 2000.

McAllister, Ian with Moore, Rhonda and Makkai, Toni. *Drugs in Australian Society*. Longman Cheshire. Melbourne. 1991.

McCoy, Alfred W. *Drug Traffic: Narcotics and Organised Crime in Australia*. Harper & Row. Sydney. 1980.

——. *The Politics of Heroin: CIA Complicity in the Global Drug Trade*. Lawrence Hill Books. New York. 1991.

McGrath, Alistar. *The Twilight of Atheism: The Rise and Fall of Disbelief in the Modern World*. Doubleday. New York. 2004.

McGrew, Roderick E. *Encyclopaedia of Medical History*. McGraw-Hill Book Company. New York. 1985.

McKenna, Terence. *Food of the Gods: The Search for the Original Tree of Knowledge: A Radical History of Plants, Drugs and Human Evolution*. Rider. London 1992.

Meadows, Graham with Singh, Bruce (eds). *Mental Health in Australia*. Collaborative Community Practice. Oxford University Press. Melbourne. 2001.

Meiksins Wood, Ellen. *Democracy Against Capitalism*. Cambridge University Press. Cambridge. 1997.

Moore, Michael. *Stupid White Men*. Regan Books. New York. 2001.

Morales, Edmundo. *Cocaine: White Gold Rush in Peru*. The University of Arizona Press. Tuscan. 1989.

Musto, David F (ed). *One Hundred Years of Heroin*. Auburn House. Westport, Connecticut. 2002.

National Drug and Alcohol Research Centre. *Australian Trends in Ecstasy and Related Drug Markets 2004*. Findings from the Party Drugs Initiative (PDI). Monograph No 57. Stafford, Jennifer et al.

National Drug Research Institute. *Australian Alcohol Indicators, 1990–2001*. Patterns of alcohol use and related harms for Australian States and Territories. Chitritzhs et al. 2003.

Naylor, R T. *Hot Money and the Politics of Debt*. Black Rose Books. Montreal. 1994.

——. *Wages of Crime: Black Markets, Illegal Finance and the Underworld Economy*. Cornell University Press. Ithaca and London. 2004.

Nevett, T R. *Advertising in Britain*. Heinemann. London. 1982.

Patrick, Ross. *Horsewhip the Doctor: Tales from our Medical Past.* University of Queensland Press. St Lucia, Queensland. 1985.

Penguin Macquarie Dictionary of Australian Politics. Penguin Books. Ringwood, Victoria. 1984.

Perrine, Daniel M. *The Chemistry of Mind-Altering Drugs: History, Pharmacology and Cultural Context.* American Chemical Society. Washington, DC. 1996.

Pilger, John. *Heroes.* Pan Books. London and Sydney. 1986.

———. *Hidden Agendas.* Vintage. Great Britain. 1998.

Porter, Roy. *The Greatest Benefit to Mankind: A Medical History of Humanity.* W W Norton & Company. New York, London. 1997.

———. (ed) *The Cambridge Illustrated History of Medicine.* Cambridge University Press. Cambridge. 1996.

———. with Bynum, W F (eds). *Companion Encyclopaedia of the History of Medicine.* Routledge. London and New York. 1994.

———. with Teich, Mikulas (eds). *Drugs and Narcotics in History.* Cambridge University Press. Cambridge. 1995.

Quinn, Susan. *Marie Curie: A Life.* Simon and Schuster. New York.1995.

Rabinow, Paul (ed). *The Foucault Reader.* Penguin Books. London. 1991.

Ranelagh, John. *The Agency: The Rise and Decline of the CIA.* Weidenfeld and Nicolson. London. 1986.

Raynack, Elton. *Not So Free: The Political Economy of Milton Friedman and Ronald Reagan.* Praeger. New York. 1987.

Ricardo, David. *Works and Correspondence.* Cambridge at the University Press for the Royal Economic Society. 1952.

Richardson, Mathew. *Imagination: 100 Years of Bright Ideas in Australia.* IP Australia. Woden, ACT. 2004.

Robinson, Jeffrey. *The Laundrymen.* Simon and Schuster. London. 1994.

———. Prescription Games. Simon and Schuster. London. 2001.

Robinson, Rowan. *The Great Book of Hemp.* Park Street Press. Rochester, Vermont. 1996.

Rogers, Paul. *Losing Control: Global Security in the Twenty-First Century.* Pluto Press. London. 2000.

Rolls, Eric. *Sojourners.* University of Queensland Press. Queensland. 1992.

Royal Commissions of Inquiry into the Activities of the Nugan Hand Group. AGPS. Canberra 1985.

Royal Commissions of Inquiry into the New South Wales Police Service. First Interim Report 1996, Final Report 1997.

Royal Commissions of Inquiry into Whether There Has Been Corrupt or Criminal Conduct by any Western Australian Police Officer. January 2004.

Ruggerio, Vincenzo with South, Nigel. *Eurodrugs: Drug Use, Markets and Trafficking in Europe.* UCL Press. London. 1995.

Sarup, Madan. *An Introductory Guide to Post-Structuralism and Postmodernism.* The University of Georgia Press. Athens, Georgia. 1989.

Schlosser, Eric. *Reefer Madness.* Houghton Mifflin Company. Boston, New York. 2003.

Schudson, Michael. *Advertising: The Uneasy Persuasion.* Basic Books Inc. New York. 1984.

Schwartz, Richard. *The Cold War Reference Guide.* McFarland & Company Inc, Publishers.

Jefferson, North Carolina. 1997.

Scruton, Roger. *A Dictionary of Political Thought.* Pan Books. London. 1983.

Sears and Roebuck 1897 Catalog. Western Australia State Library Collection.

Senate Standing Committee on Social Welfare. *Report: Drug Problems in Australia: An Intoxicate Society?* AGPS Canberra. 1977.

Sennett, Richard. *The Corrosion of Character.* W W Norton & Company. New York. 1998.

Shann, Edward. *An Economic History of Australia.* Cambridge University Press. London. 1930.

Shorter, Edward. *A History of Psychiatry.* John Wiley & Sons, Inc. New York. 1997.

Silcott, Push & Mireille. *the book. of e.* Omnibus Press. London. 2000.

Singer, Charles with Holmyard EJ, Hall AR and Williams Trevor I. *A History of Technology.* Oxford University Press. Oxford. 1958.

Smith, Adam. *An Inquiry into the Nature and Causes of the Wealth of Nations.* George Bell & Sons. London and New York. 1896.

Smith, Wilfred. *An Economic Geography of Great Britain.* Methuen & Co. Ltd. London. 1951.

Sneader, Walter. *Drug Discovery: The Evolution of Modern Medicine.* John Wiley & Sons. New York. 1986.

Sournier, Jean-Charles. *A History of Alcoholism.* Basil Blackwell Ltd. Oxford. 1990.

Sourkes, Theodore L. *Nobel Prize Winners in Medicine and Physiology 1901–1965.* Abelard-Schuman. London. 1967.

Spillane, Joseph F. *Cocaine: From Medical Marvel to Modern Menace in the United States, 1884–1920.* Johns Hopkins University Press. Baltimore. 2000.

Stevens, Christine. *Tin Mosques and Ghantowns. A History of Afghan Cameldrivers in Australia.* Oxford University Press. Melbourne. 1989.

Stewart, Mark A with Wendkos Olds, Sally. *Raising a Hyperactive Child.* Harper and Row. New York. 1973.

Stokes, Geoffrey with Chalk, Peter and Gillen, Karen. *Drugs and Democracy: In Search of New Directions.* Melbourne University Press. Melbourne. 2000.

Strauss, Maurice B (ed). *Familiar Medical Quotations.* J & A Churchill Ltd. London. 1968.

Sweezy, Paul M. *Modern Capitalism and Other Essays.* Monthly Review Press. New York. 1972.

Taylor. A J P *The First World War: An Illustrated History.* Penguin. London.1966.

Thomas, Edward with Auslander, M. Arthur (eds). *Chemical Inventions and Chemical Patents.* Clark Boardman Company Ltd. New York. 1964.

Thornton, E M. *The Freudian Fallacy: Freud and Cocaine.* Palladin Grafton Books. London. 1986.

Travers, Bridget with Frieman, Fran Locher (eds). *Medical Discoveries.* UXL. Detroit. 1997.

Trocki, Carl A. *Opium, Empire and the Global Political Economy.* Routledge. London. 1999.

Twitchell, James B. *20 Ads that Shook the World.* Crown Publishers. New York. 2000.

Tyrell, Ian. *Deadly Enemies: Tobacco and its Opponents in Australia.* UNSW Press. Sydney. 1999.

UNESCO. *Compulsory Education in Australia. A Study by the Australian Co-operating Body for Education.* Paris. 1951.

United Nations Department for Disarmament Affairs, Co-ordination and World Disarmament Campaign Section. *Armament and Disarmament. Questions and Answers.*

New York. 1985.

United Nations Office on Drugs and Crime. World Drug Report 2004. World Drug Report 2005.

United States General Accounting Office. Washington, DC. Correspondence January 8 2003. Coca Estimates in Columbia.

Unwin, Elizabeth with Codde, Jim. *Comparison of Deaths Due to Alcohol, Tobacco and Other Drugs in Western Australia and Australia.* Health Department of Western Australia. Epidemiology and Analytical Services. Health Information Centre. June 1998.

Walker, Martin. *The Cold War and the Making of the Modern World.* Fourth Estate. London. 1993.

Walker, Robin. *Under Fire: A History of Tobacco Smoking in Australia.* Melbourne University Press. Melbourne. 1984.

———. with Roberts, Dave. *From Scarcity to Surfeit: A History of Food and Nutrition in New South Wales.* New South Wales University Press. Kensington, NSW. 1988.

Walmsley, Julian. *Macmillan Dictionary of International Finance.* Second Edition. Macmillan Press. London. 1985.

Walton, Stuart. *Out of It: A Cultural History of Intoxication.* Penguin. London. 2002.

Waterhouse, Richard. *Private Pleasures, Public Leisure: A History of Australian Popular Culture Since 1788.* Longman. Melbourne. 1995.

Weatherall, David. *David Ricardo: A Biography.* Martinus Nijhoff. The Hague. 1976.

Webb, Gary. *Dark Alliance.* Seven Stories Press. New York. 1999.

Wells, Andrew. *Constructing Capitalism: An Economic History of Eastern Australia 1788–1901.* Allen and Unwin. Sydney. 1989.

Wheen, Francis. *Karl Marx.* Fourth Estate. London. 1999.

Whitton, Evan. *Can of Worms.* The Fairfax Library. Sydney. 1986.

Wilding, Michael. *Marcus Clarke.* University of Queensland Press. St Lucia. 1976.

Wilkinson, Marion. *The Fixer: The Untold Story of Graham Richardson.* William Heinemann. Melbourne. 1996.

Willis, Evan. *Medical Dominance: The Division of Labour in Australian Health Care.* Allen and Unwin. Sydney. 1989.

Wills, Gary. *Reagan's America: Innocents at Home.* Heinemann. London. 1988.

Wood, Michael. *Conquistadors.* BBC Worldwide Limited. London. 2000.

Wong, J Y. *Deadly Dreams: Opium and the Arrow War (1856–1860).* Cambridge University Press. Cambridge. 1998.

World Health Organisation. *The Tobacco Atlas.* UK. 2002.

Newspapers and Journals
Australasian Psychiatry
The Age
The Australian
British Medical Journal
The Guardian Weekly
Journal of Drug Issues
The Lancet

The Medical Journal of Australia
The Mercury
Le Monde Diplomatique
The New England Journal of Medicine
New Internationalist
The New York Times
The Sydney Morning Herald
The Washington Post
The Weekend Australian
The Weekend Australian Financial Review
The West Australian

Internet Sources
Pharmaceutical Companies — profits and advertising:
   www.familiesusa.org
   www.healthyskepticism.org
Atheists and Adherents:
   www.atheistempire.com/reference/stat
   htpp://www.adherents.com/adh_faq.html#god
World Drug Report 2004:
   htpp://www.unodc.org/unodc/world_drug_report_2004.html
World Drug Report 2005:
   http://www.unodc.org/unodc/en/world_drug_report.html

Acknowledgements

I am indebted to the helpful staff at the University of Western Australia Medical
and Dental Library, the University of Wollongong Library and the state libraries
of Western Australia, Victoria and New South Wales. I need also to thank
Margot O'Neil, who guided me through the arcane weights and measures used by
apothecaries, and Nick Koletsis who made sense of the Greek acronyms.

Paul Kaplan and George McIlroy read early drafts of the munuscript and offered
helpful advice. Peter Ewer and Mike Donaldson were enthusiastic from the start and
provided detailed comments on both text and structure. Kay and Sid Anderson were
pillars of support and Lea, Phoebe, Seamus and Conor were very understanding,
particularly during the difficult times. Stephen and Ella accepted the long absences
with typical good grace.

A special thanks to Ray Coffey and Janet Blagg at the Press. As ever, any errors or
omissions remain the sole responsibility of the author.

Index

Abel, John 52
ADHD (Attention Deficit Hyperactivity Disorder) 140–42
adrenalin 52
AFL-CIO (American Federation of Labour – Congress of Industrial Organisations) 235
Afghan (ship) 213
Afghan Cameleers 165
Air America (Air Opium) 244, 266
alchohol 27, 82, 97–106, 311–14
Alcoholics Anonymous 314
Allende, Salvador 122
Alles, Gordon 129
Alpert, Richard 180
Alzheimer, Alois 249
American Civil War (1861-5) 91, 222
American Medical Association 18, 20, 28, 129, 152
American Psychoanalytic Association 39
American Society for Experimental Pharmacology and Therapeutics 52
Amphetamines
  discovery and early history 129–30
  association with the expression 'drugs' 80
  post-Second World War drug of addiction 65
  use among armed forces 130–31
  use among prominent politicians 131
  use by writers 132
  and 'Beat Generation' 132
  as appetite suppressant 133
  use in Sweden 132–4
  use in post-war Japan 133–4
  use in Asian countries 138
  epidemics of use 133–4, 137
  growth of illicit market 134–5
  global market 138
  Australian consumption of 67, 138
  illicit production by bikie gangs 136, 138–9
  and Melbourne underworld 139
  use in treatment of ADHD 140–42
  Ice (crystal meth) 137–8
  recorded offences in Australia 169
Amytal 58
anaesthetics 27–8
analgesics 64–5
Anslinger, Harry 149–52, 154–8, 166, 175, 177, 231
APCs (Aspirin Phenacetin and Caffeine), 64–5
Armstrong, Louis 154
Aschenbrandt, Theodor 120, 130
Askin, Sir Robert 265
aspirin 50, 64, 147
Asquith, Herbert Henry, Earl of Oxford and Asquith 103–4
AstraZenica 72
Attention Deficit Hyperactivity Disorder (ADHD) 140–42
Auckland, Lord 205
Auden, Wystan Hugh 132
Australian Competition and Consumer Commission (ACCC) 32, 309
Australian Bureau of Narcotics 267
Australian Medical Association 29, 58
Australian Sports Anti-Doping Authority 304
Australian Transaction Reports and Analysis Centre (AUSTRAC) 277
Avicenna (ibn Sina) 78

Baeyer, Adolf von 57
Balzac, Honoré de 145
Bank of Credit and Commerce International (BCCI) 252
Banks, Sir Joseph 161–2
Banting, Frederick 52–3
barbiturates 40, 57–8, 147, 186, 295
Bartholdi, Frederick Auguste 109
Barwick, Sir Garfield 269
Basie, Count 154
Baudelaire, Charles 145
Bayer 50, 51, 57, 222
Beard, George 38, 112
Beat Generation 132, 135, 183

Beatniks 135, 183
Behring, Emil von 33–4, 36
Bennett, William 291, 301–2
Bentham, Jeremy 203
Bentley, William H. 115, 117
Benzedrine 130, 140
benzodiazepines 65–6
Bernhardt, Sarah 109
Berridge, Virginia 6
Best, Charles 52–3
Bhutto, Zulfikar Ali 245
Bichat, Xavier 48
Bin Laden, Osama 247–8
Binh Xuyen 241
Black, General Edwin Fahey 262
Blainey, Geoffrey 210
Blake, William: *The Marriage of Heaven and Hell* 180
Blandon, Oscar Danilo 252
Bligh, William 102
Boerhaave, Herman
    pioneering role in clinical medicine 25
    Institutiones Medicae 108
Boer War (1899-1902) 94
Boggs, Hale 155
Boland, Edward 249
Bonsack, James Albert 90
Bradley, Charles 140
Braverman, Harry 325
Brent, Charles Henry, Bishop of the Philippines 218–19, 330
Brezhnev, Leonid 281
Bridges, Harry 231–2
British Medical Association 13, 28–9
bromide 40
Browning, Elizabeth Barrett 7
Buchheim, Rudolf 48, 57
Buckley, William F. 291
Bulwer-Lytton, Sir Edward 7
Bureau of Internal Revenue 149
Burroughs, William 132
Burton, Robert: *Anatomy of Melancholy* 144
Bush, George 159–60, 191, 249, 283, 291
Bush, George W. 126, 159, 161, 184, 253, 331

Byron, George Gordon, Baron of Rochdale 7

Cade, John 40
Caen, Herb 183
caffeine 49, 64–5, 80, 82, 83–5, 105, 112, 142, 299
Calloway, Cab 155
Canadian Medical Association 28
cannabis
    early history 143–8
    history and use in Australia 161–70
    growth of Australian market 256–60
    extent of Australian consumption 67, 138
    Griffith cannabis trade 258–9, 270
    police involvement in trade 275
    international prohibition 12, 198
    international consumption 289
    patterns of use and prohibition in US 15–16, 148–61
    research on licit recreational consumption 300–301
    use among professional footballers 304
    recorded offences 306
Capone, Al 157, 233
Carter, Jimmy 159, 245
Chain, Ernst 53
Chaplin, Charlie (Sir Charles Spencer): *Modern Times* 113, 186
Charcot, Jean-Martin 38
Chiang Kai-shek 9, 230, 238–9, 282
Chinese Exclusion Act (US,1896) 216
Chinese Restriction and Regulation Act (NSW,1888) 213
Chiu Chau Triads 238–9, 244, 254
chloral hydrate 57, 147
chloroform 27, 57, 59, 164
Churchill, Sir Winston Leonard Spencer 227–8
chu ma 143
Clark, Terrence John 259–60
Clarke, Marcus Andrew Hislop
    use of cannabis 162–4
    For the Term of his Natural Life 163

Clines, Thomas 251, 263, 268
Clinton, William ('Bill') 159–61, 292
Clive, Robert, Baron of Plassey 198–9
Coburn, James 179
Coca-Cola 109–10
cocaine
  early history 107–12
  popularised by medical profession 17
  manufacture of 58, 110
  effect of *Harrison Narcotic Act* 18
  US regulation of 13–16, 125–6
  international controls 12
  eradication program in Colombia 123
  consumption in Australia 46–7, 67,
    121, 128, 304
  recreational use in US 112, 120–27
  marginalisation of users 79, 151
  use to enhance productivity 113–14
  as local anaesthetic 119, 122
  as cure for opiate addiction 115
  use among troops 120
  use in post-revolutionary Russia 319
  Freud's experiments with 116–119
  international consumption 67, 127–8,
    289
  supply by Nicaraguan Contras 250–52
  Police involvement in supply 275,
    295–6
  and psychopharmacological crime 297
cocoa 82, 84
Cocke, General Erle 262
Colby, William Egan 262, 268
Coleridge, Samuel Taylor
  opium addiction 7
  recreational use of nitrous oxide 28
  private schooling 162
  Kubla Khan 7
Collins, Wilkie: *The Moonstone* 7
Columbian Exchange 88, 108, 197
Columbus, Christopher 54, 84, 88
Commonwealth-New South Wales Joint
  Task Force on Drug Trafficking (1982)
  262, 264, 268
compound analgesics 64
Communist International 318, 324

Continental Air Services 266
Cook, Captain James 161
Corporate Affairs Commission (NSW)
  269–70
Corset Gang 254
Cortes, Hernando 84, 108
Crimean War (1853-6) 89
Critchley, Macdonald 119
Cromwell, Oliver 291
Curie, Marie and Pierre 52
Culpeper, Nicholas 144

Darwin, Charles 279–80
Davis, Angela 186
Davis, George 118
Davy, Sir Humphry 28, 305
Delysid (LSD) 176
De Quincey, Thomas
  opium use 6–7
  influence of David Ricardo on 61
  private schooling 162
  influence on Marcus Clarke 163
  Confessions of an English Opium-Eater 7
De Jerez, Rodrigo 88
Derrida, Jaques 327
Desoxyn 135
Deutscher, Isaac 229
Devine, Tilly 121
Dewey, Thomas E. 226, 229, 232
dexamphetamine 130, 140–41
Dickens, Charles
  opium use 7
  The Mystery of Edwin Drood 7
Diem, Ngo Dinh 242–3
Dien Bien Phu (battle of, 1954) 242
Direct to consumer advertising (DTCA)
  72–4
Doyle, Sir Arthur Conan: *The Adventures
  of Sherlock Holmes* 110
Drug Enforcement Agency (US) 264
drugs
  origins of term and change in usage
    78–9
  definition 80
  association with illicit substances 80

social costs of in Australia 106
Australian consumption of 63–4, 67
Dulles, Allen 177
Dumas, Alexandre 109, 145
Duong Van Ia 276

East India Company 84, 146, 197,
198–201, 203, 329
ecstasy (MDMA)
discovery and early history 188–9
chemical structure 188
effects of 191–2
similarity to Prozac 66
association with the expression drugs 80
use by clubbers 188, 190
criminalisation of use 296
use by professional footballers 304
consumption in Australia 67, 192
international consumption 192
Edeleano, L. 129
Eden, Sir Anthony 131
Eden, George, Earl of Auckland 205
Edison, Thomas Alva 109, 111
Egan, John Wesley 254, 275, 278
Ehrlich, Paul 54–5
Elgin, James Bruce, Earl of Elgin and
Kincardine 206
Eli Lilly 53, 73, 146, 178–9
Eliot, George (Mary Ann Evans) 315
Elliot, Captain Charles 205
Elliot, Admiral George 205
Ellington, Duke 155
Elizabeth I, Queen 198
Engels, Friedrich
and *Communist Manifesto* 279, 290,
326
on Communist society 322–3
*The Condition of the Working Class in
England* 193, 279
ephedrine 129, 137
epinephrine 52
Erlenmeyer, Albrecht 119
Escobar, Pablo 252
Esquirol, Jean Etienne Dominique 37
ether 27, 124

Eureka Stockade 102, 212

Faust, Beatrice: *Benzo Junkie* 68
Federal Bureau of Investigation (FBI)
150, 180, 231, 282
Federal Bureau of Narcotics (FBN)
149–50, 152, 157, 177–8, 231
Feuerbach, Ludwig: *Des Wasens des
Christentum (The Essence of Christianity)*
315–16
Fisher, Emil 57
5T gang 274
Flaubert, Gustave 145
Fleischl-Marxow, Dr Ernst von 116–19
Fleming, Alexander 53
Florey, Howard 53
Forbes magazine 252
Ford, Gerald 123, 160
Foucault, Michel 20, 24, 40, 325, 327
French, Sir John 103
Freud, Sigmund 116–20, 315–16
Friedman, Milton 283–5, 290–92, 294–5
Capitalism and Freedom 283
Free to Choose 283
Fuerza Democratico Nicaraguense
(FDN) 250
Fukuyama, Francis 279

Gagarin, Yuri 320
Galen 22–3, 78, 144
George IV, King of Great Britain 7
German Imperial Health Office 55–6
German Society for Combating Quackery
56
Gillespie, Dizzy 155
Ginsberg, Allen
cannabis use 158
first use of LSD 181
Howl and Other Poems 135
Gladstone, William Ewart 7, 202
GlaxoSmithKline 72, 76
Gore, Al 126–7, 161
Gracey, Major-General Douglas 241
Gramsci, Antonio 324
Grant, Cary 179

Grant, Ulysses S. 109
Green Gang 238–9
Greene, Graham
  The Quiet American 132, 243
  Our Man in Havana 132
  The Confidential Agent 132
  The Third Man 132
Guantanamo Bay, Cuba 217
Halsted, William Stewart 115
Hampton, Lionel 155
Hand, Michael Jon 261–70
Hare, H.A. 146
Harrison Narcotic Act (US,1914) 15, 18,
  79, 219
Harvey, William 23
Hata, Sahachiro 55
Hayek, Friedrich 283–4, 290
Haywood, William ('Big Bill') 114
Hearst, William Randolph 151, 153–4
Hegel, Georg 5, 315
Hekmatyar, Gulbuddin 246–7
hemlock 27
Herer, Jack: *The Emperor Wears No Clothes*
  153
heroin
  discovery and early use 222–3
  consumption and supply in Australia
    46–7, 67, 254–61, 264, 267, 270–78
  estimates of users in Australia 271–2
  consumption and supply in US 16,
    223–5
  and French Connection 155, 232–6
  international consumption 46, 67
  consumption in Indonesia 278
  consumption in Russian Federation 331
  intravenous use 128, 223
  supply in Manchuria 238
  manufacture in Golden Triangle 236–7,
    244
  manufacture in Golden Crescent 245–8
  'gateway' drug 155
  marketed by brand name 288
  association with crime 297
  cannabis drought and increased
    consumption 168

addicts 16, 17, 95, 125, 226, 271–2,
  299, 301
addicts in medical profession 17, 19
increased number of addicts in Pakistan
  246
control and prohibition in US 15–16
prohibition in Australia 47
international controls 12, 14
Hezbi-i Islam 246
Hippocrates 22
Hitler, Adolf 131
Ho Chi Minh 236, 240, 242
Hobsbawm, Eric 206, 325
Hoechst 50, 55
Hoffman, Abbie 58
Hoffman, Dr Albert 175–6, 179
Hoffman-La Roche 66, 225
Hollywood Independent Citizens
  Committee of the Arts, Sciences and
    Professions (HICCASP) 282
Holmes, Dr Oliver Wendell 27
Hoover, J. Edgar 150
Houghton, Bernie 263–6, 268
Hubbard, Captain Alfred M. 180
Hugo, Victor 145
Hunayn ibn Ishaq 78
Hunter, John (Governor of NSW) 102
Hunter, John (physiologist) 54
huo ma ren 143
Husak, Douglas 296–8, 300, 302–3
Huss, Magnus 314
Huxley, Aldous
  experiments with LSD and mescaline
    179–80
  The Doors of Perception 180
  Heaven and Hell 180

ibn Sina (Avicenna) 78
Ibsen, Henrik 109
Illich, Ivan 43–4
inhalants 305
insulin 52–3
Inter Services Intelligence (ISI) 246
International Workingmen's Association
  318

Inuit 80
Irish Republican Army 330

James I, King of England 88, 307
Jardine, William 8–9, 203, 206
Johnson, Lyndon Baines 160, 181
Johnstone, Christopher Martin 259–60
Journal der Pharmacie 49

Karzai, Hamid 247
Keats, John 7, 162
Kemp, Richard 187
Kennedy, John Fitzgerald 131, 157, 160,
    181, 224
Kennedy, Joseph Patrick 224
Kerouac, Jack: *On the Road* 132
Kerry, Senator John 251–2
Kesey, Ken: *One Flew Over the Cuckoo's
    Nest* 181
Keynes, John Maynard, Baron 283
Khan, Dr. Abdul Qadeer 248
King, Kermit Walker 267
King, Martin Luther, Jr. 181, 185
King, Philip Gidley 102
Koch, Robert 34, 51
Koller, Carl 119
Korean War (1950–53) 131
Korsch, Karl 324
Kremers, Edward 306
Krupa, Gene 154
Khrushchev, Nikita 281
Ku Klux Klan 157, 282
Kuomintang 9, 230, 237–9
Kuznets, Simon 294
Ky, Nguyen Cao 243–4

Laing, Ronald David 40
Lansky, Meyer 150, 155, 224–6, 232–4,
    258, 276
Lavoisier, Antoine Laurent 48
Lawn, John 301
Leary, Timothy 180, 182, 187
Leigh, Kate 121
Lenin, Vladimir Ilyich 101, 318–21
Leo XIII, Pope 109

Lepke and Gurrah 224
Levi-Strauss, Claude 327
Librium 66
Liebig, Justus von 56
Liebknecht, Karl 319
Liebreich, Oscar 57
Lin Tse-hsu 204–5
Linnaeus, Carolus 143, 194
Lipitor 73
Loan, Nguyen Ngoc 243
Locke, John 302
Long, Huey 233
L'Onorata (the Honourable Society) 258
Louis XV, King of France 24
LSD *see* Lysergic Acid Diethylamide
Luce, Clare Booth 186
Luce, Henry 186
Luciano, Charles (Lucky) 224–6, 232–4,
    276
Lukacs, George 324
Luxemburg, Rosa 318–19, 321
Lyons, Joseph Aloysius 166
Lysergic Acid Diethylamide (LSD)
    early history 175–6
    CIA experiments with 177–8
    therapeutic use 179
    use by scientists and writers in 1950's
        California 179–80
    recreational use in US 181–3
    use in Australia 187–8

McCarthy, Joseph Raymond 156–7
McCoy, Alfred W. 245
McDonald, Walter Joseph 262
McFarlane, Robert 249
Mackay, Donald Bruce 168, 259, 268,
    274–6
McKenna, Terence 81
McKeown, Thomas 35
McKinley, William 109
Macquarie, Lachlan 102
Magendie, Francois 49
ma huang 129, 143
Malcolm X (Malcolm Little) 181, 184
Mandel, Ernest 325

mandrake 27
Manor, Lieutenant-General Leroy Joseph
  262
Mao Tse-tung 9, 208, 230, 239, 323
Mariani, Angelo 109
marijuana *see* cannabis
Marijuana Tax Act (US,1937) 16, 152–5,
  166
Marshall Plan 234–5
Matheson, James 8–9, 203
Marx, Karl
  on religion as opium of the people 5, 8
  on East India Company 200–201 on
    free trade 203
  on opium trade with China 207
  as pillar of atheism 315–16
  on Communist society 322
  historical materialism 322–9
  and revenge of religion on 330
  Communist Manifesto 279, 290, 326
  Das Kapital 317
Medellin Cartel 250, 252
Melbourne, William Lamb, Viscount 205
Mellon, Andrew 149–50, 153–4
Menzies, Sir Robert 269
Merck 49, 58, 74–5, 110, 117–18, 188,
  225
Mering, Joseph von 57
mescaline 180, 188
methamphetamine hydrochloride 130
Methedrine 135
methylphenidate (Ritalin) 140–41
Mill, James: *History of British India* 203
Mill, John Stuart 203
Mindszenty, Cardinal Jozsef 177
Mitchell, Silas Weir 39, 112
Mitchum, Robert 155
MK-ULTRA 177–8, 181
Moffitt Royal Commission into
  Organised Crime (NSW, 1974) 260
Molé, Louis Matthieu, Comte 7
Monroe, Marilyn 58
Mont Perelin Society 284
Moreau de Tours, Dr. Joseph 163
morphine

discovery 49
addiction 18
women addicted by medical profession
  17, 19
use in asylums 40
international controls 12
illicit supply on D-Day 157
Mr Asia syndicate 259, 267
Musto, David 300

Nagai, Nagayoshi 129
National Association of Evangelicals 282
Negroponte, John 250, 253
Nembutal 58
Newman, John 274–6
New Economic Policy 320
Newton, Huey P. 185–6
New Yorker 328
New Zealand Medical Association 74
Nhu, Ngo Dinh 243
Nicaraguan Contras 123, 248–52
Nicholson, Jack 179
Niemann, Albert 108
Nietzsche, Friedrich 57
Nightingale, Florence 7
nitrous oxide 27–8, 305
NLF (Front for the Liberation of South
  Vietnam) 242
Nixon, Richard Milhous 122, 160, 181,
  280
North, Lieutenant-Colonel Oliver 249–51
Northern Alliance 247
Novocain 120
Nugan, Frank 261–70
Nugan Hand 261–70
Nugan, Kenneth 268, 270
Nutt, Colonel Levi 149

Ochoa, Jorge 252
Office of Naval Intelligence (ONI) 231
Office of Strategic Services (OSS) 180,
  231–3, 240, 262
Omar, Mullah 247
O'Neill, Eugene: *Long Day's Journey into
  Night* 17

opium
  early history and use 194–7
  19th century use 5–8, 215
  in proprietary medicines 13, 58–9, 196
  laudanum 6–7, 14, 195
  smoking 9, 13–14, 197, 204, 208,
      211–14, 221
  use in surgery127
  use by US troops in Vietnam 131
  use with cannabis 167
  use in China 197–202
  Opium Wars 8–9, 203–7
  effects according to De Quincey 163
  smuggled into US 226
  smuggled into Marseille 234
  production in Golden Triangle 236–44
  production in Golden Crescent 245–8
  restrictions on use 12–15, 79, 214–21,
      296
  opium growing in Australia 196, 210
Organisation for Economic Co-operation
    and Development (OECD) 73
Organisation of Petroleum Exporting
    Countries (OPEC) 281
Ortega, Daniel 248
O'Shaughnessy, William 145–6
Osler, Sir William 51
Osmond, Dr Humphry 180
Oswald, Lee Harvey 157
Ouane Rattikone, General 244

Palmerston, Henry John Temple,
    Viscount 205–6
Paracelsus (Philippus Aureolis
    Theophrastus von Hohenheim) 23, 195
paracetamol 50
Paris Commune 101, 319
Parke-Davis 14, 52, 58, 110–11, 116–19,
    146
Parkes, Sir Henry 213
Pasteur, Louis 33, 51
Paz Garcia, General Policarpo 250
Pemberton, John 109, 115
penicillin 53–5
People's World 282

Perkins, William Henry 50
pethidine 293
Pfizer 73, 76
phenacetin 50, 64
Philippines Opium Committee 218
Physiocrats 24
Phillip, Captain Arthur 162
Pinel, Philippe 37, 39
Pinochet, Augusto 122–3
Pius X, Pope 109
Pol Pot 280
Police Integrity Commission (NSW) 275
Pope Leo XIII 109
Pope Pius X 109
Porter, Roy 34, 98
Previn, Andre 179
Priestley, Joseph 28
prohibition
  Convention for the Suppression of
      the Illicit Traffic in Dangerous Drugs,
      Geneva (1936) 46
  Convention on Psychotropic
  Substances
      (1971) 134, 172
  International Conference on Opium,
      The Hague (1911-12) 15, 219
  International Opium Commission,
      Shangai (1909) 15, 219
  International Opium Conference,
      Geneva (1924-5) 12–14, 16, 46, 148,
      219–21
  Limitation Convention (On the
      Manufacture of Narcotic Drugs),
      Geneva (1931) 16, 45
  Single Convention on Narcotic Drugs
      (1961) 172
  Opium Act (South Australia 1895) 214
  Sale and Use of Poisons Act
      (Queensland 1891) 214
  Smoking Opium Exclusion Act (US
      1909) 15, 219
  Australian referendums on alcohol
      prohibition 104
  alcohol prohibition in US 16, 148–9,
      220

Gin Act (Britain1736) 100
  rationale for prohibition 296 – 303
  *See also Harrison Narcotic Act and
    Marijuana Tax Act*
proprietary medicines 6, 13, 27, 56–66,
  164–5
Proust, Marcel 58
Prozac 66, 76
psilocybin mushrooms 81, 189

Quayle, Dan 160
Quang, General Dang Van 244
Quesnay, Dr Francois 24
quinine (Jesuits bark) 50

*Racketeering-Influenced and Corrupt
  Organisations Act* (RICO) 309
Reagan, Ronald 123, 159–60, 184, 249,
  282–3
Reed, John: *Ten Days That Shook the World*
  318
Reefer Madness 151, 175
Reil, Johann 36
Ricardo, David
  and doctrine of caveat emptor 61
  work on political economy continued
    by Marx 322
  *Principles of Political Economy and
    Taxation* 61, 202
Riley, Murray Stewart 258, 264, 267
Rockefeller, Senator Jay 253
Rockefeller, John D. 225
Rodin, Auguste 109
Roesler & Fils 225
Roget, Peter Mark 28
Rolleston Report (1926) 19
Rolls, Eric 211
Roosevelt, Franklin Delano 157, 227–9
Roosevelt, Theodore 219
Rosenhan, David 40
Rossetti, Dante Gabriel 57
Rothstein, Arnold 224
Royal Commission of Inquiry into the
  New South Wales Police Service
  (1994–7) 275, 295

Royal Commission on Liquor Laws in
  New South Wales (1951–4) 273
Ruby, Jack 157
Russian Civil War (1918–20) 319
Russian Mafia 247, 273
Russo-Japanese War (1904–5), 318
Ryan, Peter 275

Saffron, Abe 265
Sandoz 175–8
Sartre, Jean-Paul 324–5, 327
Saussure, Ferdinand de: *Course in General
  Linguistics* 325, 327
Schiaparelli 232
Schmiedeberg, Oswald 48
Schultz, Arthur (Dutch) 224
Seale, Bobby 185–6
Seconal 58
Secord, General Richard 251, 262
Sennett, Richard 81–2
Sergi, Antonio 258
Sertürner, Friedrich 49, 55
Service de Documentation Exterieure et
  du Contre-Espionage (SDECE) 241
Shackley, Ted 263
Sheehan, J.C. 53
Shelley, Percy Bysshe 7
Shen Nung, Emperor 129
Shulgin, Ann and Dr.Alexander:
  PiKHAL: A Chemical Love Story;
  TiKHAL: The Continuation 189
Siegel, Benjamin (Bugsy) 224, 226
Smith, Adam
  and apothecaries' profits 24
  effect of invisible hand 203, 285–6
  on equal benefit of free exchange
    287–8
  description of exchange mechanism
    288
  work on political economy continued
    by Marx 322
  *An Inquiry into the Nature and Causes
    of the Wealth of Nations* 24, 202
Smith Kline and French 130
Smith, Robert Holbrook 314

Social Text 328
Sokal, Alan: *Fashionable Nonsense: Postmodernist Intellectuals' Abuse of Science* 328
Somoza, Anastasio 250
Sopsaianna, Prince 244
Southey, Robert 7, 28
Spanish-American War (1898) 217–18
Spencer, James Oswald 268
Squibb 146
Squires, Peter 146
Stalin, Josef 177, 227–30, 235, 281, 320–25
Stanley, Augustus Owsley 186
Stark, Ronald Hadley 187
Stevenson, Robert Louis: *The Strange case of Dr Jekyll and Mr Hyde* 110, 117, 152
Stoll, Dr Arthur 175
Stoll, Dr Werner 176
Strasser, Sir Paul 265
streptomycin 53
sugar 84–8, 105, 299
Sulphonal 57
Sun Yat-Sen 237–8
Sydenham, Thomas 20, 195
Sylvius, Franciscus 25, 99
Szasz, Thomas 40

Taft, William 218
Taliban 247
TAP Pharmaceuticals 72
Taylor, Frederick Winslow 113
tea 84–7
thalidomide 68
Thieu, Nguyen Van 244
Thompson, E. P. 325
Time magazine 181, 325, 329
tobacco 82, 88–97, 105–6, 307–11
Trimbole, Robert 258–9
Trotsky, Leon 319–21
Truman Doctrine 229–30
Truman, Harry S. 156, 229
Tu Yueh-sheng 238–9

United Nations Office on Drugs and Crime 271

Valium 66, 136, 186
Vang Pao, General 244
Verne, Jules 109
Veronal 57
Versailles Peace Treaty (1919) 219
Viagra 73
Victoria, Queen 27, 109, 146
Villa, Pancho 151
Vin Mariani 109
Vioxx 74–6
Virchow, Rudolf 54
Voltaire 26, 315

Waksman, Selman A. 53
Walker, John D. 265
Walton, Stuart 80, 98
Washington, George 152
War Communism 319–20
Weber, Max 58
Weinberger, Caspar 249
Wells, H. G. 109
Wexler, Irving (Waxey Gordon) 224
White, George Hunter 177–8
Whitton, Evan 265
Wilberforce, William 7
Wilde, Oscar
   opium use 7
   The Picture of Dorian Grey 7
Wilson, Edwin P. 263
Woolf, Virginia 58
World Health Organisation (WHO) 43, 96, 134
Wright, C.R. Alder 222
Wyeth Australia 76

Yates, Admiral Earl Preston 261, 265–6, 268

Zola, Emile 109
Zia-ul-Haq, General Muhammed 245

www.ingramcontent.com/pod-product-compliance
Lightning Source LLC
Chambersburg PA
CBHW020523270326
41927CB00006B/420